SAFETY AND RISK IN SOCIETY

REHAB, PROTECTION AND SAFETY MEASURES FOR FIREFIGHTERS AND EMERGENCY RESPONDERS

SAFETY AND RISK IN SOCIETY

Additional titles in this series can be found on Nova's website at:
https://www.novapublishers.com/catalog/index.php?cPath=23_29&seriesp=Safety+and+Risk+in+Society

Additional E-books in this series can be found on Nova's website at:
https://www.novapublishers.com/catalog/index.php?cPath=23_29&seriespe=Safety+and+Risk+in+Society

SAFETY AND RISK IN SOCIETY

REHAB, PROTECTION AND SAFETY MEASURES FOR FIREFIGHTERS AND EMERGENCY RESPONDERS

ANDREO RIOS
EDITOR

Nova
Nova Science Publishers, Inc.
New York

NOTICE TO THE READER

Library of Congress Cataloging-in-Publication Data

Rehab, protection, and safety measures for firefighters and emergency responders / editor, Andreo Rios.
p. cm.
Includes bibliographical references and index.
ISBN 978-1-60741-566-4 (hardcover)
1. Fire fighters--Health and hygiene. 2. Fire fighters--Rehabilitation.
3. Fire extinction--Safety appliances. I. Rios, Andreo.
RC965.F48R44 2010
363.37092--dc22
2010012867

Published by Nova Science Publishers, Inc. ✢ New York

CONTENTS

PREFACE

The physical and mental demands associated with firefighting and other emergency operations exceed those of virtually any other occupation. When you combine the inherent stresses of handling emergency incidents with the environmental dangers of extreme heat and humidity or extreme cold, you create conditions that can have an adverse impact on the safety and health of the individual emergency responder. When emergency responders become fatigued, their ability to operate safely is impaired. As a result, their reaction time is reduced and their ability to make critical decisions diminishes. This book examines the need for rehab operations at emergency scenes and defines the concept of emergency incident rehabilitation with a review of the historical pattern of firefighter injuries and deaths associated with the stresses of emergency operations.

Chapter 1 - The physical and mental demands associated with firefighting and other emergency operations exceed those of virtually any other occupation. Unlike many jobs, firefighters cannot pick the time or conditions these jobs must be carried out. Emergencies occur at all times and in every conceivable environmental condition. When you combine the inherent stresses of handling emergency incidents with the environmental dangers of extreme heat and humidity or extreme cold, you create conditions that can have an adverse impact on the safety and health of the individual emergency responder. Members who are not provided adequate rest and rehydration during emergency operations or training exercises are at increased risk for illness or injury, and may jeopardize the safety of others on the incident scene. When emergency respond-ers become fatigued, their ability to operate safely is impaired. As a result, their reaction time is reduced and their ability to make critical decisions diminishes. Rehabilitation is an essential element on the incident scene to prevent more serious conditions such as heat exhaustion or heat stroke from occurring.

In this chapter the authors will examine the need for rehab operations at emergency scenes and training exercises. First the authors will define the concept of emergency incident rehabilitation and then the authors will review the historical pattern of firefighter injuries and deaths associated with the stresses of emergency operations. The latter portions of the chapter will provide some case study information on injuries and deaths to firefighters as a result of failing to recognize environmental dangers or provide adequate rehabilitation during training sessions and emergency incident operations. These cases studies are not intended to criticize or embarrass those agencies and individuals who were involved. Rather, they serve to show that these incidents can occur in all fire departments and jurisdictions and they happen fast, often without warning. Lastly, the authors will review the various standards that place the requirements for conducting rehab operations on the fire service.

Chapter 2 - Firefighters are exposed to many thermal environments, both hot and cold, in the course of their duties. The firefighter responds to structural and wildland fires as well as other emergencies including vehicle, industrial, aircraft and marine accidents, hazardous materials (hazmat) incidents, and search and rescue operations during disasters such as floods, hurricanes, tornados, blizzards, and earthquakes. Exposure to environmental factors also is experienced during training activities and physical fitness programs. While environmental conditions can be considered in scheduling training activities, the critical nature of the firefighters' job often requires prolonged exposure to extreme thermal conditions during emergency operations. Defining the firefighters' environment is an important first step in developing effective work practices and strategies for protecting them from stress-related illnesses and injuries.

Severity of environmental exposure is related to several factors that influence the amount or rate of heat lost to, or gained from, the external environment. Though both environmental extremes pose hazards for firefighters, problems related to heat stress tend to be far more common and severe than those created by exposure to extreme cold. In this chapter the authors will examine the issue of heat stress on firefighters and the potential problems it may cause.

Chapter 3 - Of the two environmental temperature extremes (hot and cold) that firefighters may be expected to operate in, historically, extreme heat has been the most problematic of the two. The heavy, encapsulating equipment that is worn to perform the physically tasking jobs only adds to the problems posed by working in heat. Most jurisdictions spend a considerable amount of their effort in establishing rehab plans and programs on dealing with heat.

However, fire departments in jurisdictions subjected to cold weather must also recognize the impact that these conditions will have on its firefighters and operations. Accordingly, these departments must develop plans to deal with prolonged exposures to extreme cold temperatures during the course of training or emergency scene operations. While the threat of a systemic illness (comparable to heat exhaustion or heat stroke) is more remote in cold weather, there is an equal or greater chance for other injuries, such as frostbite and injuries as a result of slips and falls.

In this chapter the authors will examine the impact of cold weather on firefighters and fire department operations. We will highlight the physiological strains these conditions place on firefighters and the injuries that can result. Lastly, the authors will examine how to avoid these types of injuries.

Chapter 4 - Ensuring that firefighters are in good physical condition, properly hydrated, and well-fed prior to responding to an incident are important in helping to ensure their safety during operations. However, even physically fit firefighters can suffer the consequences of overexertion and exposure to harsh environmental conditions during the course of emergency operations and extended physical/practical training activities. Most of the illnesses and injuries discussed to this point in the document can be avoided by establishing and operating a proper emergency incident rehabilitation, or rehab, area.

This chapter will provide detailed information on establishing and equipping a rehab area. The chapter begins by highlighting how to determine when it is necessary to establish rehab operations at an incident or training activity. It is important that rehab operations operate under the umbrella of the Incident Command System (ICS) structure being used at the scene, so suggestions on how to do that are covered also. The latter portions of the chapter discuss selecting, organizing, and equipping rehab operations for duty.

Chapter 5 - There is much more to establishing an effective rehab area than selecting a good location and having the right vehicles and equipment. The whole purpose of establishing the rehab operation is to ensure optimum care of the firefighters and other responders who will be operating at the incident. In order to do this there must be effective means for operating the rehab area, established procedures for requiring firefighters to enter the rehab area, and a solid plan for providing the services that are required.

This chapter examines means for minimizing the amount of stress placed on firefighters during incident operations. This includes establishing safe work-to-rest ratios and monitoring personnel for signs of problems. Detailed information on performing both self-rehab and formal rehab functions is provided also. The latter half of the chapter details medical evaluation and treatment considerations for rehab operations, as well as principles of hydration and fluid and nutritional support.

Chapter 6 - The fire department's responsibility for safeguarding the well-being of their members does not end when the last firefighter leaves the rehab area at an incident. Policies and procedures must be in place to ensure that firefighters continue to receive restorative care after the incident. The fire department also must ensure that the resources used to provide rehab services are replenished and ready for the next incident where they may be needed.

This chapter briefly examines the de-escalation of rehab operations at an incident scene. It also provides information on care that firefighters should receive once they leave this incident scene. This includes medical evaluation, self-monitoring for hydration needs, and critical incident stress services, should they be required.

This is an edited, excerpted and augmented edition of a United States Fire Administration publication, dated February 2008, and edited by Andreo Rios.

INTRODUCTION

It is only in the last quarter-century that a significant portion of the fire service began to realize that the fire service's historic role as being one of the most dangerous occupations needed to be addressed. Perhaps no event in the history of the fire service brought these safety issues to the forefront more than the release of the first edition of National Fire Protection Association (NFPA) 1500, *Standard on Fire Department Occupational Safety and Health Program* in 1987. This document recognized many of the issues that were injuring and killing firefighters and provided standard methods for correcting them.

As we will detail in Chapter 1 of this document, approximately one-half of all firefighter fatalities and a significant percentage of injuries and illnesses are as a result of stress and overexertion on firefighters involved in emergency scene operations and training exercises.There is no question that despite all the advantages brought about by modern technology, the delivery of fire department services remains largely a job that requires arduous manual labor. In many cases, it is labor at the maximum extremes of human physical endurance.

One solution is to ensure that firefighters are in better physical condition prior to responding to the emergency call. In general, improvements to firefighter health, wellness, and fitness have been made in recent years, particularly in the career fire service. However, there remains considerable work to do in this area. A proactive injury prevention approach must be implemented to reduce risks in the fire service and improve personnel resistance to injuries. This proactive injury prevention program shall include the following:

- a comprehensive and effective wellness program;
- a physical fitness program;
- a strong commitment to safety from both labor and management;
- a designated Safety Officer;
- an ergonomic analysis of all aspects of the workplace to identify potential injury causes and address unsafe conditions that can be corrected by improved design;
- a program to manage medical and injury rehabilitation to decrease time loss and reduce reinjury rates;
- an educational component that begins in the fire academy and continues throughout the entire career;
- a recognition system for personnel who practice, play, and preach safety;

- a relationship between labor, management, and risk management; and
- an integrated and participatory fire department "near miss" program.

Even if we were able to achieve a high level of fitness and wellness among all firefighters, the issue of excessive stress and overexertion at emergency scenes and training sessions does not go away. Even perfectly conditioned firefighters can be extended beyond the limits of their conditioning. When this occurs, occupational illness and injuries typically follow.

There are a number of ways that we can reduce the tendency to overexert firefighters at the emergency scene or training session, regardless of the level of their physical condition. First is to assign an adequate number of personnel to perform the required tasks safely. In addition, Incident Commanders (ICs) must take the effort required to perform tasks into consideration prior to assigning them. These same principles must be extended to training settings. The old militaristic "run them until they drop and then build them up again" mentality needs to be eliminated. If there is one thing more tragic than losing a firefighter in an uncontrolled emergency scene setting, it is losing one in a training setting that should have been totally under control.

Even if reasonable assignments are made, at some point all firefighters will become exhausted and need a break. This realization was noted in the first edition of NFPA 1500. The standard required fire departments to develop policies and procedures for emergency incident rehabilitation, simply referred to as "rehab," operations at emergency scenes and training exercises. The purpose of rehab operations is to provide rest for firefighters who have been working for extended periods of time. In addition to rest, firefighters receive medical evaluations or attention as required and are given the opportunity to replace fluids and eat as necessary.

Though NFPA 1500 placed the requirement on fire departments to perform rehab, it provided little in the way of guidance in how to set up and operate a rehab area. It also did not establish much in the way of criteria for evaluating firefighters when they enter the rehab area. In fact, even though some organizations had been performing at least some aspects of a rehab operation for many years, there really was no definitive source of information on the topic available. Several articles had been written and fire departments shared Standard Operating Procedures (SOPs), but no single source of comprehensive information was available.

The first significant effort at providing comprehensive information on the topic of rehab occurred in July 1992 when the U.S. Fire Administration (USFA) released report FA-114, *Emergency Incident Rehabilitation*. This document provided basic information on performing rehab operations at emergency scenes and also included a sample SOP. A more comprehensive text, bearing the same title as the USFA report, was also released in 1997 by Brady and Fire Protection Publications. This was the first, and the only, full-length text dedicated to the topic of providing rehab services at emergency scenes and training exercises.

This increased level of interest in rehab operations led the NFPA Standards Council to direct the NFPA Fire Service Occupational Safety and Health technical committee to develop a new document devoted entirely to rehab operations. The new document, titled NFPA 1584, *Recommended Practice on the Rehabilitation of Members Operating at Incident Scene Operations and Training Exercises*, was released in early 2003. At the time this chapter was being written, the NFPA was in the process of developing a 2008 edition of NFPA 1584 and was changing the document from a recommended practice to a formal standard.

The USFA is committed to working with the major national level fire service organizations in reducing firefighter fatalities in the U.S. Numerous programs, research efforts, and other work are being done to support/ reach this goal. As part of the effort, the USFA determined that the 1992 FA-114, *Emergency Incident Rehabilitation* report needed to be updated to ensure that the latest information on the care of firefighters engaged in emergency scene and training operations was made available. In order to facilitate the revision, the USFA entered into a cooperative agreement with the International Association of Fire Fighters (IAFF), Division of Occupational Health, Safety and Medicine, to provide this revised report.

In: Rehab, Protection and Safety Measures or Firefighters ... ISBN: 978-1-60741-566-4
Editor: Andreo Rios

Chapter 1

THE NEED FOR REHAB OPERATIONS AT INCIDENTS AND TRAINING EXERCISES

The physical and mental demands associated with firefighting and other emergency operations exceed those of virtually any other occupation. Unlike many jobs, firefighters cannot pick the time or conditions these jobs must be carried out. Emergencies occur at all times and in every conceivable environmental condition **(Figure 1.1).** When you combine the inherent stresses of handling emergency incidents with the environmental dangers of extreme heat and humidity or extreme cold, you create conditions that can have an adverse impact on the safety and health of the individual emergency responder. Members who are not provided adequate rest and rehydration during emergency operations or training exercises are at increased risk for illness or injury, and may jeopardize the safety of others on the incident scene. When emergency respond-ers become fatigued, their ability to operate safely is impaired. As a result, their reaction time is reduced and their ability to make critical decisions diminishes. Rehabilitation is an essential element on the incident scene to prevent more serious conditions such as heat exhaustion or heat stroke from occurring.

In this chapter we will examine the need for rehab operations at emergency scenes and training exercises. First we will define the concept of emergency incident rehabilitation and then we will review the historical pattern of firefighter injuries and deaths associated with the stresses of emergency operations. The latter portions of the chapter will provide some case study information on injuries and deaths to firefighters as a result of failing to recognize environmental dangers or provide adequate rehabilitation during training sessions and emergency incident operations. These cases studies are not intended to criticize or embarrass those agencies and individuals who were involved. Rather, they serve to show that these incidents can occur in all fire departments and jurisdictions and they happen fast, often without warning. Lastly, we will review the various standards that place the requirements for conducting rehab operations on the fire service.

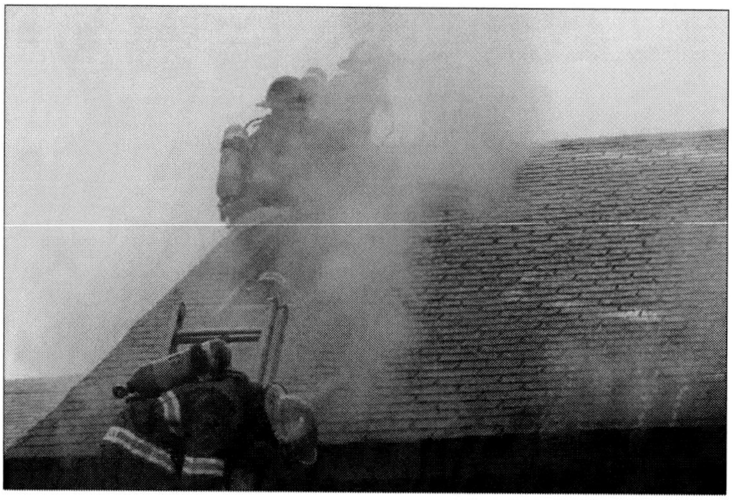

Figure 1.1.

Rehab Defined

If one looks up the word "rehabilitation" in the dictionary, numerous variations of definitions will be noted. However, the variation that is most pertinent to the concept of caring for firefighters and other emergency responders during emergency and training operations reads "to restore or bring to a condition of health or useful and constructive activity."

The formal term applied to caring for emergency responders during incident and training activities is emergency incident rehabilitation. In daily use this is shortened to simply rehab. The term rehab is used to describe the process of providing rest, rehydration, nourishment, and medical evaluation to responders who are involved in extended and/or extreme incident scene operations (Figure 1.2). The goal of rehab is to get firefighters either back into the action or back to the station in a safe and healthy condition. When rehab operations are implemented properly, they go a long way towards making sure that the physical and mental conditions of responders operating at the emergency scene do not deteriorate to a point that affects the safety of any responder or that jeopardizes the safety or effectiveness of incident operations.

Stress-Related Injuries and Deaths in the Fire Service

The dangers of firefighting and emergency scene operations have long been documented and recognized. Though firefighters spend a considerable amount of time training to deal with the physical hazards of fire-fighting operations, such as fire conditions or building construction hazards, in truth, the most credible hazard that firefighters will face is the stress that their job places upon their own bodies. This fact can be emphasized by looking at historical data showing the causes of firefighter injuries and deaths.

The latest data on firefighter injuries and deaths that were available at the time this chapter was written was for the calendar year 2005. Information on injuries was obtained from *U.S. Firefighter Injuries*, 2005, by the National Fire Protection Association (NFPA). Information on firefighter fatalities was obtained from *Firefighter Fatalities in the United States* in 2005 (FA-306) by the U.S. Fire Administration (USFA).

Before looking at some of the specific numbers found in these reports, it is important to keep in mind that the U.S. fire service is not particularly adept at capturing vital statistics and information. This is particularly true of the injury statistics. The available injury statistics likely represent only a portion of the true total of firefighter injuries that occurred. These statistics, however, are valuable in terms of comparing various types of injuries and the settings in which they compare to each other for an overall understanding on the likelihood in which injuries may occur.

The available statistics on firefighter fatalities are more reliable. This is because there are lesser occurrences of deaths than there are injuries, these occurrences generally are well-publicized, and numerous agencies document and report the fatalities.

In reviewing firefighter injuries statistics for 2005, it was noted that were 3,555 reported injures related to thermal stress (either hot or cold), which accounted for 4.4 percent of the total reported injuries. This was the fifth highest cause of injuries in the 10 areas that were listed. Table 1.1 shows a breakdown of the activities the firefighters were engaged in at the time of the thermal injury.

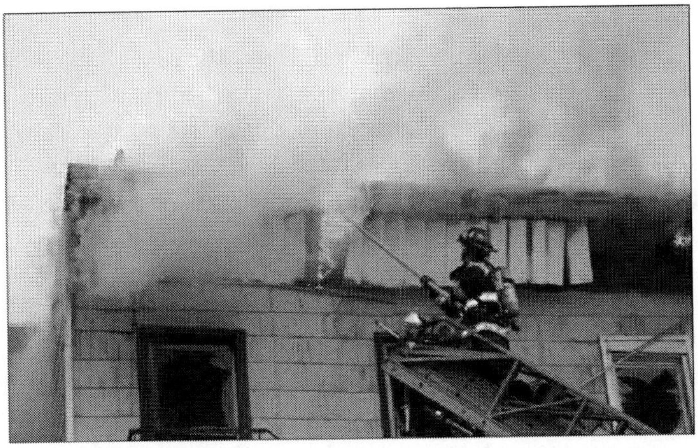

Figure 1.2. Courtesy of Ron Jeffers, Union City, NJ.

Table 1.1. Duties at the Time of a Thermal Injury - 2005

Duty	Number of Injuries	Percent of Total
Fireground	2,480	70
Training	380	11
Nonfire Emergency	285	8
Responding/Returning	255	7
Other Onduty Activity	155	4
TOTAL	3,555	100

Table 1.2. Duties at the Time of a Cardiac Event – 2005

Duty	Number of Injuries	Percent of Total
Fireground	315	41
Other Onduty Activity	185	24
Training	125	16
Nonfire Emergency	85	11
Responding/Returning	55	8
TOTAL	**765**	**100**

Clearly, the most likely place for a thermal injury to occur is on the fireground. This is most likely due to the heavy protective gear worn by firefighters during these operations, the amount of strenuous activity being performed while wearing this gear, and the heat generated by the incident itself.

It also should be noted that while reducing the risk of thermal illness is one major objective for rehab operations, reducing the occurrence and impact of cardiac events is another prime motivator for effective rehab operations. Firefighters who are overstressed and physically expended are at a greater risk for suffering a heart attack or stroke. However, when reviewing the injury statistics for firefighters it is noted that in 2005 they accounted for only one percent of all firefighter injuries. Table 1.2 shows a breakdown of the activities the firefighters were engaged in at the time of the cardiac event.

Again, it is clear that the fireground is the most likely place for a cardiac event to occur.

The USFA reported that there were 115 firefighters who died in the line of duty in 2005. The manner in which the USFA categorizes deaths and when they occurred differs from the NFPA injury statistics. The USFA uses a category called "stress/overexertion" into which it combines deaths caused by heart attacks, strokes, and thermal exposures. In 2005, 62 firefighters died as a result of stress or overexertion.This represented 55 percent of the total firefighter fatalities. Of these 62 deaths, 55 were as a result of heart attacks, 6 were due to strokes, and 1 was a result of heat exhaustion. The USFA report does not list what the people who died of stress/overexertion were doing at the time of their deaths.

The most glaring fact that becomes immediately evident when reviewing both the injury and death statistics is the severity of heart attacks when they occur. While cardiac events account for only 1 percent of all firefighter injuries, they account for more than half of all firefighter deaths. Clearly, the best way to minimize the impact of these events is to prevent them from happening. While much of this has to due with the lifestyle and conditioning of firefighters prior to operating at an event or in a training exercise, it also shows the need for, and importance of, proper rehab procedures during incident and training functions.

CASE STUDIES

Much can be learned by looking at past incidents that have affected the well-being of fire service personnel. When reviewing the following cases studies, note the varied geographical locations of the incidents and the range of conditions under which they occurred. This should impress upon the reader that the need for proper firefighter rehabilitation operations is not limited to areas of the country prone of frequent extreme weather conditions. Rather, having good policies and procedures for training and emergency scene rehabilitation operations are needed by all fire departments.

The case studies that are provided highlight the important facts that led to the firefighter injury or illness. Lessons learned from each incident are noted also. The information in each of these studies will then form the basis for the information that follows throughout the rest of the report. Additional case studies are provided further back in the report to highlight specific concerns where they are addressed.

Case Study 1

Name: Todd David Colton
Age: 25
Rank: Firefighter
Status: Career
Years of Service: 9 months
Date of Incident: September 6, 1990
Time of Incident: 1155 hours
Date of Death: September 6, 1990
Weather: Extremely hot, humid, and windy, temperature of 97 °F (36.1 °C) and wind at 24 miles per hour (mph), gusting to 35 mph.

On September 6, 1990 just before noon, the Sedgwick County, Kansas Fire Department was dispatched to a brush fire at the rear of a manufactured home in a wooded section of the county. The fire began when an occupant of the home set a trash pile on fire and let it get out of control. The occupant tried unsuccessfully to control the fire with a garden hose for about 20 minutes before calling the fire department.

By the time the first fire units arrived, the fire had spread to adjacent yards and to an auto salvage yard behind the yard of origin. Sedgwick County Engine 6, staffed by Firefighter Colton and his captain, was the first unit to arrive on the scene, at 1155 hours. They maneuvered the engine behind the house and down an incline close to the fire and began suppression operations. The captain called for additional units and, as Command, assigned them to adjacent properties to surround and contain the fire's spread. At about 1220 hours the captain radioed that he and Firefighter Colton needed relief because they were exhausted. He radioed for relief again at 1227 hours and at 1241 hours.

Another Sedgwick County firefighter arrived in a tanker (tender) and saw the captain and Firefighter Colton some time between 1227 and 1241 hours. That firefighter and a volunteer firefighter on mutual aid pulled lines from the tanker (tender) and began suppression operations. When the tanker (tender) ran out of water, the pair left the scene to refill it. When the tanker (tender) returned to the scene, Firefighter Colton and his captain were no longer with their apparatus.

By this time, a Sedgwick County assistant chief had arrived and assumed Command. He could not see or locate the Engine 6 crew. After several attempts to explain Engine 6's location to the chief, the captain decided to go to the Command Post to accompany the chief into the fire scene. He instructed Firefighter Colton to remove his personal protective equipment (PPE), get a drink of water, and rest on the rear step of Engine 6 until he returned with firefighters to relieve them.

The chief had established the Command Post on the road in front of the salvage yard. An ambulance was parked next to the Command Post with emergency medical technicians (EMTs) standing by to treat injuries or exhaustion. As the captain approached the Command Post, exhaustion overcame him, and the chief ordered him to the ambulance for rehabilitation. He advised the chief that Firefighter Colton also needed relief. At approximately 1335 hours, Firefighter Colton was ordered by radio to report to the Command Post and the receipt of the order anonymously was acknowledged.

At this point, Firefighter Colton and his officer had been working for approximately 90 minutes in full structural firefighting protective clothing including protective trousers, protective coat, gloves, rubber boots, and a helmet. Firefighter Colton was not wearing a Personal Alert Safety System (PASS) device.

While the captain was in rehab in the ambulance, a request to assist a downed firefighter came over the radio. The captain attempted to leave the ambulance, believing that the downed firefighter was Firefighter Colton, but the medical quality control officer stopped him. The downed firefighter turned out not to be Firefighter Colton. When the captain left rehab, he inquired about Firefighter Colton's status and was told that he had been assigned to drive a tanker (tender). The captain was then assigned as a sector commander and assumed that role in the suppression operation.

There were conflicting reports that Firefighter Colton visited rehab or was provided with water by other firefighters some time around 1430 hours.

Just after 1600 hours, a volunteer firefighter discovered Firefighter Colton's body. Firefighter Colton was still in his full personal protective clothing in a brush-covered, unburned area which sloped away from the house of origin. That slope may have prevented other firefighters from seeing him. He was laying supine on a car wheel and EMS assessment revealed rigor mortis. The Sedgwick County coroner ruled that his death was caused by heat stroke.

A National Institute of Occupational Safety and Health (NIOSH) investigation of the incident cited several factors that contributed to Firefighter Colton's death including lack of a Safety Officer on the incident, lack of a coordinated system of rehab between fire and EMS agencies on the scene, lack of an onscene accountability system, understaffmg of Firefighter Colton's engine company, and the lack of a PASS device.

The occupants of the house where the fire started pled guilty to charges of not obtaining a rubbish fire permit and failure to watch properly over their burning trash pile. They were sentenced to 30 days in jail, fined, required to do community service, and put on probation for a year.

Case Study 2

Name: Karl K. Kramer, IV
Age: 22
Rank: Firefighter Recruit

Status: Career
Years of Service: Less than a year
Date of Incident: May 19, 2005
Time of Incident: 1600 hours
Date of Death: May 28, 2005
Weather: 79 °F (26.1 °C)

On May 19, 2005, Firefighter Recruit Karl Kramer reported to the Jacksonville, Florida Fire Department's training academy at 0630 hours. A second generation firefighter, he was under pressure to be successful in completing recruit training. At 6 feet 4 inches tall and 305 pounds, he was considered obese, but had been cleared medically to participate in recruit training.

The day's training began at 0700 hours and included a high angle rope drill comprised of multiple ascents and descents from a three-story rappelling tower. Class instructors told recruits to take rest breaks as needed; a lunch break was scheduled at noon. Firefighter Kramer made no complaints during the day and ate a full lunch at noon. At 1600 hours, physical training began. Led by an instructor, it included stretching, light aerobics, abdominal crunches, and a 2-1/2- to 3-mile run off of the training grounds.

Firefighter Kramer, known as a poor runner, led the run. In previous exercises, he had been forced by fatigue to walk, and other members of the class were told to run in a circle around him until he could run again. He exhibited fatigue in this run also and complained of blurred vision to another student but did not stop until he stumbled and fell about 300 to 500 yards from the training offices. Instructors told fellow students to pick him up; he ran a short distance and collapsed again. After this second collapse, he was picked up and carried inside the gate of the training compound, at approximately 1719 hours.

Inside the training compound, Firefighter Kramer was found to be pale, perspiring profusely and mumbling incoherently. One instructor ran to the office and ordered staff to call 9-1-1; he returned in his truck, into which he and other instructors loaded Firefighter Kramer and took him to the office. Once he was in the office, they started two IV lines, supplied oxygen via a nonrebreather mask, elevated his extremities, and removed his clothing as a cooling measure.The ambulance arrived at 1729 hours and Firefighter Kramer was transported. En route to the hospital, his vital signs were: pulse of 180 beats per minute; breathing rate of 40 per minute; blood pressure 96/41 mmHg. His oxygen saturation was 97 percent (normal), blood sugar was elevated slightly at 168 (normal is 70 to 110), and a cardiac monitor showed supraventricular tachycardia (an abnormal heart rhythm). He vomited during the transport and was laid on his side for suction. The ambulance arrived at the emergency department at 1745 hours.

The emergency department staff found Firefighter Kramer to have a rectal temperature of 108.6 °F. He was intubated successfully; emergent cooling treatments and vigorous hydration were instituted until he was transferred to the intensive care unit at 2100 hours with a core body temperature of 98.6 °F. He was hospitalized for nine days but never regained consciousness and died on May 28, 2005. The cause of death was listed as severe heat stroke with multisystem organ failure and sepsis with multiple complications.

A NIOSH Firefighter Fatality Investigation and Prevention Program report was prepared on this incident (F2005-26).The report made four recommendations to reduce the future incidence of this type of death. The recommendations were:

- Formulate and institute a heat stress program.
- Create a training atmosphere that is free from intimidation and conducive for learning.
- Use physical training staff who have fitness training instruction and are knowledgeable about all aspects of a heat stress program.
- Use trail vehicle and/or equip training instructors with portable radios for offsite runs.

The report is available for review and downloading at the following url: www.cdc.gov/niosh/fire/reports/face200526.html

Case study 3

Name: Stephen Joseph Masto
Age: 28
Rank: Firefighter/Paramedic
Status: Career
Years of Service: 8 months
Date of Incident: August 27, 1999
Time of Incident: 1030 hours
Date of Death: August 27, 1999
Weather: 105 °F (40.6 °C)

On August 27, 1999, the Santa Barbara, California Fire Department responded to a call from the U.S. Forest Service (USFS) for EMTs at the scene of a wildland fire. Probationary Firefighter/Paramedic Stephen Masto was assigned to his first wildland fire, along with a 15-year-veteran firefighter.The two gathered wildland gear and reported to the base camp in Los Padres National Forest, where 180 acres already had burned in a fire sparked by lightning.The temperature at 1030 hours was 103 °F (39.4 °C), and ground temperatures were approximately 120 to 130 °F (48.9 to 54.4 °C).

The two firefighters were instructed to meet up with different crews and the pair were taken several miles from the base camp. Firefighter Masto was dropped off to begin his uphill hike of about 1-1/2 miles to meet the division to which he was assigned. The veteran firefighter made sure Masto drank plenty of water before he started up a well-marked trail. The experienced firefighter also advised Firefighter Masto to alert the division supervisor by radio that he was on his way.

At 1330 hours, about an hour after he started up the trail and about halfway to his destination, Firefighter Masto encountered the division supervisor, who was on his way downhill. The supervisor directed him to take a shortcut from the main trail to the fire crew's new location. Firefighter Masto followed the supervisor's directions until he was close to the crew. Then, mysteriously, he turned and began climbing an 80-degree slope instead of staying on the gradual incline leading up to the ridge where the crew was located.

The supervisor was the last to see Firefighter Masto alive and may have witnessed, but not recognized, the early stages of heat stress, in that he was not visibly sweating, despite the strenuous climb and being heavily clothed in full wildland protective equipment. Other firefighters who met Firefighter Masto on the trail before he encountered the supervisor also failed to recognize any problems.

No one from the base camp, or the fire crew he was headed to, tried to make contact with Firefighter Masto. The hike from where he was dropped off to the fire crew's location should have taken 1-1/2 to 2 hours. The fire crew should have tried to contact him by 1430 hours; investigators speculated that the crew did not know he was coming. In fact, no one tried to communicate with him until the veteran firefighter he had gone out with attempted to at 1800 hours.

Firefighter Masto's body was found at 0800 hours the next morning, slumped on his knees and one hand clinging to a clump of brush. His backpack still had two full bottles of water and his radio was operational. The coroner determined that his death was due to heat stroke.

As a result of his death, his fire department was fined by California Occupational Safety and Health Administration (OSHA) and the USFS updated its training and operating procedures for EMTs.

Case Study 4

Name: Wayne Mitchell
Age: 3 7
Rank: Firefighter Recruit
Status: Career
Years of Service: 3.5 months
Date of Incident: August 8, 2003
Time of Incident: 1000 hours
Date of Death: August 8, 2003
Weather: 87 °F (30.6 °C), with 80-percent humidity

On August 9, 2003, Miami-Dade, Florida Fire Department Recruit Class 93 was scheduled to participate in a live-burn exercise at the Resolve Marine Fire School at Port Everglades, Florida.

The facility was a series of shipping containers put together to simulate a ship; it was not certified by the State Bureau of Fire Standards and Training, nor was it approved for liquefied petroleum gas (LPG) use or designated to have any type of fire outside the burn box. The facility was being used under a memorandum of agreement with the local fire department because the Miami-Dade Fire Department did not have an approved burn facility operational at the time.

The training scenario involved five recruits following a fire hose through two stories of the ship simulator into a section designated the fire box, where they took turns operating a nozzle in various patterns without extinguishing the fire. The firefighter recruits were then assigned to follow the fire hose through a series of three watertight hatches and to "duck walk" across an open-grated floor over the engine room fire, down a ladder and through the simulated engine room. Each squad of five recruits was accompanied by three instructors who had walked through and made themselves familiar with the facility. The recruits were not given the opportunity to walk through the prop prior to the drill, even though this is a requirement of the NFPA 1403, *Standard on Live Fire Training Evolutions.*

Firefighter Mitchell was wearing full structural firefighting protective clothing, including a self-contained breathing apparatus (SCBA). He was in the fourth group of recruits to go through the exercise on an extremely hot day. When his squad arrived at the burn box, one firefighter recruit accidentally sprayed the fire, causing the intensity to drop. The instructor waited a couple of minutes to allow the intensity to build again; then he decided that the squad should have a second rotation at the nozzle. After the first two recruits completed their second rotation, the incident commander transmitted a 15-minute time stamp, indicating that it was time for the squad to begin exiting. Because of the incomplete second nozzle rotation, the recruits were out of order as they turned around and began to exit. The lead instructor exited because he was overheated; the second instructor already had exited because of problems with his SCBA. In the third compartment, the third instructor had difficulty in getting the recruits to exit because of confusion over the proper exit order.

Visibility in compartments one and two was much lower than in compartment three, and the instructor and recruits did not follow the fire hose but went directly across the compartments to the faint outline of the exit doors.

Once out, the chief instructor asked the Incident Commander (IC) for a Personnel Accountability Report (PAR). At that point, the instructors realized that Firefighter Mitchell was missing. The IC alerted staff and began opening all the doors on the second floor. Instructors from the earlier squads donned their SCBA and entered the structure. One instructor entered compartment two from compartment one just as another entered from compartment three. They both saw Firefighter Mitchell lying prone next to the hose. His PASS device was not sounding.

The IC, who had just opened to exterior door to compartment two, and the first instructor pulled Firefighter Mitchell to the outside deck and began assessing his condition. They took off his facepiece and noted the sound of compressed air rushing out. Once his protective clothing was stripped off, Firefighter Mitchell was found to be unresponsive with no pulse or respirations and hot to the touch. Cardiopulmonary resuscitation (CPR) was initiated, and cold water and ice rushed to him.

An onduty firefighter from the neighboring fire department saw Firefighter Mitchell being pulled from the structure and called his station's engine company and medical rescue unit to the scene. Paramedics with advanced life support (ALS) equipment arrived and proceeded with intubation, cardiac monitoring, and intravenous medications. The medical rescue unit arrived at the local hospital's emergency department at 1030 hours and ALS procedures continued until 1054 hours, when Firefighter Mitchell was pronounced dead. The autopsy concluded his death was caused by cardiac arrhythmia due to exposure to heat.

A NIOSH Firefighter Fatality Investigation and Prevention Program report was prepared on this incident (F2003-28).The report made a number of recommendations to reduce the future incidence of this type of death. The recommendations were

- Ensure the Fire Department's Occupational Safety and Health Bureau (OSHB) provides oversight on all Recruit Training Bureau (RTB) safety issues, including live-fire training.

- Provide the Training Division, and specifically the RTB, with adequate resources, personnel, and equipment to accomplish their training mission safely.
- Create a training atmosphere that is free from intimidation and conducive for learning.
- Conduct live-fire training exercises according to the procedures of the most recent edition of NFPA 1403, *Standard on Live Fire Training Evolutions*.
- Ensure that SOPs specific to live-fire training are developed, followed, and enforced.
- Ensure that team continuity is maintained during training operations.
- Ensure that fire command always maintains close accountability for all personnel operating on the foreground.
- Ensure coordinated communication between the IC and firefighters.
- Equip all live-fire participants, including recruits, with radios and flashlights.
- Establish an onscene rehabilitation unit consistent with NFPA 1584, *Recommended Practice on the Rehabilitation of Members Operating at Incident Scene Operations and Training Exercises*.
- Report and record all work-related injuries and illnesses.

Case Study 5

Name: David Michael Ray
Age: 21
Rank: Firefighter
Status: Career
Years of service: Unknown
Date of Incident: May 29, 1997
Time of Incident: 1430 hours
Date of Death: May 30, 1997
Weather: 98 °F (36.7 °C) with 30-percent relative humidity, calm winds

Just before noon on May 29, 1997, a fire crew from the California Department of Forestry, La Cima Fire Center, California Conservation Corps was assigned to dig a fire break to help contain a 20-acre brush fire in the Lakeside Fire Protection District, located in San Diego County. The fire had started at 1030 hours that morning. The crew was away from the fire, working in a steep canyon with no shade or breeze. They constructed 1,300 feet of fire line, gaining approximately 320 feet in elevation.

The crew began work at noon. At 1345 hours, they took a 10- to 15-minute break to rest and hydrate. At 1415 hours, a firefighter fell and injured his shoulder. He received first aid and was walked down the hill and transported to the hospital. Subsequently, he was diagnosed as suffering from heat exhaustion.

At about 1430 hours, Firefighter Ray wandered off the line, apparently disoriented. Five minutes later he collapsed, and the fire crew captain came to his location. He was semiconscious and apparently suffering from acute heat stress symptoms. Fire-break construction ceased as the crew administered first aid by removing clothing, applying water to his skin, treating for shock, and applying cold packs to neck and armpits. EMTs arrived at

1450 and paramedics at 1457. They continued treatment and carried Firefighter Ray approximately 510 feet in a scoop stretcher to an ambulance.

Upon his arrival at the hospital, Firefighter Ray was found to have a body temperature of 107 °F with a pulse of 180 and respirations of 14. Despite treatment in the hospital, Firefighter Ray never regained consciousness and was pronounced dead at 0106 hours on May 30, 1997. The cause of death was listed as hypoxic encephalopathy secondary to hyperthermia (heat stroke).

Firefighter Ray had been out of work for four days, returning to duty the day before the incident occurred. He mentioned to other crew members that he was feeling unwell but did not say anything to the crew captain. There had been a history of recurrent contagious illnesses among crew members. It is possible that a preexisting illness contributed to the inability of Firefighter Ray's body to regulate his body temperature.

Case Study 6

Name: Michelle Smith
Age: 23
Rank: Firefighter
Status: Career
Years of service: 3
Date of **Incident:** June 9, 1996
Time of **Incident:** 0900 hours
Date of Death: June 9, 1996
Weather: Ambient temperature of 94 °F (34.4 °C) with 11-percent humidity

On June 9, 1996 at 0915 hours, 16 members of the Globe Interagency Hot Shot crew, a Federal firefighting team assigned toTonto National Forest, Arizona, began a training run through Six Shooter Canyon. The temperature in the canyon was 94 °F and the relative humidity was 11 percent. Firefighter Smith lagged behind at about 1.7 miles into the 3.4 to 4.2 mile run.The other crew members thought she had returned to the station and, therefor, were not concerned until they arrived back and she was not there.

A search was organized when the crew realized she was missing. Her body was spotted about 1030 hours on June 10, 1996 by the crews of two news helicopters. She was one-tenth of a mile off the path of the run, having passed several homes where she could have gotten water or help. The Gila County sheriff noted that it appeared she sat down and laid back and attempted to get back up. Her body was found supine.

Firefighter Smith was described as being in excellent physical condition and neither her supervisors nor close relatives knew of her having any medical problems. Her death was determined to have been caused by heat stroke.

Case Study 7

Name: Andrew James Waybright
Age: 23
Rank: Firefighter
Status: Career
Years of service: 3 days
Date of Incident: July 3, 2002
Time of Incident: 0810 hours
Date of Death: July 3, 2002
Weather: Hot, starting at 75 °F (23.9 °C), and humid

July 3, 2002 was the third day for Frederick County, Maryland, Recruit Class 6. The temperature at 0700 hours was 75 °F, with humidity of 94 percent. The temperature climbed throughout the morning. The class of 12 assembled at 0700 hours and started with physical training.

The physical training instructor, who had a degree in biology and physiology but no certification as a physical fitness instructor, led the class walking for 1/2-mile, along with an assistant instructor. The class then jogged at the pace of 10 minutes per mile for about 2.7 miles.The jog ended at a park.The instructor had the class perform calisthenics, including jumping jacks, pushups, sit ups, squats, leg raises, and crunches, for 15 to 20 minutes. After the calisthenics, the class ran uphill through the park to return to the park entrance. Three of the recruits, including Firefighter Waybright, fell out of formation at this point and began lagging behind.

At the park entrance, when the group reassembled, the instructor had the class run two sets of uphill wind sprints, approximately 300 feet in length. A couple of the recruits experienced dizziness and dry heaves and were told to sit down and take a break. When the class was done with the sprints, they started back to the academy, jogging as a group. During this jog, 6 or 7 of the 12 fell out of formation, including Firefighter Waybright, and lagged behind. Firefighter Waybright remained in the middle rear of the pack. At approximately the 3.5 mile mark of the jog, Firefighter Waybright stumbled and fell to the ground. He told both instructors he wanted to finish the run, and the assistant instructor helped him to his feet. Firefighter Waybright then became dizzy and was told to sit down. He tried to continue by crawling several feet before collapsing on his stomach.The assistant instructor stated Firefighter Waybright was cold and clammy to the touch when he collapsed.

The physical training instructor left the assistant instructor with Firefighter Waybright and led the rest of the class back to the academy. The instructor sent two of the academy staff to the assistant instructor to help him with Firefighter Waybright. Meanwhile, Firefighter Waybright lost consciousness and went into cardiac arrest. The assistant instructor began CPR and told the staff to call 9-1-1.

Emergency medical units were dispatched at 0813 hours; the paramedic supervisor arrived at 0817 hours and reported that Firefighter Waybright was in cardiac arrest. ALS procedures were initiated immediately and continued throughout the transport to the hospital. The ambulance arrived at the hospital at 0840 hours. Firefighter Waybright's core body temperature was reported to be 107 °F on arrival in the emergency department.

Resuscitation efforts continued for about 40 minutes, until the attending physician pronounced Firefighter Waybright dead at 0922 hours. The autopsy listed hyperthermia as the cause of death.

Lessons Learned From These Case Studies

When one reviews the facts surrounding the case studies presented in this section, a number of important factors become immediately obvious. The first is the age of the seven firefighters who died in these cases. We normally associate the hazards of high heat situations with the elderly. As emergency medical responders we do see increased call volumes on elderly heat illness patients when the weather is hot. However, in reviewing the case studies it is noted that six of the seven fatalities were young people in their twenties. The seventh victim was 37 years of age. This flies in the face of convention.

Young people in the fire service typically are very enthusiastic about what they are doing and in many cases have somewhat of a sense of invincibility. These two factors, combined with inexperience in recognizing signs of danger, are probably instrumental in the likelihood of young firefighters exceeding their own limits in high heat stress situations.

Another significant factor in the case studies that becomes obvious is that four of the seven deaths occurred during training exercises. As stated earlier in this chapter, training deaths are perhaps the most unfortunate, as these are situations that should be totally under our control. There is a fine line between building up the physical capabilities of firefighters and harming them by taking the exercise too far. In most of these cases, obvious warning signs were ignored, often multiple times. Instructors must be trained thoroughly in the hazards of heat illnesses and departments should have policies that prohibit or reasonably limit physical activities in potentially harmful conditions.

Another factor that relates to both the young age of the victims and the training setting of the deaths that cannot be overlooked is the pressure that these young people often feel to succeed. This comes in the forms of both peer pressure among the other firefighters and the desire to please their instructors and succeed in their training. Peer pressure is a powerful thing. Several of the firefighters in the case studies showed remarkable, and ultimately fatal, perseverance in trying to continue on with their activities after they clearly were already suffering severe effects of heat illness. Many of these young people probably wanted to be firefighters their whole lives and feared that buckling to the heat would endanger their opportunity to do that. In reality it endangered their lives.

Typically young firefighters (or young people in general) are more susceptible to peer pressure than are more mature individuals. Leaders and instructors must be cognizant of this fact and step in before it is too late. This is not only true of training setting, but also in emergency scene operations. It would appear that peer pressure to keep up with the rest of a group was also a factor in a couple of the incident-related case study fatalities.

PERTINENT LAWS, STANDARDS, AND GUIDELINES

There is no question that taking good care of firefighters is the right thing to do from an ethical standpoint. Most fire departments do not need any further reason or push to develop and implement policies and procedures that ensure the safety and well-being of their firefighters. However, to ensure that all fire departments have these procedures in place and that the procedures they develop are reasonable and effective, there are a variety of laws, standards, and guidelines that provide information on the need for rehabilitation and give guidance on how to do it.

However, before getting into a discussion on specific documents that impact the provision of rehab operations on fire departments, it is important to understand the differences in these documents. Specifically, it is important to understand the differences between laws and standards and how they may be enforced on fire departments and other emergency service organizations.

Laws are rules of society that have been adopted formally by some governmental agency, typically referred to as an "authority having jurisdiction" or AHJ. AHJs are governmental agencies at the Federal, State, county, and local levels. Adherence to laws is enforced by agents of the government, including law enforcement agencies, district attorney's offices, and regulatory agencies such as the Department of Labor, health departments, etc. Criminal penalties apply to individuals or organizations who fail to comply with laws. Criminal penalties include fines, incarceration, and other forms or punishment.

Standards are consensus positions on some aspects of a particular area or discipline that are developed by a group of people with a common interest in that area or discipline. Unless formally adopted into law by a governmental body (AHJ), there is no criminal penalty for failing to obey a standard. This does not mean, however, that organizations have no reason to follow standards (other than ethical concerns). On the contrary, fire departments have very valid reasons for adhering to certain standards, particularly those developed by the NFPA. NFPA standards have been recognized routinely in civil courts as nationally-accepted, consensus-developed practices. Thus, while failure to establish a rehab area at an emergency scene will not lead to criminal penalties, failure to follow the standard can lead to civil liability for the department. In a lawsuit situation the fire department could be forced to pay monetary damages for "failure to meet accepted standards of practice." For this reason, fire departments need to follow standards as much as possible.

It is realized that virtually no fire department has the resources or capability to follow every single provision of every standard that may apply to their operation. However, fire departments should attempt to identify standards that are pertinent to their operations and attempt to meet as many provisions of those documents as is realistically possible. As long as they can show a reasonable attempt at meeting the standards, their risk of liability will be reduced considerably.

OSHA REQUIREMENTS

In response to increasing numbers of occupational injuries and deaths across a wide variety of occupations, including firefighting, the United States government passed legislation titled the Occupational Safety and Health Act of 1970. Among the many provisions of this legislation was the creation of the Occupational Safety and Health Administration (OSHA). Organizationally, OSHA is located within the U.S. Department of Labor and is responsible for developing and enforcing workplace safety and health regulations.

Provisions within the OSHA legislation allow individual States to develop their own occupational safety and health programs rather than be bound to the Federal government's OSHA. To date, 26 States have adopted their own standards and enforcement policies and have had those programs approved by OSHA. For the most part, these States adopted standards that are identical to OSHA's, although in some cases each State has its own requirements and enforcement policies in particular areas. The OSHA regulations require State-approved programs to have requirements that are at least as restrictive as the Federal OSHA requirements. Both OSHA regulations and State-regulated programs fall into the category of laws that must be followed to avoid criminal penalties.

Heat and cold stress hazards are addressed in specific standards for general industry. Section 5(a)(1) of the OSHA Act, often referred to as the General Duty Clause, requires employers to "furnish to each of his employees employment and a place of employment which are free from recognized hazards that are causing or are likely to cause death or serious physical harm to his employees." Section 5 (a) (2) requires employers to "comply with occupational safety and health standards promulgated under this Act."

While there are a wide variety of OSHA regulations that may be applied to fire departments, two in particular stand out. 29 Code of Federal Regulations (CFR) 1910.156, Fire Brigades, sets forth safety and health regulations for fire brigades and fire departments.There are no specific requirements in this regulation related to firefighter rehabilitation. However, requirements to wear certain types of protective clothing and other requirements do affect the need to provide rehabilitation services at incidents.

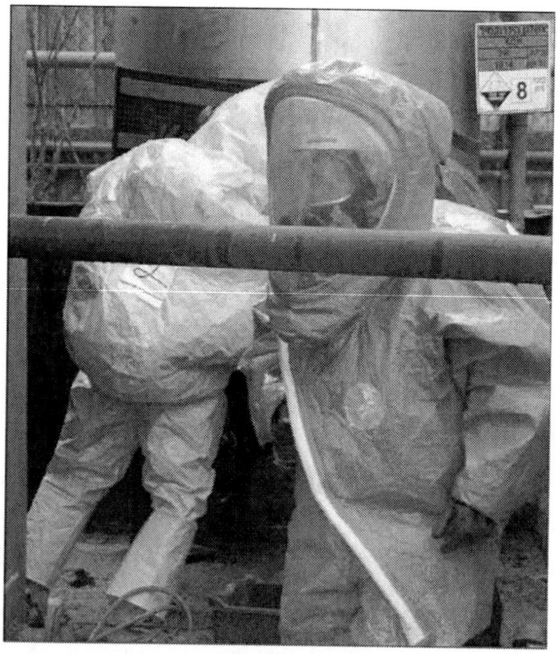

Figure 1.3. Courtesy of IFSTA/Fire Protection Publications.

The second OSHA regulation that greatly affects fire departments is 29 CFR 1910.120, Hazardous Waste Operations and Emergency Response. All fire departments that respond to hazardous materials (hazmat) incidents (and virtually all fire departments do) are bound by the requirements of this section (Figure 1.3). This document has specific language that requires fire departments to address the issue of rehabilitation. Requirement 1910.120(g)(5)(x) requires fire department operation plans and procedures to address limitations during temperature extremes, heat stress, and other appropriate medical considerations.

Although it is not in the category of a regulation, fire departments may choose to consult an excellent document on the topic of heat stress that is provided by OSHA. *The OSHATechnical Manual* (OTM) is an expansive document that provides information on a wide variety of occupational safety and health issues. Section III, Chapter 4 of the OTM is dedicated entirely to heat stress issues. The information in this Chapter includes

- Introduction;
- Heat Disorders and Health Effects;
- Investigation Guidelines;
- Sampling Methods;
- Control;
- Personal Protective Equipment; and
- Bibliography.

Most OSHA requirements and documents can be downloaded from its Web site at www.osha.gov

NIOSH

The National Institute for Occupational Safety and Health (NIOSH) was also created by the Occupational Safety and Health Act of 1970. Organizationally, NIOSH is located within the Centers for Disease Control and Prevention (CDC), which is under the U.S. Department of Health and Human Services. Unlike OSHA, NIOSH is not a regulatory agency. NIOSH was established to help assure safe and healthful working conditions for working men and women by providing research, information, education, and training in the field of occupational safety and health.

Among the myriad of special programs within NIOSH is the Firefighter Fatality Investigation and Prevention program. This program conducts investigations of firefighter line-of-duty deaths to formulate recommendations for preventing future deaths and injuries. The program does not seek to determine fault or place blame on fire departments or individual firefighters, but to learn from these tragic events and prevent future similar events. Separate divisions within this program investigate traumatic deaths and cardiovascular deaths. The results of these inquiries are made available to the public and can be used as the basis for improving programs and services in the future to avoid further firefighter injuries and deaths.The program also develops informational bulletins and documents on pertinent safety and health issues. For more information on the program and to see reports related to rehabilitation issues, go to www.cdc.gov/niosh/fire/

There are two NIOSH documents related to the topic of this chapter that should be of particular interest to firefighters. *Criteria for a Recommended Standard: Occupational Exposure to Hot Environments* (1986) provides a template for organizations to use in developing plans and procedures for dealing with working in environmental extremes. Another useful publication is *Protecting Emergency Responders, Volume 3: Safety Management in Disaster and Terrorism Response* (NIOSH Publication 2004-144).This document provides direct information on rehabilitation, work-to-rest ratios, and other pertinent information when operating at large-scale incidents. These documents also may be downloaded from the NIOSH Web site.

NFPA 1500

While safety is an aspect that can be tied to virtually any fire service standard that has been promulgated by the NFPA, certainly no standard has had more of an impact on the safety and health of firefighters than NFPA 1500, *Standard on Fire Department Occupational Safety and Health Program* (Figure 1.4). The first edition of this standard was adopted in 19 8 7 and it immediately had a profound effect on the manner in which fire departments operated and how they approached safety in the programs and operations. The most recent version of the standard at the time this chapter was written had been adopted in June 2006.

NFPA 1500 provides information on safety and health issues in all aspects of fire department operations, including training, emergency response, station safety, and related safety and wellness programs for members of the department. The standard does contain specific requirements for fire departments to provide rehabilitation services during emergency operations. Section 8.9 of the 2006 edition of NFPA 1500 is titled "Rehabilitation During Emergency Operations" and it lists a number of requirements for fire departments to implement.

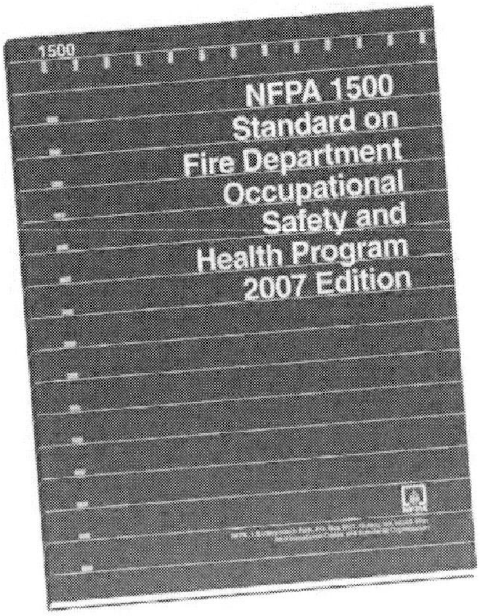

Figure 1.4.

Section 8.9 requires fire departments to develop a systematic approach to rehab operations and to include these procedures in the department's SOPs. It requires the IC to consider the need for rehab at each incident and to establish rehab operations in compliance with the SOPs when the need is evident. It also requires each member on the scene to be responsible for monitoring their own need and communicating their need to rehab when it arises. NFPA 1500 specifies that rehab operations should have a number of fixed components when it is established at an emergency scene, including rest, hydration, active cooling (when required), basic life support (BLS) operations, food (when required), and protection from extreme environmental elements. Fire departments also must establish a plan for replenishing drinking supplies at the incident and wildland firefighters must be supplied with at least 2 quarts of water.

Within NFPA standard, only the information that is contained or referenced within the actual chapters of the document is considered requirements of the standard. These documents also provide a considerable amount of annex (appendix) information, that while not formal requirements of the standard, provide explanation and guidance on implementing the requirements of the chapters of the document. Section 8.9 of NFPA 1500 has a considerable amount of annex information referenced to it to help fire departments develop rehab SOPs. Included in the annex information are considerations for operations in hot and cold weather, information on locating rehab sites, and recommendations for food and water supply at rehab operations.

NFPA 1582 AND 1583

Though not related directly to requirements for rehabilitation operations in training and emergency scene operations, NFPA 1582 and 1583 are important from the standpoint of firefighter fitness. NFPA 1582, *Standard on Comprehensive Occupational Medical Program for Fire Departments* provides details on the preservice and inservice medical exams and testing that firefighters should be capable of passing before being allowed to participate in fire department operations. Meeting the requirements of this standard will help ensure that the firefighter is physically sound to participate in the rigors of emergency operations and thus is related to rehabbing firefighters in training and at incidents. Firefighters who are physically sound will have less of a chance of being impaired during training and emergency operations and also will be easier participants in the rehab operation.

NFPA 1583, *Standard on Health-Related Fitness Programs for Fire Fighters*, provides guidelines on proper fitness programs for fire department members (Figure 1.5). Again, members who participate in a properly managed fitness program will be in better physical condition prior to strenuous activities and will less likely become incapacitated for extensive periods of time during training and emergency scene operations.

NFPA 1584

Though the requirements for providing rehabilitation operations at emergency scenes contained within NFPA 1500 were ground breaking and helpful, they were by no means comprehensive or complete enough to develop a thorough rehabilitation plan for fire departments. The NFPA responded to numerous inquiries for more detailed information on rehab operations by tasking the NFPA 1500 committee with developing a complete document that specifically addressed rehab operations more thoroughly. For this purpose the committee developed NFPA 1584, *Recommended Practice on the Rehabilitation of Members Operating at Incident Scene Operations and Training Exercises* in 2003.

Before discussing NFPA 1584, it is important to note that the first edition of that document was developed as a recommended practice, not a standard. Recommended practices are advisory in nature and do not hold the same legal weight as a standard. The purpose of a recommended practice is to provide guidance and direction on an important topic without being regulatory in nature. It should be noted that at the time this chapter was being developed, a 2008 edition of NFPA 1584 was in the process of being developed. The draft of the new document showed the 2008 version to be released as a standard versus a recommended practice. This will change the level of importance that fire departments will need to place on this document.

NFPA 1584 (2003 ed.) provides comprehensive guidelines on developing rehab SOPs and performing the duties during emergency operations and training exercises. The major sections of NFPA 1584 (2003 ed.) include

- Chapter 1: Administration;
- Chapter 2: Referenced Publications;
- Chapter 3: Definitions;
- Chapter 4: Pre-Incident Response;
- Chapter 5: Rehabilitation Area Characteristics;
- Chapter 6: Incident Scene and Fireground Training Rehabilitation; and
- Chapter 7: Post-Incident.

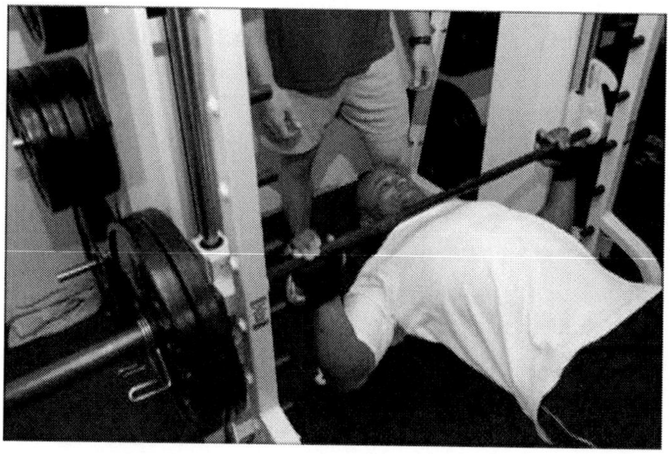

Figure 1.5. Courtesy of IFSTA/Fire Protection Publications.

There is also annex (appendix) information that provides detail on integrating rehab operations into the department's accountability system and a list of other sources of information on the topic. Fire departments must ensure that new or current rehab SOPs are checked against this document to ensure compliance as much as possible.

In: Rehab, Protection and Safety Measures or Firefighters … ISBN: 978-1-60741-566-4
Editor: Andreo Rios

Chapter 2

HEAT STRESS AND THE FIREFIGHTER

Firefighters are exposed to many thermal environments, both hot and cold, in the course of their duties. The firefighter responds to structural and wildland fires as well as other emergencies including vehicle, industrial, aircraft and marine accidents, hazardous materials (hazmat) incidents, and search and rescue operations during disasters such as floods, hurricanes, tornados, blizzards, and earthquakes. Exposure to environmental factors also is experienced during training activities and physical fitness programs. While environmental conditions can be considered in scheduling training activities, the critical nature of the firefighters' job often requires prolonged exposure to extreme thermal conditions during emergency operations. Defining the firefighters' environment is an important first step in developing effective work practices and strategies for protecting them from stress-related illnesses and injuries.

Severity of environmental exposure is related to several factors that influence the amount or rate of heat lost to, or gained from, the external environment. Though both environmental extremes pose hazards for firefighters, problems related to heat stress tend to be far more common and severe than those created by exposure to extreme cold (Figure 2.1). In this chapter we will examine the issue of heat stress on firefighters and the potential problems it may cause.

HEAT STRESS TERMS AND CONCEPTS

Before we can enter into a detailed discussion on heat stress, it is important to define some important terms and concepts as they relate to heat stress. In most cases these terms also have application when discussing cold injuries.This section will focus on their relationship to heat stress situations and also note applications to cold weather considerations so that this information does not have to be repeated in Chapter 3: Cold Stress and the Firefighter.

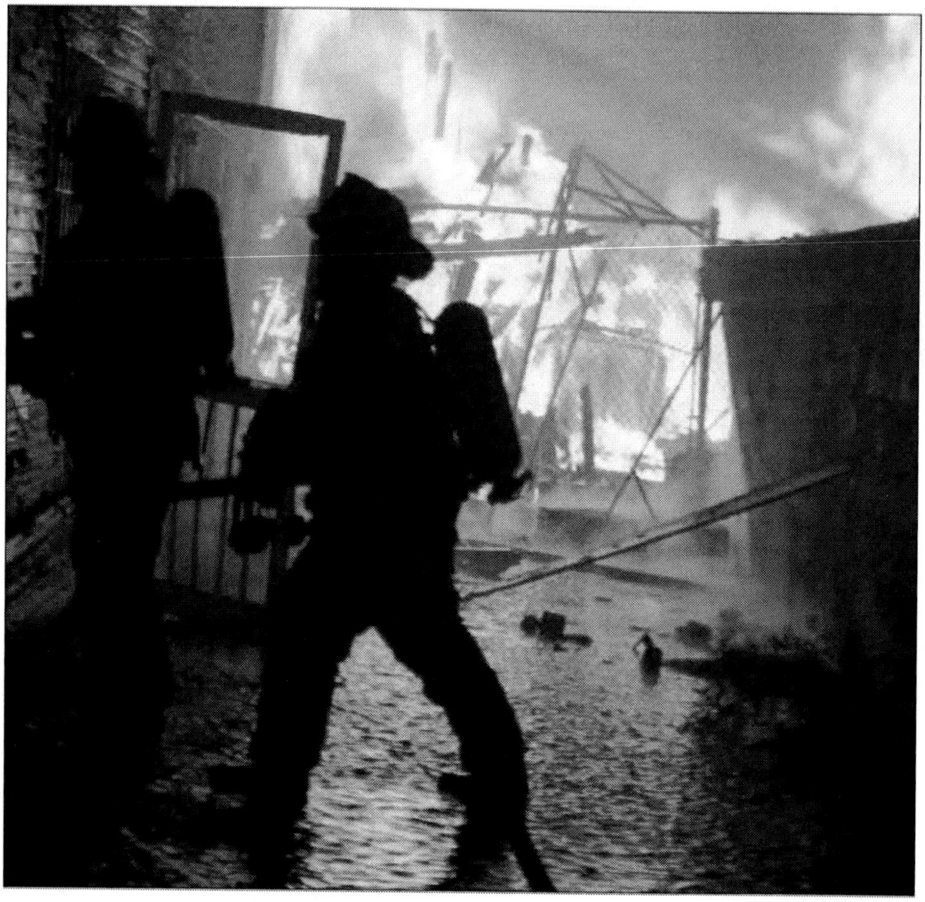

Figure 2.1 —Courtesy of Chris Mickal, New Orleans Fire Department.

The most obvious factor influencing heat stress is the **environmental temperature**, which can be defined **as a measure of how hot the material or objects surrounding the body are**. This is sometimes also referred to as the ambient temperature. Environmental temperature is measured in degrees (°) in reference to standard temperature scales such as Fahrenheit (°F) or Celsius (°C).

Another important factor is **thermal radiation, which occurs between objects of unlike temperature via invisible infrared rays and is related only to the difference in temperature between the objects, such as firefighters' protective clothing and a flame front**. Measurement of thermal radiation is made of the rate of heat transferred per unit area per unit time and is expressed in watts per square centimeter (watts/cm^2) or calories per square centimeter per second (cal/cm^2/sec), where 1.0 watts/cm^2 equals approximately 0.24 cal/cm^2/sec.Thermal radiation can transfer heat from hot objects to the body or from the body to cold objects depending upon object temperatures. Research suggests that thermal radiation is the most important component of heat exposure during actual interior structural firefighting **(Figure 2.2)**.

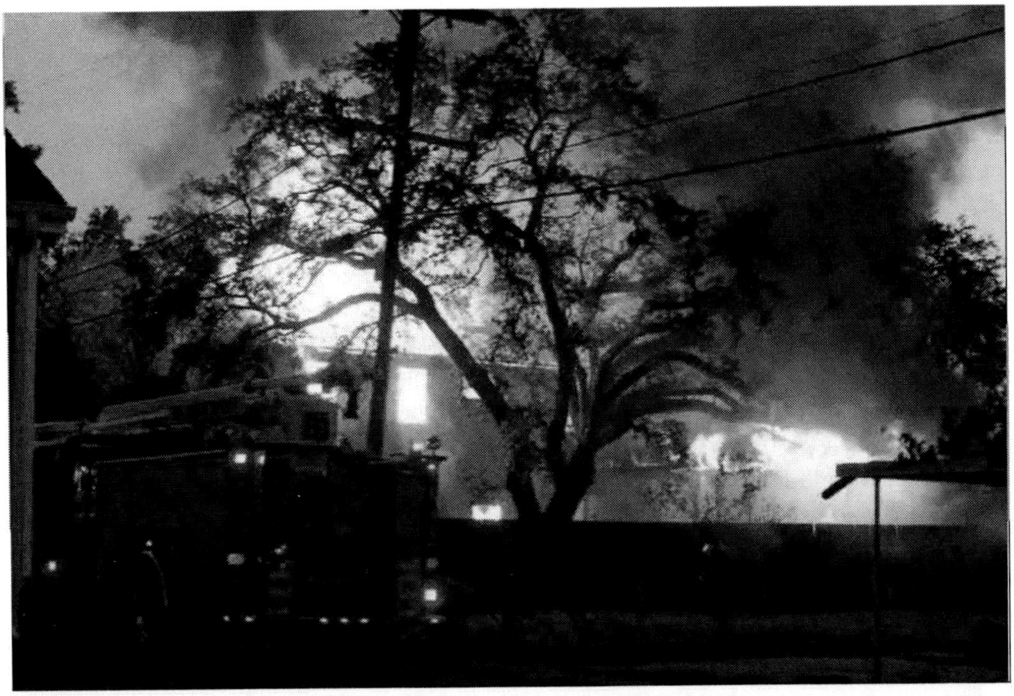

Figure 2.2. Courtesy of Chris Mickal, New Orleans Fire Department.

Heat also can be transferred between objects of different temperatures by **conduction**. **Transfer of heat by conduction requires direct contact between materials**. Examples relevant to firefighters include kneeling or crawling on a hot or cold surface or touching hot or cold objects. It must be noted that the heat transferring ability of materials can vary greatly. For example, water and steam transfer heat many times faster than air; metals transfer heat faster than nonmetals.

Another component of heat transfer is by convection. If the conducting medium surrounding the body, such as air or water, is moving, significantly more heat transfer can occur than in still conditions. A commonly used example of convective heat transfer is the wind chill Index. The wind chill Index is a system that attempts to express the cooling effect of air movement on humans exposed to cold temperatures in terms of equivalent wind chill temperatures. For example, for an environmental temperature of 32 °F (0 °C) with a wind velocity of 40 miles/hour, the equivalent wind chill temperature is 2 °F (-16.7 °C).This means that although the skin temperature does not fall below the environmental temperature, the body loses heat at the same rate as it would at the equivalent wind chill temperature. More information on the wind chill Index is contained in Chapter 3 of this book.

A similar effect occurs at high environmental temperatures. Above about 100°F (37.8°C), air movement above 10 mph can significantly increase heat transfer to the body. In general this is the concept by which a convection oven operates and is the reason this type of oven cooks food much more quickly than a standard oven.

It should be noted that regardless of the type of heat transfer that is occurring, heat **always** travels from the warmer object to the colder object. It is physically impossible to transfer "cold" to a warmer object. The warmer object always loses heat as it transfers some of its heat to the colder object.

Relative humidity is also a contributory factor because it determines the rate of heat transfer by **evaporation.** When liquid water changes to steam or water vapor, heat is dissipated. Relevant examples include the cooling that occurs from the evaporation of sweat and the vaporization of water by thermal radiation from a fire when a fog nozzle is in service.The higher the relative humidity, the less evaporation can occur to remove heat. Relative humidity is measured in terms of the amount of humidity contained in the air relative to the maximum amount that can be contained at that temperature. For example, if the air temperature is 60 °F (15.6 °C) and the relative humidity is 50 percent, the air contains one-half of the total water vapor that it can hold at that temperature.

The Steadman Apparent Temperature Index expresses the combined effect of environmental temperature and humidity, sometimes referred to as the humiture, on the body **(Figure 2.3).** It should be noted that exposure to direct sunlight will also increase apparent temperature by about 10 °F (-12.2 °C).The apparent temperature is determined in a manner similar to wind chill. For example, with an environmental temperature of 90 °F (32.2 °C) and a relative humidity of 90 percent, the apparent temperature is 122 °F (50 °C). Thus, the firefighter exposed to these conditions will experience discomfort similar to that associated with an environmental temperature of 122 °F at low humidity.

SOURCES OF HEAT EXPOSURE

Firefighters are exposed to varying levels of heat in two basic contexts: environmental conditions and fire exposure conditions. Understanding the role and impact of both of these situations is important.

Environmental Heat Exposure

Environmental heat exposure is related directly to interaction with climatic and seasonal conditions. Firefighters are subjected to environmental heat conditions during everything they do. Though the U.S. covers an expansive land area and contains various types of climates, most fire departments operate in locations that can subject them to at least occasional summer environmental temperatures in excess of 90 °F. Many locations in the south and southwestern U.S. regularly endure temperatures over 100 °F for extended portions of the year. Unlike sports enthusiasts or industrial workers, the critical nature of emergency operations does not allow curtailment of environmental exposure during climatic extremes. No matter how hot it is, the firefighters' job must be done. Perhaps the only other occupation with similar climatic exposures is the military, which has done extensive research into human performance under climatic extremes. The U.S. military classifies climatic exposure into four categories: Hot-Wet, Hot-Dry, Cold-Wet, and Cold-Dry.

Dry Bulb Temperature (°F)	Relative Humidity (percent)										
68	61	62	63	64	65	66	67	68	69	70	70
70	63	65	66	67	68	69	70	71	72	72	73
72	66	67	68	69	70	71	72	73	74	75	76
74	68	69	70	71	72	73	74	75	76	77	78
76	71	72	73	74	75	76	77	78	79	80	81
78	74	75	76	77	77	78	79	80	81	83	85
80	76	77	78	79	80	81	82	83	85	87	90
82	78	79	80	81	82	83	85	87	89	92	96
84	79	80	81	83	84	86	88	90	93	97	103
86	81	82	83	85	86	89	91	95	99	105	113
88	82	84	85	86	89	91	95	99	105	114	
90	84	85	87	89	92	95	99	104	112		
92	85	87	89	92	95	99	104	112			
94	87	89	91	95	98	103	110	120			
96	88	91	94	97	102	108	117				
98	90	93	96	100	105	113					
100	92	95	98	103	109	119					
102	93	96	100	106	114						
104	95	98	103	110	120						
106	96	100	106	114							
108	97	102	109	118							
110	99	104	112	122							
112	100	106	115								
114	102	108	118								
114	102										

Figure 2.3.

- **Hot-Wet** conditions are characterized by environmental temperatures exceeding 68 °F (20 °C), but rarely exceeding 100 °F. Relative humidity is in excess of 75 percent and rain is experienced regularly, especially in the form of thundershowers. Hot-wet conditions are experienced commonly in much of North America during the summer months.
- **Hot-Dry** conditions are characterized by environmental temperatures exceeding 68 °F and regularly exceeding 100 °F. Relative humidity is less than 75 percent, and is commonly less than 25 percent. Long periods without precipitation are common. Hot-dry conditions are experienced commonly in areas of the southwestern U.S.

- **Cold-Wet** conditions are characterized by environmental temperatures of between 14 °F (-10 °C) and 68 °F. Temperatures can change rapidly and daily freeze/thaw cycles can occur. Precipitation in the form of rain, freezing rain, sleet, or snow can be experienced regularly. Most areas of North America experience cold-wet conditions at some time during the year. Even tropic, desert, and polar areas regularly experience conditions of this type.

- **Cold-Dry** conditions are characterized by environmental temperatures of less than 14 °F. Below-zero and windy conditions are often experienced and temperatures of less than -60 °F (-51.1 °C) have been recorded in many areas. Above-freezing conditions are uncommon. Precipitation is in the form of dry snow. Areas of North America commonly experiencing cold-dry conditions include the north-central U.S., portions of the northeastern U.S., central and northern Canada, Alaska, and areas with mountainous terrain such as the Rockies and Sierras.

It is important to remember that the above descriptions identify climatic conditions, not areas or climate types. Many areas experience two or more climatic conditions on a regular basis depending on the short-term weather cycles and the day-night or seasonal variations. Additionally, unusual conditions of weather or geography can prevail that will cause an area to experience conditions far more severe than normal. Since the firefighter is required to function efficiently at all times, it is important that equipment and training appropriate for the most severe conditions is provided.

Fire Exposure

The most critical thermal exposure faced by firefighters, fire exposure, occurs during actual fire suppression and fire rescue activities. Research by the National Bureau of Standards (NBS; they would later change their name to the National Institute of Standards and Technology or NIST) and the U.S. Fire Administration (USFA) examined the fire environment both in simulated laboratory fires and by placing thermocouples and heat-sensitive tape on firefighters while they were engaged in interior structural firefighting. In general, four conditions are faced by structural firefighters.

Class I conditions occur when a small fire is burning in a room. Environmental temperatures up to 140 °F (60 °C) and thermal radiation up to 0.05 watts/cm^2 are encountered for up to 30 minutes **(Figure 2.4).**

Class II conditions occur in a room that has been totally involved after the fire has been "knocked down." In this case, environmental temperatures from 105 to 203 °F (40.6 °C to 95 °C) and thermal radiation from 0.050 to 0.100 watts/cm^2 are encountered for up to 15 minutes.

Class III conditions exist in a room that is totally involved. Environmental temperatures from 204 to 482 °F (95.6 °C to 250 °C) and thermal radiation from 0.175-4.2 watts/cm^2 are encountered for up to 5 minutes.

Class Iv conditions occur during a flash-over or backdraft, where environmental temperatures from 483 to 1,500 °F (250.6 to 815.6 °C) and thermal radiation from 0.175-4.2 watts/cm^2 are encountered for about 10 seconds.

Firefighters face particularly severe exposures during combustible/flammable liquid fuel and chemical fires **(Figure 2.5).** Research by the U.S. Air Force found that environmental temperatures of 2,000 °F (1,093.3 °C) and thermal radiation of 5.0 watts/cm^2 can be approached.

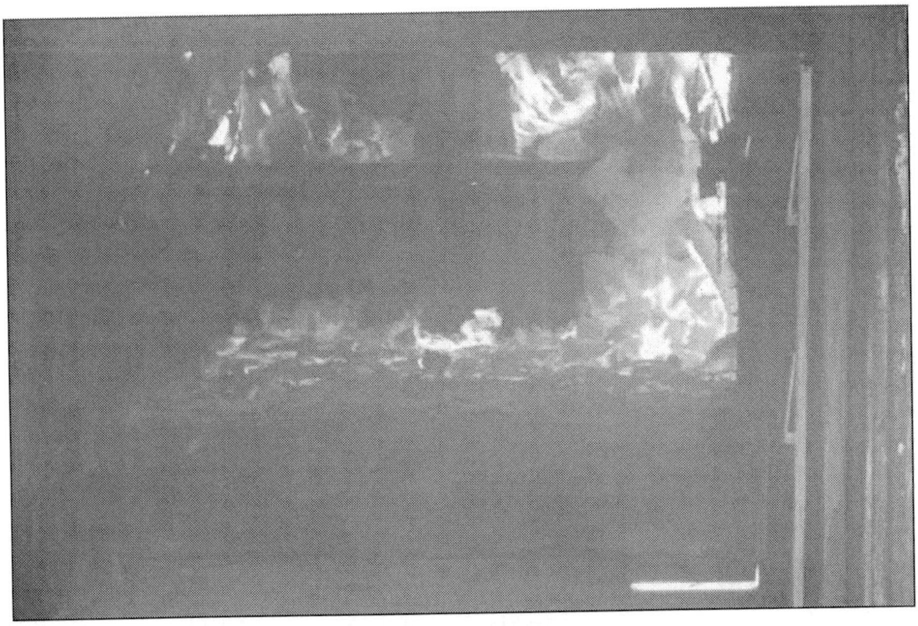

Figure 2.4.

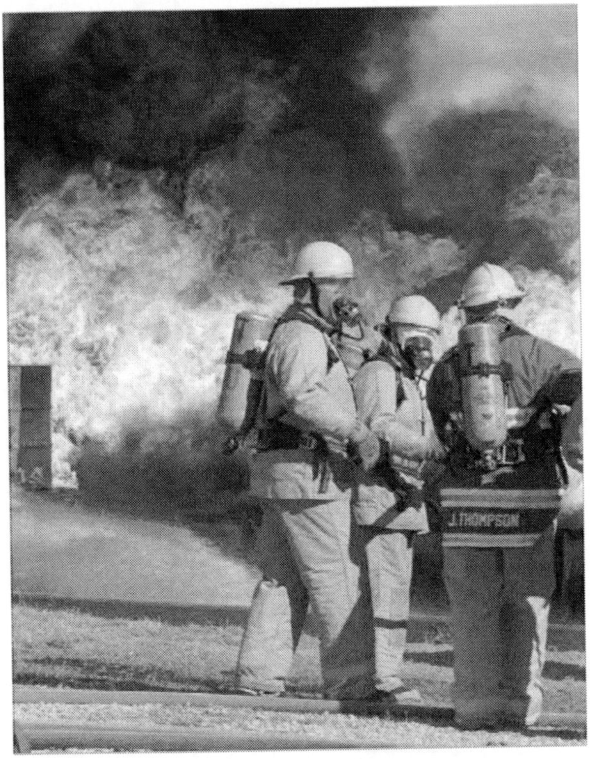

Figure 2.5. Courtesy of Chris Mickal, New Orleans Fire Department.

Long-Term Exposure to Heat

For the vast majority of municipal firefighters, exposure to extreme heat situations will occur in limited, short doses. Career firefighters and many volunteers typically will spend the majority of their time in a climate-controlled setting, such as the fire station, home, or workplace.There are several exceptions to this, including:

- Career firefighters who have been involved in training exercises or repetitive calls during high temperature conditions.
- Volunteer firefighters who work outdoor or otherwise hot atmospheric jobs and respond to fire calls after extended periods exposed to heat.
- Wildland firefighters who operate for long periods of time in high temperature conditions and may not be able to retreat to climate-controlled facilities during down periods.

Research conducted by the U.S. Army shows that the effects of high heat on personnel are cumulative. The Army uses the HEAT acronym to outline the concerns of repetitive exposure to heat:

- High heat conditions, especially on several sequential days. For the Army, wet-bulb globe thermometer (WBGT) ambient temperatures over 75 °F are considered high heat for training and hard work situations. In the fire service, acceptable temperature levels will vary depending on the location and normal atmospheric conditions encountered by the firefighters.
- Exertional level of work or training, especially on several sequential days. Continued periods of heavy work will negatively impact the firefighter's ability to cool down on subsequent days.
- Acclimatization and other individual risk factors. Both of these will be discussed in more detail later in this chapter.
- Time. The length of heat exposure and amount of recovery time will impact the firefighter's ability to recover on subsequent days of exposure to high levels of heat.

The longer the prolonged period of exposure to conditions of elevated temperature, the greater the chance that personnel will fall victim to heat-related illnesses and injuries. Incident Commanders (ICs) and supervisors must monitor conditions and personnel continuously for the purpose of taking action before injuries begin to occur. Clusters of minor heat-related problems must be taken as a warning sign of impending serious injuries and personnel should be rotated out of action or otherwise treated to prevent the situation from worsening. Even if the heat problems were on a previous day, the cumulative effect of the heat buildup could increase the chance of serious problem on this new day. Key personnel failed to recognize these signs in several of the cases studies discussed in the previous chapter of this manual and this ultimately led to firefighters suffering fatal heat stress injuries.

EFFECTS OF PERSONAL PROTECTION EQUIPMENT ON HEAT STRESS

Firefighters wear a variety of protective ensembles that consist of protective clothing and equipment items to provide protection against a variety of hazards. Typical ensembles include protective garments, helmets, eye/face protection, hoods, gloves, footwear, and respiratory protective devices. Ensembles are configured differently depending on the application—structural or proximity firefighting, wildland firefighting, technical rescue, hazardous materials operations, and emergency medical services (EMS) all include different materials and components in items designed for specific levels of protection. The clothing and equipment provide protection by placing materials and components between the person and the hazards in the environment. For example, for structural firefighting, one of the principal functions of the clothing is to insulate from high heat. This insulation is accomplished by layered clothing, gloves, and footwear which attenuate the radiant and convective foreground heat; additional layers often reinforce the clothing for extended contact with hot surfaces. Structural firefighting protective clothing also includes barrier layers to prevent firefighter contact with harmful fireground liquids that can include hot water, certain chemicals, and blood or body fluids. This same barrier material technology is implemented in garments, gloves, and footwear for other types of applications, sometimes using higher performing barriers such as in the case of hazardous materials (hazmat) protective ensembles.

The provision of protection comes at the expense of human factors, particular in placing an additional burden on the firefighter that lead to increased physiological stress. Firefighter protective ensembles significantly impact the normal mechanisms of body heat loss that occur primarily through conduction and evaporation of sweat, given the encapsulation or near encapsulation of the firefighter's body. Simply stated, personal protective equipment (PPE) inhibits the transfer of heat between the firefighter and the external environment. In cold atmospheres this works to the firefighter's advantage, as the PPE keeps the body heat trapped within the ensemble and helps keep the firefighter warm. However, in high heat, high humidity, or high work activity conditions, the protective ensembles increase the thermal strain on the wearer's body exponentially. While in one sense it is protecting the firefighter from exposure to hazardous chemicals or the extensive heat from a fire, the thermal strain being placed on the body by inhibiting its natural cooling process can accelerate the development of heat-related injuries and illnesses. Thus, the decision for wearing protective ensembles and the specific selection of minimum performance must take into account the balance or tradeoff between providing protection from the environment and overburdening the firefighter's capacity to lose heat through normal heat transfer mechanisms.

Firefighters are required to wear different protective ensembles based on Federal regulations that require employers (the fire department) to provide PPE that is appropriate for the hazards faced by their employees (the firefighters). In the case of structural firefighters, there are specific Occupational Safety and Health Administration (OSHA) regulations provided in Title 29 Code of Federal Regulations (CFR) Part 1910.156, which require fire brigades to provide suitable protective clothing and equipment. Similar regulations exist for the provision of hazmat protective ensembles as specified in 29 CFR 1910.120 and PPE to protect against bloodborne pathogens (29 CFR 1910.1030). For those States that use their own regulations, State criteria must dictate equal or higher levels of protection.

Unfortunately, these regulations are either based on outdated industry standards or include ambiguous criteria for specification of PPE.

The fire service uses standards developed by the National Fire Protection Association (NFPA) to define the minimum PPE requirements for design and performance of protective clothing and equipment. NFPA 1971, *Standard on Protective Ensembles for Structural Fire Fighting and Proximity Fire Fighting,* is the product standard that covers structural firefighting protective ensembles. Additional NFPA standards directed to the end user specify that department use PPE that meets these "product" standards. In each product standard, criteria exist that address specific clothing designs for covering portions of the firefighter's body combined with performance criteria that set specific levels for insulation, physical hazard resistance, and hold out of hazardous liquids. For example, clothing and gloves used for structural firefighting must meet a minimum thermal insulation requirement called thermal protective performance (TPP). TPP testing is conducted to ascertain the insulation provided by the major three layers of the structural firefighting clothing garments and must meet a minimum level that has been established to allow firefighters to escape emergency fireground conditions (such as occur during a flashover and backdraft) without injury. Similar requirements address other areas of performance, which affect the choice of materials and the overall bulk of the clothing and equipment worn by the firefighter. A typical structural firefighting protective ensemble is shown in **Figure 2.6.** Other types of protective ensembles incorporate similar requirements that result in clothing and equipment with varying degrees of body coverage and encapsulation.

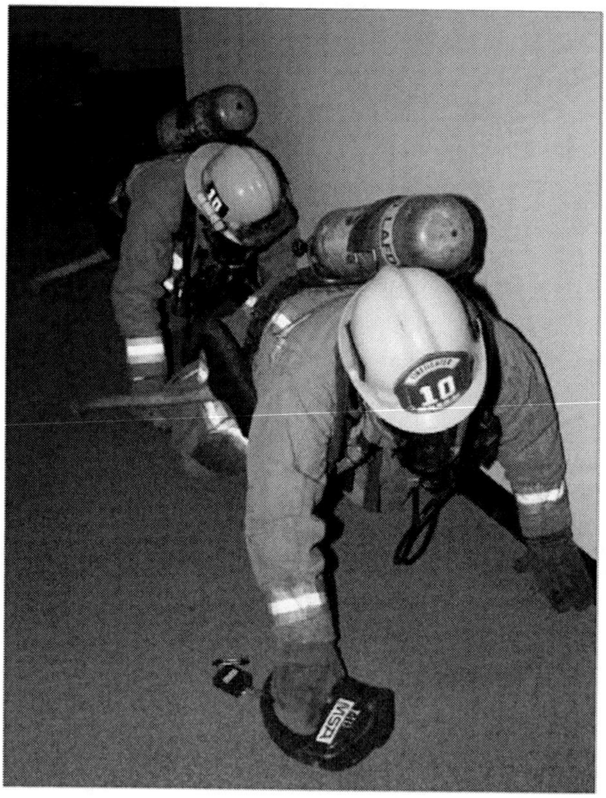

Figure 2.6.

While these requirements of NFPA product standards are intended to achieve the necessary protective function for firefighting, the clothing does interfere with heat dissipation during nonfire exposure such as overhaul, hazmat incidents, and rescue operations. For this reason, later editions of several product standards have included a new test to help balance clothing stress effects with protective requirements. Total heat loss is used to measure how well garments allow body heat to escape. The test assesses the loss of heat both by the evaporation of sweat and the conduction of heat through the garment layers, as these mechanisms are considered the two primary forms of heat loss while wearing encapsulating clothing. As clothing is made more insulative to high heat exposures, there is a tradeoff with how well the heat buildup in the firefighter's body (that can lead to heat stress) is alleviated. Garments that include nonbreathable moisture barriers or very heavy thermal barriers prevent or limit the transmission of sweat moisture, which carries much of the heat away from the body. If this heat is kept inside the ensemble, the firefighter's core temperature can rise to dangerous levels if other efforts are not undertaken (i.e., limiting time on scene, rotating firefighters, providing rehabilitation at the scene).

Thus the total heat loss (THL) test has been included in several NFPA standards to provide a balance between thermal insulation for protection and evaporative cooling insulation for stress reduction. For structural firefighting protective clothing, the minimum THL requirement was first set of 130 watts per square meter when it was introduced as part of NFPA 1971 in 2000. The new 2007 edition of NFPA 1971 raised this requirement to 205 watts per square meter. Less insulative US&R operations, wildland firefighting and emergency medical garments are subject to a requirement of 450 watts per square meter. Work for setting the level for structural firefighting was based on a major study of clothing effects on firefighter heat stress that was conducted by the International Association of Fire Fighters (IAFF). This study showed that using material composites with higher values of THL create less stress on firefighters and physiological effects of clothing on the firefighter (namely core temperature rise) could be correlated with the garment material system THL value. Thus, the study showed how the total heat loss test was able to predict the stress-related effects of clothing on the firefighter.

The THL requirement in NFPA 1971 provides a tool for examining the tradeoff between thermal insulation (from heat) and the stress-related aspects of clothing materials. In general, as the material composite thickness increases, higher levels of thermal insulation (measured using TPP testing) are obtained. At the same time, thicker composites typically create more stress on the firefighter. With the advent of total heat loss testing, fire departments can now choose to optimize the selection of their composites by balancing composite THL values with thermal protective performance values (while still meeting the minimum performance for both areas of performance). Moisture barriers have the greatest impact on THL, but THL also is affected by the choice of outer shell and thermal barrier. For TPP testing, thermal barriers usually have the greatest impact, but like THL, the TPP value for a composite is based on the contribution from each layer.

The result of adding the THL requirement to NFPA 1971 in 2000 was to eliminate nonbreathable moisture barriers such as Neoprene coated polycotton. The THL requirement now mandates only highly breathable moisture barriers that, nonetheless, can be overwhelmed by very hot conditions, high humidity, and rigorous work activity. However, material suppliers and manufacturers of turnout clothing have undertaken a number of clothing material and design improvements that are aimed at minimizing the stress on firefighters. This work began through the National Aeronautics and Space Administration (NASA) to assist in the development state of the art protective clothing and equipment for structural firefighting. The resulting effort was called Project FIRES (Firefighters Integrated Response Equipment System) and its purpose was to design, fabricate, and laboratory and field test an integrated protective clothing ensemble for firefighters that would address the known limitations of their available equipment including heat stress, interference with movement, and adequate protection during fiashover or backdrafts.The IAFF and other research efforts have further contributed to an advancement in lightweight clothing systems with an emphasis on stress reduction without any penalties in protective performance.

The sections below discuss the state-of-the-art in clothing design and material technology as applied to firefighter PPE for structural firefighting.

Turnout Clothing

Conventional firefighter protective clothing consists of three layers, in the order of an outer shell, moisture barrier, and with a thermal barrier, which is next to the wearer's skin:

1. The outer shell is the exterior layer of the turnout clothing and is intended to offer the primary physical and flame protection to the wearer. Because it is on the exterior of the clothing, it generally will have the greatest exposure and take more abuse compared to other parts of the clothing. This means that it is more likely to be soiled or stained and subject to tears, punctures, cuts, and abrasions even though the material is the most rugged layer and also is treated with a repellent finish. As a consequence, outer shells are heavy, woven fabrics made of intrinsically flame-resistant fibers and treated with finishes to provide water shedding or repellency of the outer layer.
2. The moisture barrier is typically the middle layer of the three-layer composite. It consists of a film that is laminated to a substrate fabric or a fabric that has been coated with a rubber material. This layer's prin cipal purpose is to prevent the passage of liquids (hot water, chemicals, blood, and other contaminants) into the clothing interior. The material must be both flame and heat resistant and maintain its barrier performance under high heat conditions. As a layer of the overall clothing composite, it provides a small contribution to the overall clothing insulation. In most clothing configurations, the film or coating faces towards the interior of the clothing liner to protect it from physical damage. In order to provide continuous barrier protection throughout the clothing, the sewn moisture barrier seams are covered with tape that are heat sealed onto the film side of the material. Moisture barrier material also is placed on the inside of the shell at the front closure for this purpose for complete moisture protection (this use of moisture barrier is called facings). Both the film/coating and tape must remain intact in order for the moisture barrier to perform its liquid barrier function.
3. The thermal barrier is the innermost layer of the composite and the primary layer contributing to over all clothing thermal insulation. It is essential that this layer remain intact during extreme or emergency conditions because its loss of thermal

integrity will permit faster heat transfer and increase the potential for burn injury. Most thermal barriers contain lightweight, low-density materials to trap air for increaseing the insulation of the overall clothing material composite. Many thermal barriers also consist of two parts—a woven face cloth that is next to the wearer's body and a nonwoven batting or layers that are oriented towards the moisture barrier. The face cloth is quilted to the batting to provide physical support for the overall material. In order to maintain their insulative qualities, thermal barriers must retain their "loft" or fluffmess. Thinning of the thermal barrier will cause greater heat transfer through those parts of the garment.

Collectively, these three materials are referred to as a "composite." However, composites may include other material layers, such as reinforcements, as described below.

Firefighter protective clothing consists of several other important components that function to provide protection to the firefighter. These include high visibility materials consisting of bands of striping sewn on the clothing exterior called trim that provide conspicuity of the wearer during daytime and nighttime conditions, various types of hardware that are located throughout the coat and pants primarily in the openings or closures of garments, hook and loop fastener tape (Velcro) that also is used throughout some turnout clothing for closure and pocket flaps, knit materials provided in wristlets at the end of the coat sleeves and as a comfort strip in the collar closure area.

Firefighter protective clothing also is designed with several design features, which may vary among manufacturers. For example, reinforcements are used for adding physical or thermal protection to critical areas of the clothing.Typically reinforcements are placed in the shoulders, upper back (often referred to as the yoke), and elbows of coats, and knee and seat areas for pants. Other reinforcements may be placed at pant cuffs and coat sleeve hems (in an area called "water wells" by some manufacturers). Since reinforcements generally come in contact with the ground more frequently than other parts of the clothing, they tend to experience relatively higher amounts of soiling and damage compared to other parts of the clothing.

The majority of outer shell materials are composed of meta-aramid (Nomex®), PBI®, Basofil®, and a few newer inherently flame-resistant fibers. Nearly all shell fabrics include some proportion (5 to 60 percent) of para-aramids such as Kevlar® for increased strength and thermal stability. The range of weight for shell materials generally is limited between 6 and 7.5 ounces per square yard. Lighter materials tend not to provide needed durability (they either abrade or otherwise wear out quickly), while heavier materials are too stiff leading to increased stress in clothing movement. Also affecting the choice of shell material is the weave construction. Many shell materials are offered in twill or plain-weave construction (a simple overlap fiber configuration), or duck weave (heavier fiber construction), while some materials need to be in a rip-stop construction (using intermittently heavier fibers) to provide adequate strength and durability. Twill fabrics tend to be more flexible but less durable than duck weave or rip-stop constructions.

Early moisture barriers were flame-resistant fabrics coated with Neoprene or similar flame-resistant polymers. However, owing to their high relative weight and bulk, alternative moisture barriers were developed based on microporous film technology. Microporous films offer the further benefit of promoting clothing breathability while maintaining barrier performance. Film products are either based on a form of Teflon (GoreTex® or Crosstech®) or flame-retardant polyurethanes (Porelle®) or polyester (Sympatex®). Substrate choices are usually Nomex® or flame-retardant treated fabrics; however, an increasing number of alternative choices such as Kermel® are offered, especially in Europe. These substrate fabrics can be woven or nonwoven materials such as Dupont's E89 Nomex® fabric. Moisture barriers, especially those based on microporous films, are intended to be a relatively lightweight layer in the composite or component assembly with fabric weights ranging from 3.5 to 5 grams per square meter.

Lining systems or thermal barriers typically have been multiple layers of fabric to provide bulk and air layers. Many modern thermal barriers use nonwoven batt materials that entrap air for more effective insulation. The batting is quilted to a woven face cloth to hold the thermal barrier together. Batting materials include fibers based on Kevlar®, Nomex®, Kermel®, Basofil® or other flame-resistant materials. Alternative thermal barrier or liner fabrics use multiple layers (two or three) of a nonwoven fabric, such as Nomex E89®, quilted to the face cloth fabric. Face cloths for the thermal barrier provided the inner most surface of the clothing and tend to be durable, but lightweight woven fabrics consisting of Nomex® or other flame-resistant fiber materials. Over the past several years, low friction face cloth materials (i.e., fabrics that are very smooth to the touch) such as low denier (small diameter) filament Nomex® are being used increasingly for easy clothing donning and wear.

The fire service is likely to see continued development of new fabrics and fibers with a focus on material systems and whole systems testing, particularly towards stress reduction. Future standards will move towards more composite and manikin testing making it necessary for the market place to consolidate material offerings but provide better characterized protective clothing. Manufacturers have been investigating new material technologies such as phase change materials (fabrics that contain polymers that have increased heat storage capacity) that offer similar performance but at lower weight and bulk, but numerous several developmental issues first must be addressed. The trend for testing completed garments will shift the emphasis for examining design improvements to clothing, especially in demonstrating less stress effects on firefighters.

Helmets

Historically helmets have been made of leather, and today, many still prefer the traditional style of leather helmets, despite the availability of lighter weight, more protective composites. Indeed, leather helmets have had to incorporate certain changes to reflect the standardized protection needs sought for firefighting. These helmets must now include impact caps and other devices to absorb the expected top or side impact blows that can occur to the firefighter's head. Additional concerns include electrical insulation, overall heat and flame protection, and how well the helmet stays on the firefighter's head during impact.

The key components of the firefighter helmet are the shell, energy-absorbing system, and retention system. The shell is the outer material that forms the main portion of the helmet. Other than leather, lighter weight materials are now used commonly in helmets such as fiberglass and high performance composites, reinforced with Kevlar®. The energy-absorbing system is an insulating material inside the shell in combination with the suspension system (headband and crown strap), and helps to attenuate the energy from an impact. The sweatband helps to absorb sweat from the firefighter's head. The retention system consists of the chin strap and nape device (at the rear of the helmet) for positioning the helmet on the firefighter's head. Most helmets use a ratchet on the headband for easily adjusting helmet size.

Other components include fluorescent and retroreflective markings, ear covers, and either a faceshield or goggles or both. Markings are used for both increased firefighter visibility or for identification. While many departments use the helmet colors to depict certain roles on the fireground, markings can help, particularly for nighttime operations. Fluorescent markings provide increased daytime contrast while retroreflective markings make the firefighter more conspicuous at night by reflecting light back to the source. Firefighter helmets are required to use ear covers. These single or multilayer textile coverings extend down from the sides (and sometimes back) of the helmet to provide additional protection to the firefighters' ears and neck, which may be left unprotected by the garment collar, helmet, or breathing apparatus mask.

Many firefighter helmets are provided with faceshields. This has created considerable controversy. On one hand, proponents of faceshields contend that additional eye and face protection is needed for situations, like overhaul, when breathing apparatus facepieces are not used (e.g., during victim extrication in automobile accidents). Many firefighters also complain that faceshields affixed to the helmet are rendered useless quickly by melting under high heat exposures. They also contend that faceshields do not provide primary eye protection since their coverage of the face and eyes is limited. Some of these firefighters prefer to wear goggles when their breathing apparatus mask is not in use, even though many goggles easily melt and do not use flame- and heat-resistant components.

Hoods

Protective hoods are a relatively new item of the structuring firefighting protective ensemble. Intended as an interface item of protective clothing, separate hoods typically are constructed of knitted material with a face opening to fit around the breathing apparatus mask and "bib" extensions of the material to remain tucked under the firefighter's coat. Per NFPA 1971, protective hoods have a lower thermal insulation requirement than garments, but still have to meet all of the flame- and heat-resistance requirements typically associated with garment materials. As a consequence, protective hoods are heavy single-ply or double-ply materials using Nomex®, PBI®, P84, Basofil®, Kevlar®, and FR rayon fibers.

Owing to their knit constructions, hoods are typically "one size fits all" but must be selected to fit properly with the other equipment, primarily the breathing apparatus facepiece. Because hoods are stretched repeatedly over the facepiece and the wearer's head, some hoods quickly lose their shape and can fail to properly protect the firefighter. NFPA 1971 attempted to address this requirement with a test for measuring the hood face opening size after repeated donnings and doffmgs of the hood on a manikin headform.

Features for hoods are relatively simple. These usually consist of the type of face opening (some hoods are designed to accommodate specific respirator facepieces), the length of the sides, front, and back (sometimes referred to as "bibs"), and ventilation areas. Some heavyweight hood materials use mesh materials in the ear region to permit easier communication, but this feature also reduced protection. One style of hood in North America provide a mesh on the top of the hood (sitting underneath the helmet) to provide a means for heat to escape the hood.

Some of the reluctance to use hoods has included resistance by some firefighters for total encapsulation of the body. Many more traditional firefighters claim that they use their ears as "early warning" sensors to detect excessive heat and know when to leave. Unfortunately, the sensitivity of ears to heat also makes them very vulnerable to high heat and ears are prone to burn readily.

Gloves

Other than hoods, gloves are considered to be the commodity item of the firefighter protective ensemble and perhaps one of the largest problem areas for providing adequate protection to the firefighter. On a cost basis, gloves are relatively cheaper than garments, footwear, or helmets, and thus can become a "throw away" item. Gloves represent a difficult protection problem for the hands because the hands have a very high surface area to volume ratio (only the ears are higher). This means it is difficult to provide the same level of protection to the hands in five-fingered gloves as compared to the torso and other parts of the body. Providing the same level of protection as the garment usually results in relatively bulky, difficult-to-use gloves. In fact, this practice, standardized under NFPA 1971, has caused a significantly large proportion of firefighters to use noncompliant gloves or engage in practices that endanger their hands (e.g., removing their gloves to operate a radio while on the fireground). Nevertheless, failure to adequately protect the hands can be cause for increased burn and other injuries. The hands are very susceptible to several fire scene hazards.

Most firefighter gloves are leather, using cowhide, goat, elk, moose, or pig hides. While leather provides a durable and physical hazard-resistant shell for firefighter glove use, it is also prone to shrinkage at high temperatures, and the thicker leathers required for providing adequate thermal shrinkage resistance, puncture resistance, and heat insulation, also inhibit hand function (i.e., dexterity and tactility). Leather glove shells are supplemented with various lining systems, usually a flame-resistant knit or nonwoven material, or wool. Gloves manufactured in accordance with NFPA 1971 also incorporate a coating or moisture barrier to prevent water penetration. As the number of layers increase, the level of protection improves at the expense of hand function. Some relief in diminished hand function is obtained by using alternative materials to leather such as knit Kevlar® or other high heat composite materials. Other manufacturers have sought various design practices to optimize the glove material composites while reducing bulk.

Glove features include the type of materials, the general construction design, the length, and type of glove end (straight, gauntlet, or knit wristlet). The former two features significantly affect hand function and protection, while the latter features relate to the issue of interface between gloves and garment sleeves. Glove materials also relate to hand comfort. For example, breathable glove layers will result in better comfort to the hand. Some glove manufacturers are also treating glove palm areas with special finished or raised surfaced for improved grip.

Boots

Structural firefighters have a number of footwear choices available. In general, there are a variety of different features for footwear uppers, soles, barriers, and lining packages, but much of this footwear is usually classified as rubber versus leather footwear. While both types of footwear are required to meet the requirements of NFPA 1971, the two different types of footwear achieve compliance through different ways attributable to their materials and designs. For example, rubber footwear by virtue of its overall construction provides integrity against liquid leakage by the exterior rubber coating on its outer surfaces. In contrast, leather boots must use a barrier layer underneath the leather to provide continuous liquid protection to the foot. The construction methods used in both types of footwear vary dramatically. While both footwear types are constructed using a last, a mold or form in the shape of a foot, footwear manufacture differs in how materials are joined together and the overall steps in preparing finished footwear. Firefighter preferences for footwear take into account a variety of factors that include overall weight, comfort and fit, styling appeal, protective performance, durability, and cost. As with the selection of any firefighter footwear, the determination of the most important characteristics involves a series of tradeoffs.

The weight of footwear has become a topic to some as the fire service seeks to find ways of reducing the stress imposed on firefighters. Stress reduction already has been identified as a principal goal in firefighter PPE selection as consideration is given to products being breathable and lighter. For footwear, the argument is that items of PPE that are worn farthest from the firefighter's center of gravity impose the greatest potential stress to the firefighter in terms of weight and burden. Some research has indicated that a reduction in one pound of footwear is equivalent to reducing a pound of weight from the firefighter's back. In general, rugged tall boots are heavier than boots that are form fitting that are made of lighter materials. In a 1980's study commissioned by the IAFF, the University of Delaware found higher energy expenditure by firefighter test subjects wearing then available rubber footwear compared to leather footwear. Nevertheless, not all field studies have shown relatively little differences in subjective ratings between leather and rubber footwear. Furthermore, both rubber and leather footwear providers have endeavored to find ways of lightening the relative weight of their products. For example, certain rubber formulations and the design features on rubber footwear help reduce weight. In the case of leather footwear, the use of nonleather upper textile materials with lighter weight reinforcement has made some footwear products lighter. Both types of footwear benefit from improved composite hardware inside toes and outsoles.

Fit and comfort are probably some of the more closely perceived factors associated with the choice of footwear. A firefighter that has uncomfortable footwear is not likely to be an effective firefighter. While the NFPA 1971 standard remains progressive in requiring that footwear manufacturers provide footwear products in a full range of sizes for both men and women, including half sizes and three widths, footwear fit is a matter of personal preference and experience. For some firefighters, rubber footwear which may tend to be less form fitting compared to leather footwear, is considered perfectly adequate in terms of its ankle support and comfort. Yet other firefighters might require closely conforming footwear to prevent blisters and wearing discomfort. The relative flexibility of leather combined with lace up designs and other footwear features enable leather footwear to often better conform to the firefighter's feet, but some rubber footwear manufacturers have developed innovative designs to close this gap.

The key aspects of footwear performance include insulation from heat (and cold), maintenance of liquid integrity, and physical durability. The levels of insulation provided by footwear that keep the feet warm in the winter or cool on the fireground has less to do with the general type (rubber versus leather) than it does the actual construction for that specific style of footwear. In both types of footwear, the primary insulation is provided by linings. The thickness and placement of these linings will affect insulative qualities, though both styles of footwear generally perform extremely well as compared to other PPE items. Problems can occur when extremely thin insulation packages are chosen or the insulation is non uniform over the entire boot. Rubber boots tend to provide more consistent liquid integrity only because the liquid integrity usually coincides with the height of the footwear. In contrast, leather footwear that uses a barrier on the boot interior may not extend to the full height of the boot depending on the extension of the barrier layer and the closure features used in the design of footwear. For example, where a gusset is used to aid in footwear donning, the lowest points of the gusset may be the where the overall height of liquid protection stops. It is further important that pull tabs and other donning aids not be sewn through the barrier layer creating pathways for liquid leakage. Rubber boots tend to be more durable than leather boots being able to withstand abrasion, cuts, and puncture more readily, but leather boots that are properly maintained also provide long service life.

Station Uniforms

The clothing worn beneath firefighter turn out clothing is just as important as the turnout clothing itself. This clothing should be capable of absorbing perspiration and should not add to the thermal stress of the wearer. Certainly, this clothing should be heat resistant (by resisting melting and dripping) and not create additional hazards to the wearer in the event of catastrophic failure. While it is not intended to provide additional thermal insulation, the presence of additional clothing underneath the primary turnout clothing does create additional protection in the event that dangerous levels of heat or other fire products breach the turnout clothing. If exposed to heat, synthetics such as nylon or polyester or cotton/synthetic blends have been known to melt and damage the underlying skin. Most career fire departments have specific requirements for the clothing that is worn while on duty and require it to meet the specification of NFPA 1975, *Standard on Station/ Work Uniforms for Fire and Emergency Services*. Consideration of both comfort and flame resistance should also be a factor in selection of undergarments worn beneath the station uniform. Flame resistance is now currently an option in NFPA 1975 that must be specified.

The issue of what is worn beneath turnout clothing becomes much more difficult when addressing the volunteer fire service. In most cases the volunteers will show up to the station or the event in whatever they were wearing at the time the call for service was received. Volunteer fire department should have standard operating procedures that specify what is and is not acceptable for volunteers to wear when reporting for duty. These SOPs should include a minimum of clothing that most be worn. At a very minimum the firefighters should have a t-shirt, shorts, and socks beneath their turnout clothing. Depending on theTPP factor of the protective trousers, long pants may be required. Firefighters who are not wearing socks may soon be rendered ineffective by blisters. Those without shirts have nothing to absorb perspiration beneath their turnout clothing. Encourage volunteer members to keep spare clothing in their station lockers or personal vehicles in the event that they are not wearing appropriate clothing at the time of a call.

Project HEROES®

Earlier in this section we mentioned the Project FIRES research that led to the modern protective ensemble worn by today's firefighters. At this time this chapter was written, significant research was being conducted on the next generation of structural firefighter protective clothing. The new research is known as Project ®, which stands for Homeland Emergency Response Operational and Equipment Systems.This project was initiated by the IAFF and it now includes numerous other fire service and governmental agencies, as well as research universities and protective clothing manufacturers.

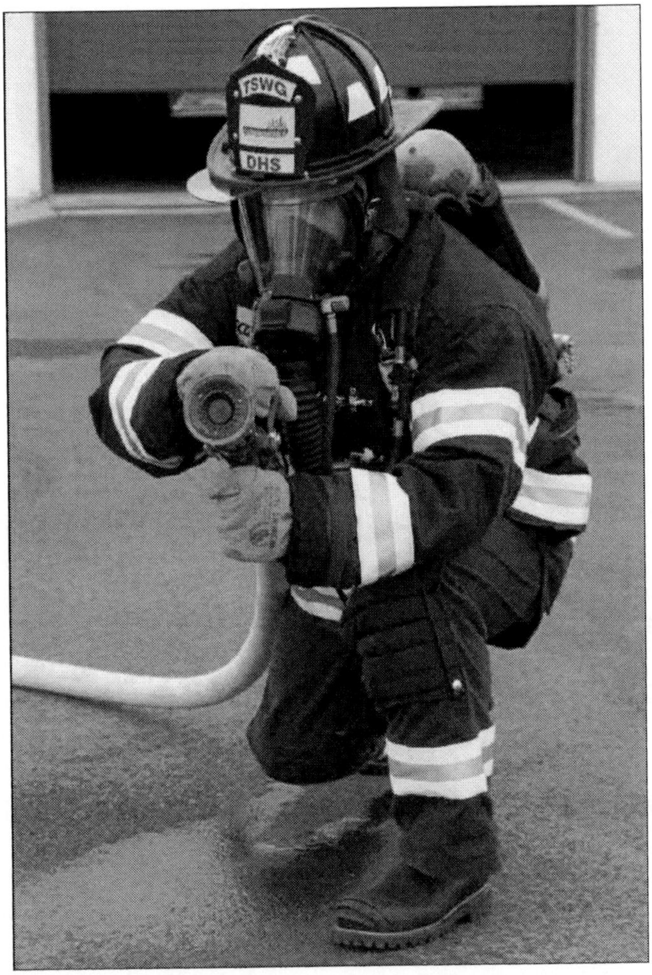

Figure 2.7. Courtesy of Total Fire Group/Morning Pride.

The goal of this research is to develop a new turnout ensemble that not only protects firefighters from the "traditional" byproducts associated with firefighting, but also to provide some level of protection against chemical, biological, radiological, and nuclear (CBRN) hazards that may be present at different types of incidents, including terrorist attacks. While it is relatively easy to develop turnout clothing for structural fire-fighting and also develop special clothing for exposure to CBRN incidents, it is not so easy to develop one ensemble that works for both applications. The challenge in this project has been to develop an ensemble that prevents inward leakage of CBRN products beneath the protective clothing, without vastly increasing the thermal stress on the wearer during "routine" structural firefighting and other incidents **(Figure 2.7).** This has been a particularly challenging task as the more sophisticated barrier materials are required that will retard not just penetration, but permeation of chemicals on a molecular scale.

Project HEROES® research was still ongoing at the time of this chapter. However, significant progress had been made at developing better insulating cooling systems and vapor-excluding closures between the various pieces of the ensemble. These new interfaces have the effect of creating greater encapsulation of the firefighter, but in conjunction with the use of redirect exhalation air from the SCBA facepiece into the upper torso area of the ensemble, some convective flow and consequent cooling effects are achieved. A new selectively permeable membrane has been developed that offers breathability at NFPA 1971 requirements but effectively stops permeation of CBRN chemicals. It is likely that all these advances will find their way into standard firefighter protective clothing in the years to come.

Effects of Heat Stress on the Human Body

In order to understand the need for firefighter rehabilitation and how to effectively perform it, it is important that responders have a firm understanding of the effects of heat stress on the human body. In this section we will examine both the physiological and psychological impacts of heat stress on our well-being. We will also look at various factors that increase the negative impact of heat stress and thus the further endanger the firefighter.

Physiological Effects of Heat Stress

Humans are "warm-blooded" animals, which means that regardless of external conditions, our bodies attempt to maintain a nearly constant internal core (head, neck, and internal organs of the torso) temperature of approximately 98.6 °F (37 °C). The figure of 98.6 °F is an average among all humans and it is not uncommon for an individual's "normal" body temperature to be as much as 2 °F above or below this figure.

The body, like any machine, burns fuel and produces heat as a byproduct of producing energy from food. To maintain body temperature within safe limits, body functions are regulated to conserve or dissipate heat, depending on the external thermal environment. For a nude resting human, the range of environmental temperature for which no physiological compensation is needed is only about 6 °F (14.4 °C). When exposed to air temperatures lower than about 80 °F (26.7 °C), body heat must be conserved; for temperatures in excess of about 86 °F (30 °C), body heat must he dissipated.

Physiological body temperature regulation is accomplished mainly by automatic responses controlled by the brain, which monitors body temperature by continuously measuring skin temperature and the temperature of the circulating blood. When the brain determines that body temperature has deviated from normal, temperature control mechanisms are activated. For heat stress these include dilation of the blood vessels in the skin and extremities (arms and legs), increase in heart and respiratory rates, and initiation of the sweating mechanism. When these mechanisms are not able to cope with the thermal stress imposed upon the body, the body temperature deviates from normal.

Performance of almost any task becomes impaired when the temperature of the heart and brain drops below 95 °F (35 °C). Below 85 °F (29 °C) the heart is highly susceptible to cardiac arrest (ventricular fibrillation); above 105 °F (41 °C) the brain can suffer irreparable cellular damage.The head and neck are particularly sensitive to external environmental conditions and have very limited mechanisms for local thermoregulation. Thus, full blood flow to the head is maintained despite the external thermal conditions; during cold exposure an unprotected head can lose as much heat as the whole rest of the body. Most local tissue is much more resistant to thermal stress. Many cells can survive temperatures from below 40 °F (4 °C) to above 120 °F (49 °C), although function may be temporarily or permanently compromised or lost. For example, even very short exposure of the hands to cold water can cause almost complete loss of sensation and function, even though actual cold injury may not occur.

Immediately after an exposure to an environmental extreme, the body uses all of its adaptive mechanisms in an attempt to regain normal temperature. Each person has an individual tolerance to heat or cold, which may vary depending on previous exposure, overall physical condition, and other factors. Persons with a higher percentage of body fat may be less affected by cold exposure than individuals with leaner builds, while the opposite may be true during heat exposure. Racial variations also appear to exist. For example, U.S. Army studies suggest that African-Americans may be especially vulnerable to cold injury, particularly of the hands and feet, due to variations in circulatory response.

Inextricably linked with heat stress is the impact of dehydration on the firefighter's body. Most internal heat stress illnesses are due in major part to failure to maintain adequate hydration on the part of the firefighter. Research by the U.S. Army indicates that each 1 percent of the body's fluid that is lost will raise the core temperature by about 0.25 (-17.6) to 0.5 °F (-17.5 °C). A 4 percent loss of fluid volume will decrease the person's performance by as much as 50 percent. Research at the University of Pittsburgh School of Medicine shows that a person's ability to sweat (and thus cool oneself) is impaired when as little as 5 percent of the person's body mass is lost in fluid weight. The resulting decrease in plasma volume will result in a reduced heart stroke volume, leading to a compensatory increase in heart rate. The body's ability to thermoregulate will be impaired at this point also. Strategies for avoiding this situation will be discussed later in this document.

Psychological Effects of Heat Stress

While the major focus of this work will certainly be focused on the physiological effects of heat stress on firefighters, one should also not overlook the psychological impact of high heat situations. To some extent, acclimation to high heat situations will affect the responder's ability to maintain reasonable mental function under these conditions. In other words, firefighters who are used to, or like, working in hot weather will not be affected as quickly as those who are not used to it or do not prefer those conditions. This will be discussed in more detail in the next section on acclimatation.

Regardless of acclimation, eventually heat stress will reduce mental performance at some point. While there is little detailed research on mental performance degradation to graded levels of heat stress and strain, it is clear that some does exist. It may be mediated by thermal discomfort, including high skin temperature, high skin wettedness, and cardiovascular strain. Heat stress slows reaction time and decision time.Tasks that require attention to detail, concentration, and short-term memory and are not self-paced may degrade from heat stress **(Figure 2.8).** Routine tasks are done more slowly and errors of omission are more common. Research by the U.S. Army indicates that vigilant task performance will start to degrade slightly and markedly after 2 to 3 hours. Of course, keep in mind that this research is based on soldiers in top physical condition. Firefighters of a lesser condition may be affected much quicker than that. The U.S. Army research showed that dehydration greater than 2 percent of body weight will adversely affect mental function of simple tasks such as serial addition and word recognition. These performance decrements probably increase with the level of dehydration.

Increased Risk Factors

No one, regardless of the level of their fitness and/or physical condition, is immune from the possible effects of heat stress. However, there are individuals who are more likely to be susceptible to heat-related problems for one reason or another. Fire departments should identify these people before an incident and prior to the chance they might fall victim to the heat. The following is a summary of various conditions that increase the risk factor of individuals operating in high heat conditions.

- **Dehydration and salt depletion**—This was discussed previously in this section. People who are already at some level of dehydration prior to the incident stand an increased chance of falling victim to the heat.

- **Lack of heat acclimatization**—This will be discussed in greater detail in the next section.

- **Poor physical fitness/excessive body weight**—Proper physical condition will decrease the effects of heat on the body to some extent. U.S. Army research indicates that the effects of heat on poorly-conditioned soldiers may be magnified by as much as 9 times of that of properly-conditioned soldiers.

- **Skin problems**—Skin irritations such as rashes, prickly heat, sunburn, and poison ivy will increase a person's susceptibility to internal heat illness.

- **Minor illness**—Firefighters who were already suffering from a minor illness, inflammation, or fever will have an increased chance of heat injury due to a previously compromised autoimmune system. Subjects with some form of gastroenteritis are particularly at risk because they may already be dehydrated and have salt and mineral imbalances within their bodies.

- **Medications, both prescription and nonprescription**—Certain medications will affect the body's hydration level, ability to process fluids, and other bodily functions relative to dealing with the heat. Table 2.1 gives a brief summary of these concerns.

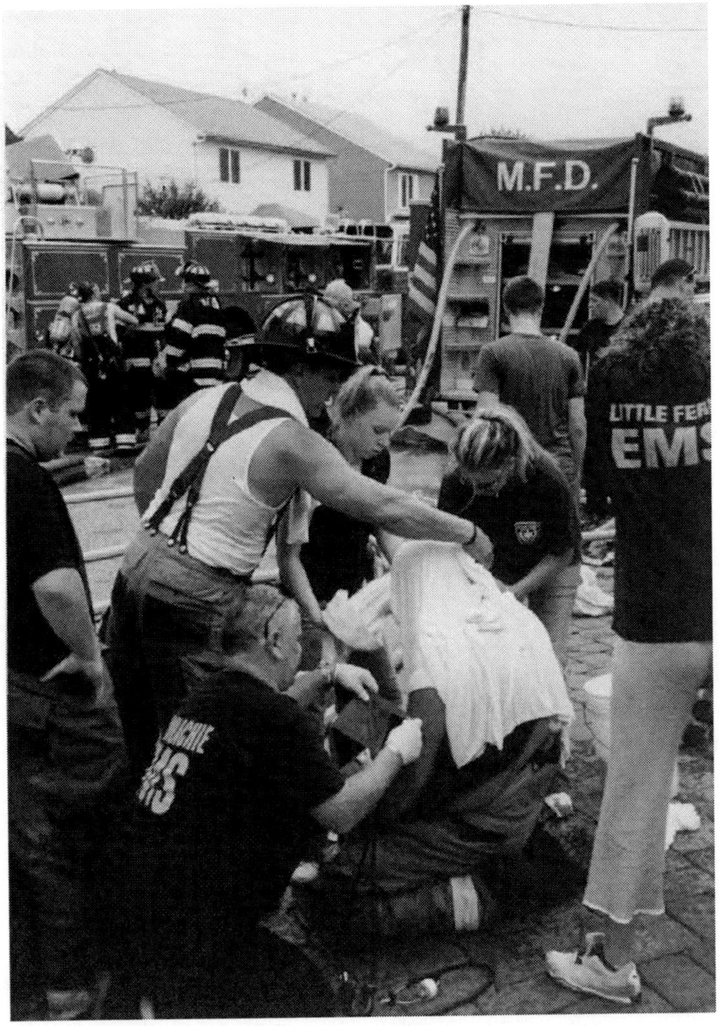

Figure 2.8. Courtesy of Ron Jeffers, Union City, NJ.

Table 2.1. Effects of Various Medications on Heat Stress Susceptibility

Drug or Drug Class	Mechanism of Impact on Heat stress
Anticholinergics (Atropine)	Impaired sweating
Antihistamines	Impaired sweating
Gluthemide (Doriden®)	Impaired sweating
Phenothiazines (antipsychotics; including Thorazine®, Stelazine®, and Trilafon®)	Impaired sweating, disturbed hypothalamic temperature regulation
Tricyclic antidepressants	Impaired sweating, increased motor activity
Amphetamines, cocaine, Ecstacy	Increased psychomotor activity, activated vascular endothelium
Ergogenic stimulants (ephedrine/ephedra)	Increased heat production
Lithium	Nephrogenic diabetes insipidus and water loss
Diuretics	Salt depletion and dehydration
Beta-Blockers	Diuresis, possible effects on intestinal permeability

- **Chronic disease**—Diseases such as diabetes mellitus, cardiovascular disease, and congestive heart failure affect overall patient condition and may result in enhanced heat illness potential.

- **Recent alcohol use**—Recent alcohol use can impair the person's judgment and also will increase the likelihood of dehydration.

- **Prior heat injury**—Heat stress and injuries are additive and can take a long time to fully recover from. Future exposures to high heat situations may result in expedited heat injury or illness.

- **Age**—U.S. Army research shows that people over 40 years of age, even those in relatively good physical condition, have an increased potential for heat illness versus people who are under that age.

- **Highly motivated people**—People who are highly motivated and committed to performing given tasks at all costs may overlook the signs of heat illness and increase their chance of overextending themselves. Firefighters engaged in highly-charged emergency scene operations clearly can fall victim to this problem.

- **Genetics**—People who have genetic mutations, such as cystic fibrosis and malignant hyperthermia, should be monitored closely in high heat situations.

ADAPTATION/ACCLIMATIZATION

Why does a fire on a 90 °F day in July place extra strain on firefighters in Massachusetts, yet not adversely on firefighters in Arizona? The easy answer is to say that the Arizona firefighters "are used to" temperatures like that. They experience them all the time. In fact, to the Arizona firefighters a 90 °F day in July would be viewed as a cold snap. Are the firefighters in the south really different than those in the north? The answer to that question is really yes and no. All humans are basically equipped the same way to deal with climatic conditions. However, humans do have the ability to adapt and become more proficient in handling extreme environmental conditions when they are accustomed to them over a period of time.

The process of adapting to environmental extremes is often referred to as acclimatization.

In general, people who grow up living in a certain environment naturally acclimatize to that environment. That is how Eskimos deal with Arctic weather and Bedouins deal with desert heat. People who move from one climate to another, such as a person who retires in Minnesota and moves to Florida, also will begin to acclimatize over time.

Historically, in the fire service acclimatization has not been a major issue. The vast majority of firefighters serve in the same geographical location and climate in which they grew up or have at least lived for a long period of time. The number of firefighters who move from one climate extreme to another is relatively small. Exceptions to this rule are wildland firefighters who move around the country and fight fires in a variety of conditions and urban search and rescue (US&R) teams who may be deployed to a different environment at a moment's notice. Methods for dealing with acclimatization issues will be discussed a little later in this section.

It is important to recognize that issues of acclimatization are becoming more and more important in today's society because of changes in lifestyle and culture. Just because an individual has grown up in a particular part of the country does not always mean that they are prepared to operate as firefighters in moderate or extreme environmental conditions. Athletic coaches and fire service officers have noted that many young athletes and firefighters do not seem to deal with the heat as well as their predecessors did. Incidences of heat-related injuries, illnesses, and deaths have been on the rise in recent years. Many have struggled as to why this is occurring.

The answer is acclimatization, or lack thereof. Young people who grew up 20, 30, or 40 years ago were more likely to do so in homes and schools that were not air-conditioned. They spent much of their free time engaging in outdoor activities. Thus, they were acclimated naturally to functioning in the prevailing atmospheric conditions. Young people today spend considerably more of their time in air-conditioned homes and schools. They spend much more of their free time in front of computers and televisions. Thus, when they enter into rigorous physical activities outdoors, their bodies may not be up to handling the conditions as recruits were in the past **(Figure 2.9).** In today's fire service, officers and instructors must give consideration to properly acclimating personnel to the conditions, particularly if the conditions are extreme, when planning any rigorous activities.

Probably no organization deals more with the issue of climatic adaptation and acclimatization than the military. They must prepare soldiers to perform in a variety of extremes found in virtually every part of the world. The U.S. military has done an extraordinary amount of research on acclimatization and the fire service can pull valuable information and practices from the military's experience. Preparing firefighters and soldiers is not all that much different. Both involve rigorous training to perform stressful, physical activities, and that can place the individual in life-threatening situations.

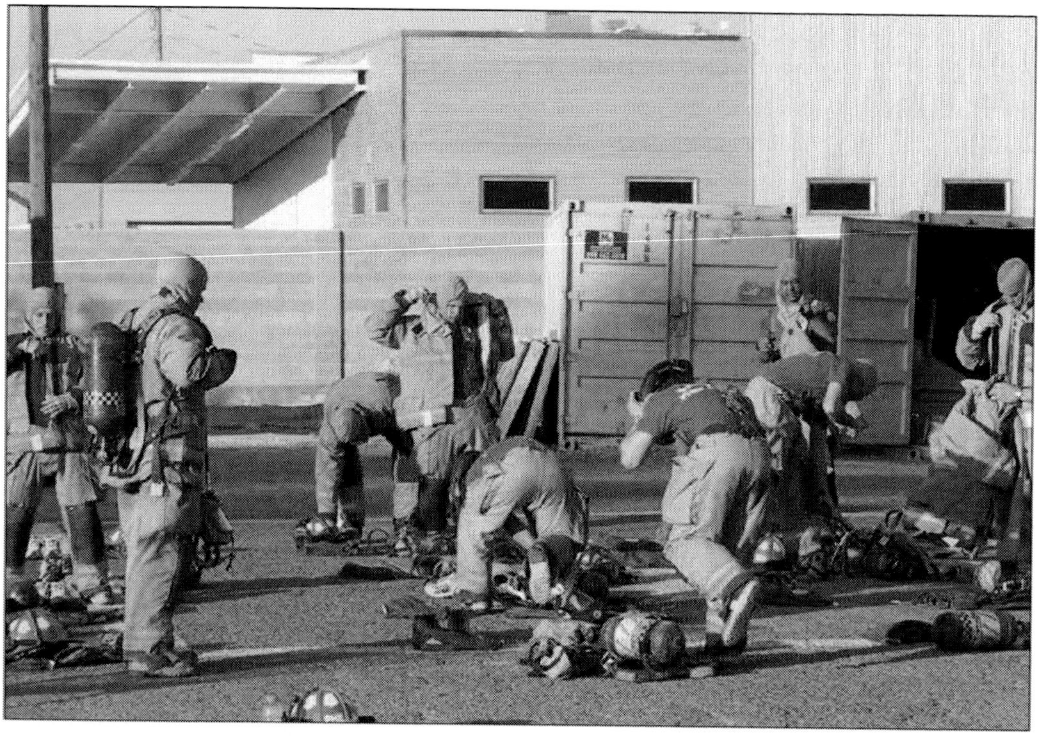

Figure 2.9.

The military has found that biological adaptations to repeated heat stress include both heat acclimatization and acquired thermal tolerance. The magnitude of both adaptations depends on the intensity, duration, frequency, and number of heat exposures. These two adaptations compliment each other as heat acclimatization reduces physiologic strain and acquired thermal tolerance improves tissue resistance injury for a given heat strain.

The military has noted that heat acclimatization is necessary even for very fit soldiers. A systematic process of heat acclimatization dramatically improves comfort and physical work capabilities. Acclimatization requires aerobic exercise in a warm environment. Simply being outside doing normal activities is not sufficient. Heat acclimatization is induced when repeated heat exposures are sufficiently stressful to elevate core and skin temperatures and provoke profuse sweating. Physiologic strain will be greatest during the initial part of the acclimation process. The magnitude of physiological strain will decrease each subsequent day of heat acclimatization.

The military process for building heat acclimation in soldiers involves having them perform increasingly rigorous activities in the high heat conditions for about 2 hours per day over a period of about 2 weeks. These activities can be split into two 1-hour sessions. Missing a day or two during the process does not adversely affect the results. The military studies show that after one week about 5 0 percent of the physiologic adaptations are complete, rising to about 80 percent after two weeks. At that point several weeks of living and working in the new climate are required to maximize acclimation. If no further heat exposures are experienced, the effect of the acclimatization process will be retained in full for about one week. By the end of three weeks they will be reduced by as much as 75 percent.

Acquired thermal tolerance refers to cellular adaptations induced by heat exposure that protect tissue and organs from heat injury. This allows an individual to become more resistant to heat injury or illness with subsequently more severe heat exposures. The process of heat acclimatization described above will help to induce this tolerance in the individuals. In short, acquired thermal tolerance is associated with heat shock proteins (HSPs) which provide protection and accelerate repair of cells from heat exposures and other stressors. The acclimatization process will increase the HSP's ability to protect the body from a heat injury or illness. **Table 2.2** provides an overview of the benefits of a heat acclimatization program on the individual firefighter.

MINOR HEAT-RELATED ILLNESSES AND INJURIES

Fortunately, the vast majority of heat-related injuries and illnesses that will be encountered during emergency incident rehabilitation operations will fall into the category of minor problems. In this section we will overview the three most common of these illnesses: miliaria, heat syncope, and heat cramps. Some medical personnel and publications also lump sunburn into this category. Because of the protective clothing that is worn by firefighters, sunburn is rarely an issue in rehab operations and therefore is omitted from this discussion.

Table 2.2. Actions of Heat Acclimatization

Factor	Action
Thermal comfort	Improved
Exercise performance	Improved
Body core temperature	Reduced
Sweating	Improved (earlier onset, higher rate, redistribution, hidromeiosis resistance)
Skin blood flow	Improved (earlier onset, higher rate)
Metabolic rate	Lowered
Cardiovascular stability	Improved
Heart rate	Lowered
Stroke volume	Increased
Blood pressure	Better defended
Myocardial compliance	Improved
Fluid balance	Improved
Thirst	Improved
Electrolyte loss (sweat and urine)	Reduced
Total body water	Increased
Plasma (blood) volume	Increased and better defended

Miliaria

Miliaria, commonly referred to as "prickly heat," is an acute inflammatory disease of the skin. It occurs especially in hot, humid environments where sweat is not removed easily from the surface of the skin which remains wet most of the time. The sweat ducts become plugged, and a rash appears. This might occur after wearing personal protective clothing, particularly hazardous chemical suits, for extended periods of time. This affliction falls more into the category of being annoying rather than debilitating. Prevention of miliaria can be achieved by resting in a cool place for portions of the work cycle, by bathing and drying the skin, and changing regularly into clean, dry clothes.

Heat Syncope

Heat syncope usually occurs in individuals who are not accustomed to hot environments and who have usually undergone prolonged standing, usually with the knees straight and locked. Heat can cause dilating of large blood vessels and pooling into the lower extremities. This results in less blood flow to the brain which causes fainting. Once supine, the individual usually recovers. By moving around and thereby preventing further pooling, the patient can prevent further fainting.

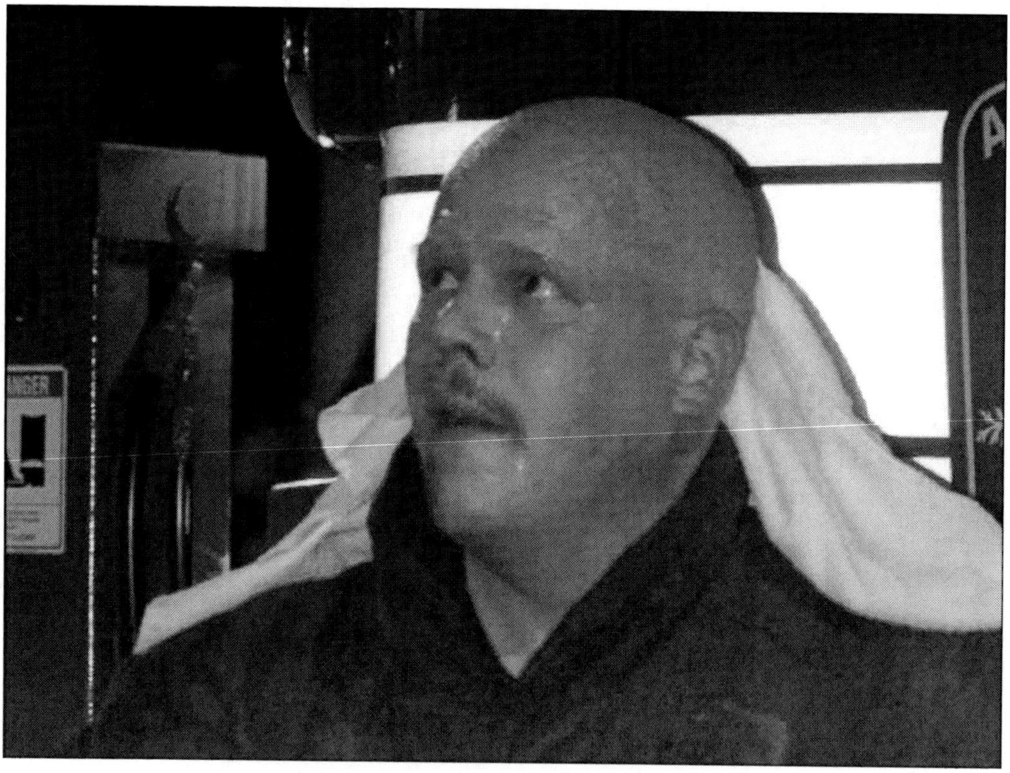

Figure 2.10. Courtesy of DennisWetherhold, Jr., Allentown, PA.

Heat Cramps

Heat cramps most commonly occur during strenuous activity in a hot environment. In these conditions the firefighter is subject to excessive sweating which results in loss of electrolytes (especially sodium) **(Figure 2.10).** Even if the firefighter drinks copious quantities of water, failure to replace the lost electrolytes (salts) may result in muscle cramping.

Heat cramps typically affect the voluntary muscles of the extremities and in some cases the abdominal wall. These cramps in the abdominal wall are referred commonly to as "side stickers." Cramps in any of these locations may be quite severe and painful. Heat cramps can occur alone or in the presence of heat exhaustion. Body temperature is usually normal unless the cramps are accompanied by heat exhaustion.

In and of themselves, heat cramps usually are not a serious problem. They respond well to rest in a cool environment and replacement of fluids by mouth. Heat cramps should be recognized as an early warning sign of a potentially more serious situation if caution is not exercised. Heat exhaustion may eventually develop in a person with heat cramps if they are left untreated and continue to lose fluid from sweating.

Recommended Treatment

Heat cramps usually are relieved by rest and replacement of salt and water lost from the body. Saline solution (0.1 percent) by mouth and/or saline solution (0.9 percent) intravenous should be administered with the route of saline administration determined by local procedure and regulations. Care should be taken not to give excessive amounts of saline solution; if saline has been administered, serum sodium levels should be monitored at a hospital emergency department to determine the patient's electrolyte status.

Heat Exhaustion

Firefighters who engage in structural and wildland fire suppression without adequate rehabilitation may eventually fall victim to heat exhaustion. The condition is also common in hazardous materials operations in which firefighters wear encapsulating suits **(Figure 2.11).**

Heat exhaustion occurs when excessive sweat loss and inadequate oral hydration cause depletion of the body's fluid volume. This results in peripheral vascular collapse and hypoperfusion of the body's organs. While heat exhaustion often is related to excessive dehydration, it can also occur from fatigue and overheating alone.

Symptoms of heat exhaustion many include any of the following:

- fainting;
- profuse sweating;
- headache;
- tingling sensations in the extremities;
- pallor (ashen color of the face);

- dyspnea (shortness of breath);
- nausea; and
- vomiting.

Heat cramps may or may not be present with heat exhaustion. Trembling, weakness, and poor coordination, often coupled with disorientation and/or momentary loss of consciousness also may be noted. National Institute for Occupational Safety and Health (NIOSH) studies stress that impairment of judgment may occur well before other symptoms are noted.

Physical examination of a possible heat exhaustion victim typically will reveal a mild to severe peripheral circulatory collapse with pale, moist, cool skin and a rapid (100 to 200 beats/minute), thready pulse. Systolic blood pressure generally will have been quite elevated (130 mm Hg or higher) prior to onset of heat exhaustion, followed by a rapid drop and commonly reaches the normal range by the time of examination. However, the pulse pressure (the difference between systolic and diastolic blood pressure) usually will remain decreased and this is a clue indicating possible heat exhaustion at the time of physical examination. The oral temperature may be subnormal due to hyper ventilation, or slightly elevated, but the rectal temperature is usually slightly elevated. It is not uncommon in heat exhaustion cases to find rectal temperatures in the range of 99 to 104 °F (3 7.2 to 40 °C) depending on the type and duration of physical activity prior to onset.

If the condition is unrecognized and untreated, a firefighter with heat exhaustion may develop more classic signs of shock or hypoperfusion. These signs include increased heart rate, increased respiratory rate, and—eventually—reduced blood pressure. If allowed to progress the firefighter may evolve into a deadly heat stroke situation.

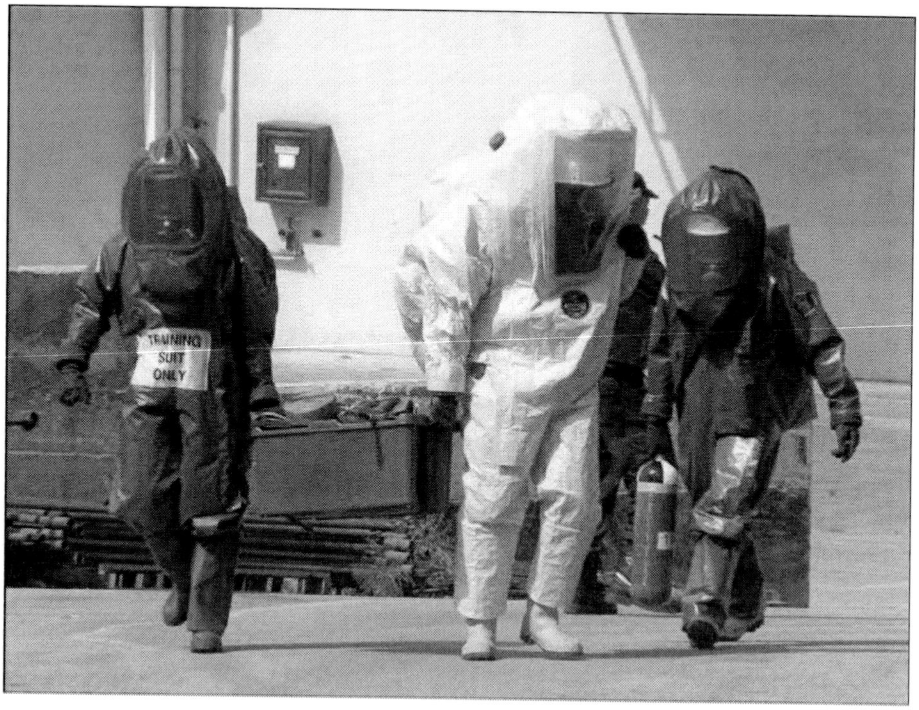

Figure 2.11. Courtesy of IFSTA/Fire Protection Publications.

Recommended Treatment

It must be remembered that heat exhaustion can develop rapidly into heat stroke, therefore continuous patient monitoring must be maintained. Elevation of the patient's legs and removal from heat stress to a cool place is indicated. Water and/or salt replacement should be undertaken as described above for heat cramps. When at all possible, replacement of fluid using intravenous methods should be used. Continuous monitoring of the patient's condition in the field and subsequent evaluation of the patient's electrolyte status at a hospital emergency department should be mandatory. Recovery from heat exhaustion usually is rapid, but immediate return to duty is not advisable.

HEAT STROKE

Heat stroke is the most severe of the three types of heat-related injuries. Heat stroke victims have a high probability of permanent disability or death as a result of this injury. Heat stroke results when the body's temperature regulating and cooling mechanisms are no longer functional. Immediately prior to onset of heat stroke, fainting, disorientation, excessive fatigue, and other symptoms of heat exhaustion may be present. Onset of heat stroke may be rapid with sudden delirium, loss of consciousness, and convulsions occurring. Typically, the skin is hot, flushed, and dry, although the skin may be wet and clammy in later stages of the condition when shock may be present. Any emergency personnel found in a hot environment with altered mental status and skin that is hot and dry, or moist to the touch, should be presumed to have a life-threatening heat-related emergency.

Rectal temperatures associated with heat stroke are elevated, frequently in excess of 106 °F. A special high-temperature reading rectal thermometer may be needed to document actual internal core temperature. A rectal temperature of 108 °F is not uncommon and indicates a poor prognosis. Pulse is full and rapid, while the systolic blood pressure may be normal or elevated and the diastolic pressure may be depressed to 60 mm Hg or lower. Respirations are rapid and deep. As a patient's condition worsens, symptoms of shock including low blood pressure, rapid pulse, and cyanosis occur. Incontinence, vomiting, kidney failure, pulmonary edema, and cardiac arrest may follow.

Even if effective treatment is initiated and the patient survives the initial episode, severe relapses can occur for several days, while rectal temperatures of 102 to 103 °F (33 to 39°C) will persist along with disorientation, delirium, and headache. If effective treatment was not initiated, brain cell damage caused by a high temperature may persist even if the patient survives. It is important to note that even after apparent recovery, temperature regulation may be impaired for some time, perhaps permanently in severe cases. Research by the U.S. Army indicates that about 10 percent of surviving heat stroke patients have long-term reduced tolerance to heat following their initial injury.

Recommended Treatment

The lowering of the body's temperature as rapidly as possible is the most important objective in the treatment of a suspected heat stroke patient. The longer the body temperature remains at the raised level, the greater the threat to a favorable outcome. Some reports indicate that aggressive, active cooling of heat stroke patients can reduce mortality rates from 50 percent to 5 percent.

Aggressive measures to lower the individual's body temperature should be started as soon as possible. In the field, the patient's clothing should be removed. If cold or ice water is available, the patient should be doused with and/or immersed in the water. An effective alternative is to cover the nude patient with a cotton sheet, continuously douse the sheet with water from a booster line or garden hose, and fan them with an electric smoke ejector. In addition, cold packs should be applied to the carotid arteries on the sides of the neck. The patient's legs should be elevated in a shock recovery position.

Patient transport to a hospital emergency department should be initiated as soon as possible, with aggressive cooling measures maintained during transport. Blood pressure, pulse, rectal temperature, and respirations should be monitored continuously. Normal saline (0.9 percent) should be cautiously administered intravenously, if advanced life support (ALS) providers are available. Oxygen should be administered if cyanosis, pulmonary congestion, or breathing difficulty is present.

Procedures used by the U.S. Army to treat heat stroke patients stipulate that active cooling procedures should be discontinued once the patient's rectal temperature reaches 101 °F. Further active cooling below this point may actually result in the patient becoming hypothermic. In most cases this temperature will not be achieved until the patient is in a medical facility.

AVOIDING HEAT-RELATED ILLNESSES AND INJURIES

There is little that firefighters can do about the atmospheric conditions in which they are forced to operate. Simply stated, there is nothing we can do to change the weather hand we are dealt. However, we have total control of how we deal with those conditions and respond to the challenges we are presented. By implementing and enforcing proper preventive and operating procedures, fire departments can minimize the impact of high heat conditions on their personnel and virtually eliminate the onset of serious heat-related injuries and illnesses.

Fire departments that operate in some of the hottest climates of the U.S., such as the deserts of Arizona, seldom, if ever, experience heat-related injuries to their members. They are able to maintain this record of safety by having and enforcing aggressive fitness, hydration, and rehabilitation policies. This section briefly outlines some of that information, with much more additional information found in later chapters of this document.

Physical Condition

As discussed earlier in this chapter, the general physical condition of the individual has a significant bearing on his/her reaction to heat stress. Individual susceptibility to heat may be enhanced by a large number and variety of conditions including: infection, fever, immunization reactions, vascular diseases, diarrhea, skin trauma such as heat rash or sunburn, use of alcohol in the last 24 hours, previous heat injury, dehydration, lack of sleep, fatigue, obesity, and drugs which inhibit sweating such as atropine, scopolamine, antihistamines, tranquilizers, cold medicines, and some antidiarrheal medications.

The risk of heat injury is much higher in overweight, unfit firefighters than in fit ones. Physical fitness programs designed to develop both cardiovascular and muscular fitness can be of great benefit in reducing heat casualties **(Figure 2.12).** However, the effects of heat eventually will wear down even a well-conditioned firefighter unless other measures, such as proper hydration and acclimatization, are followed.

Acclimatization

The benefits and procedures for achieving acclimatization to operating in high heat conditions were covered in extensive detail earlier in this chapter. By following these recommendations, fire departments can better prepare their personnel to operate more effectively and safely in high heat conditions.

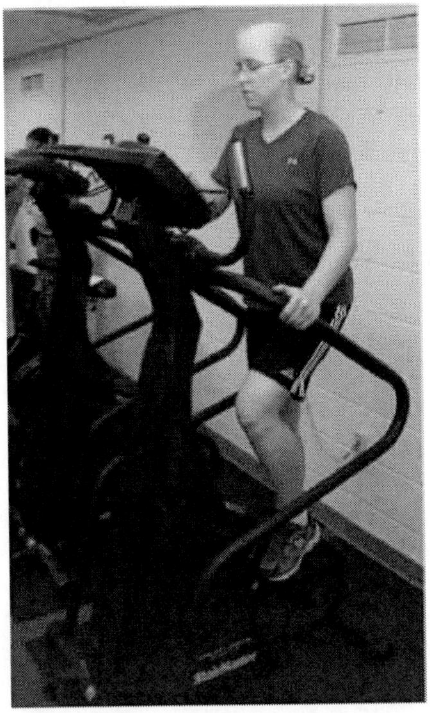

Figure 2.12. Courtesy of IFSTA/Fire Protection Publications.

The major part of this acclimatization process is thought to be due to increased effectiveness of the sweating mechanism. Thus, while significant benefits can be expected from acclimatization, firefighters wearing protective clothing will still be affected severely by heat stress due to the impairment of evaporative cooling mechanisms by the clothing. Of course, any physical fitness or acclimatization training must be coordinated with the department and firefighter's personal physician and managed with great care to ensure that each firefighter's individual physical and physiological capabilities are not exceeded. The individual is the best judge of his/her capability during actual exercise periods.

A firefighter experiencing abnormal fatigue, dizziness, nausea, or other signs of stress must not be forced beyond his/her capacity or heat injury may result. Based on available information, it is believed that drills and exercise should be monitored carefully when apparent temperature exceeds 90 °F and modified or suspended when apparent temperature exceeds 105 °F. If turnout clothing is worn, an adjustment factor of 10 °F should be added to the environmental temperature before the apparent temperature is calculated.

Hydration

Perhaps the most critical factor in prevention of heat injury is proper hydration. Even though evaporation of sweat is impaired by protective clothing, sweating still occurs. Water must be replaced, both during exercise periods and at emergency scenes. Firefighters generally drink less fluid than they should, especially during emergency operations. Thus, thirst should not be relied upon to stimulate drinking. This is even important during cold weather operations where heat stress may occur during firefighting or other strenuous activity when protective clothing is worn. Cool water and cups must be readily available at both exercise areas and emergency scenes and drinking encouraged (**Figure 2.13**). For example, during interior structural firefighting a firefighter should have water available at the site where self-contained breathing apparatus (SCBA) cylinders are changed. Care must be taken to assure that water, cups, and drinking areas are not contaminated by hazardous materials from the emergency scene.

More detailed information on prehydration and hydration for firefighters is covered in Chapter 5 of this document.

Rehabilitation Procedures

Obviously, the purpose of this overall document is to stress the importance of proper rehabilitation procedures on fire service personnel. By developing and implementing these procedures, the vast majority of training program and incident scene heat-related illnesses and injuries can be prevented. Chapters 4 and 5 of this document provide indepth details on how to establish and operate emergency incident rehabilitation areas.

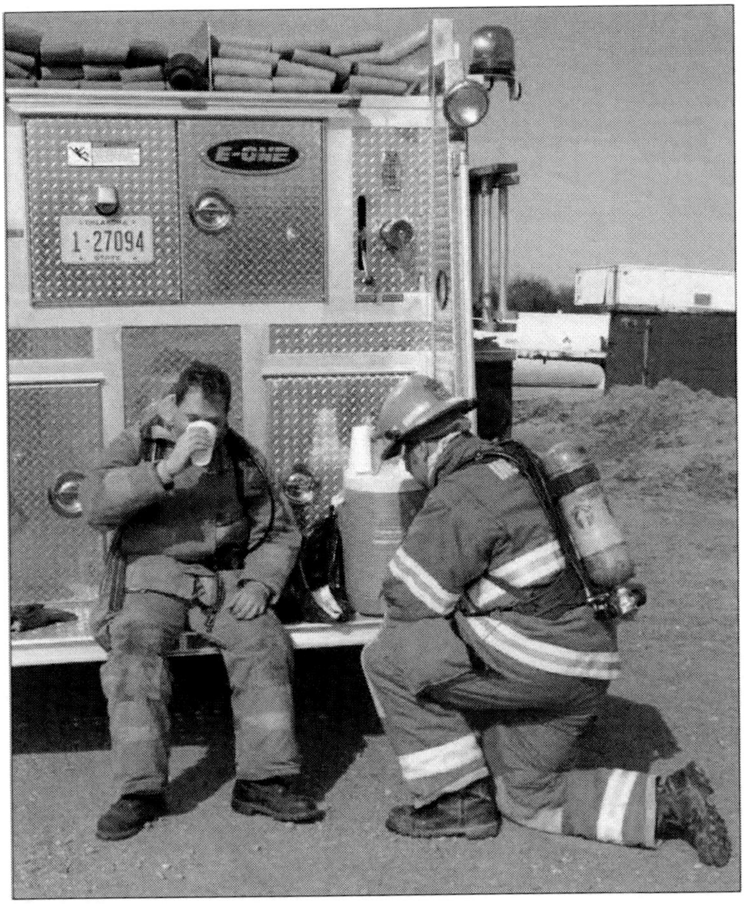

Figure 2.13. Courtesy of IFSTA/Fire Protection Publications.

In: Rehab, Protection and Safety Measures for Firefighters ... ISBN: 978-1-60741-566-4
Editor: Andreo Rios

Chapter 3

COLD STRESS AND THE FIREFIGHTER

Of the two environmental temperature extremes (hot and cold) that firefighters may be expected to operate in, historically, extreme heat has been the most problematic of the two. The heavy, encapsulating equipment we wear to perform our physically tasking jobs only adds to the problems posed by working in heat. Most jurisdictions spend a considerable amount of their effort in establishing rehab plans and programs on dealing with heat.

However, fire departments in jurisdictions subjected to cold weather must also recognize the impact that these conditions will have on its firefighters and operations. Accordingly, these departments must develop plans to deal with prolonged exposures to extreme cold temperatures during the course of training or emergency scene operations **(Figure 3.1).** While the threat of a systemic illness (comparable to heat exhaustion or heat stroke) is more remote in cold weather, there is an equal or greater chance for other injuries, such as frostbite and injuries as a result of slips and falls.

In this chapter we will examine the impact of cold weather on firefighters and fire department operations. We will highlight the physiological strains these conditions place on firefighters and the injuries that can result. Lastly, we will examine how to avoid these types of injuries.

COLD STRESS TERMS AND CONCEPTS

Most of the basic terms and concepts associated with cold stress were covered in Chapter 2 dealing with heat stress. To avoid duplication they are not repeated here and typically all of these terms have the same application in a discussion of cold weather operations; we are simply looking at the other end of the temperature scale.

In Chapter 2 we discussed the U.S. military's process for defining four distinct types of climates. Two of the four apply to cold weather operations: cold-wet and cold-dry climates. Cold-wet conditions are characterized by environmental temperatures of between 14 °F (-10 °C) and 68 °F (20 °C). Temperatures can change rapidly and daily freeze/thaw cycles can occur. Precipitation in the form of rain, freezing rain, sleet, or snow can be experienced regularly. Most areas of North America experience cold-wet conditions at some time during the year. Even tropic, desert, and polar areas regularly experience conditions of this type.

Cold-dry conditions are characterized by environmental temperatures of less than 14 °F. Below-zero and windy conditions often are experienced in these areas and temperatures of less than -60°F (-51°C) have been recorded throughout history. The colder that air becomes, the less moisture it is capable of holding, thus many of these areas tend to be rather arid and any precipitation they do receive is in the form of dry, powdery snow. Areas of North America commonly experiencing cold-dry conditions include the north-central U.S., portions of the extreme northeastern U.S., central and northern Canada, Alaska, and areas with mountainous terrain such as the Rockies and Sierras.

It is somewhat unusual for a particular region to be capable of having both of these cold weather climates on a regular basis. Most jurisdictions have only one or the other during their winter season. However, it is extremely common for all jurisdictions that have one of these cold weather climates to also have one or both of the warm weather climates during other times of the year.

In Chapter 2 we talked about the combined effects of heat and humidity on the firefighter. The more water contained in the air (humidity), the greater the heat impact on the firefighter. The combination of cold air and humidity is not an issue for firefighters.This is due primarily to the previously-stated fact that as air gets colder its ability to contain water in suspension is reduced. That is why you find dew on your yard or car in the morning. As the air cooled overnight its ability to maintain moisture decreased; the excess water "dropped" out of the air in the form of dew on surfaces.

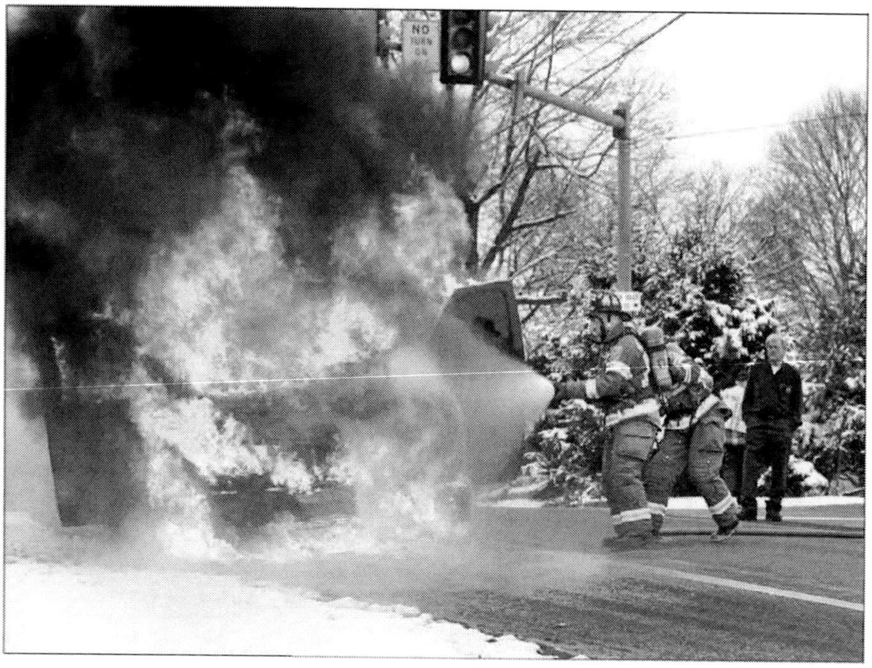

Figure 3.1. Courtesy of Bob Esposito.

More troubling to firefighters is the combination of cold and wind. The presence of wind increases the transfer of heat by the forces of convection. In this case the wind is increasing the transfer of heat away from the person's body. Although the environmental temperature is fixed at a certain degree, the person loses body heat at a rate that is comparable to a lower actual temperature in the absence of wind. This effect is referred to as the Wind Chill Index. The Wind Chill Index is a system that attempts to express the cooling effect of air movement on humans exposed to cold temperatures in terms of equivalent wind chill temperatures.

The most commonly used Wind Chill Index was called the Siple and Passel Index **(Table 3.1).** This system was developed in 1945 and both the U.S. National Weather Service (NWS) and the Meteorological Services of Canada (MSC) used it for many years.

However, advances in research and technology led to the development of a new Wind Chill Index in 2000. A consortium of governmental agencies and educational institutions formed the Joint Action Group for Temperature Indices (JAG/TI). Their advanced research techniques, coupled with clinical trials, resulted in a new system that was adopted formally for use in the U.S. and Canada in 2001. The new formula and the resultant wind chill chart **(Table 3.2)** are based on the following criteria:

- Wind speed is calculated at an average height of 5 feet from the ground, the average height of a human head, on the basis of wind speed readings taken from standard anemometers, which typically are mounted 33 feet off the ground.
- The factors are based on a human face model and a standard skin tissue resistance.
- The latest information in human heat transfer theory was used.
- Winds between 0 and 3 miles per hour (5 km/h) are considered to be calm.
- The wind chill chart assumes no impact from the sun.

Table 3.1. Wind Chill Index

	Temperature, °F												
Wind Speed, mph	**45**	**40**	**35**	**30**	**25**	**20**	**15**	**10**	**5**	**0**	**-5**	**-10**	**-15**
5	43	37	32	27	22	16	11	6	0	-5	-10	-15	-21
10	34	28	22	16	10	3	-3	-9	-15	-22	-27	-34	-40
15	29	23	16	9	2	-5	-11	-18	-25	-31	-38	-45	-51
20	26	19	12	4	-3	-10	-17	-24	-31	-39	-46	-53	-60
25	23	16	8	1	-7	-15	-22	-29	-36	-44	-51	-59	-66
30	21	13	6	-2	-10	-18	-25	-33	-41	-49	-56	-64	-71
35	20	12	4	-4	-12	-20	-27	-35	-43	-52	-58	-67	-75
40	19	11	3	-5	-13	-21	-29	-37	-45	-53	-60	-69	-76
45	18	10	2	-6	-14	-22	-30	-38	-46	-54	-62	-70	-78

Wind Chill Temperature	**Danger**
Above 25 °F (– 3.9 °C)	Little danger for properly clothed person
25 to –75 °F (– 3.9 to –59.4 °C)	Increasing danger; flesh may freeze
Below – 75 °F (–59.4 °C)	Great danger; flesh may freeze in 30 seconds

If you compare similar figures on both charts you will note that the newer figures are not as severe as the older Siple and Passel figures. This may allow fire departments to make some adjustments to Standard Operating Procedures (SOPs) and policies that were based on the old information. More information can be obtained at http://www.nws.noaa.gov/om/windchill/

PHYSIOLOGICAL RESPONSE TO COLD

Firefighters participating in training and emergency operations in many parts of the country often will encounter cold stress conditions that require management for successful mission accomplishment **(Figure 3.2)**. Excessive cold stress degrades physical performance capabilities, significantly affects morale, and eventually may cause cold casualties.

Cold stress environments include not only exposure to extremely low temperatures, but also cold-wet exposures in warmer ambient temperatures. Examples of these would be extended diving operations in cool water, performing urban search and rescue (US&R) operations in cool, wet locations, and performing searches in swamps and bogs. Fire departments certainly have the ability to perform successfully in all types of cold weather conditions and firefighters can be protected easily from these extreme elements. However, the cold weather conditions can have some other implications that influence the health and safety of firefighters and emergency operations that must be accounted for:

- Food and water requirements may be higher than expected, as people burn more calories in cold weather **(Figure 3.3).** Yet supplying these resources to the scene in adequate amounts can be difficult, resulting in inadequate nutrition and hydration during extended incidents.
- Maintaining proper field sanitation and personal hygiene in rehab operations is more difficult.
- Sick and injured individuals (emergency service providers or incident victims) are susceptible to medical complications produced by cold.
- Operational problems often arise in cold weather, including physical performance decrements, equipment malfunctions, and slow movement of vehicles and personnel.

The concepts of radiation, convection, and conduction were discussed in Chapter 2. Convection of heat occurs by the movement of a gas or liquid over the body, whether induced by body motion or natural movement of air (wind) or water, when air/water temperature is below body temperature. This movement decreases the boundary layer over the skin that insulates against heat loss. In cold air environments, convective heat transfer can be increased significantly by wind (if clothing does not create a barrier), and for firefighters wading/operating in water, convective heat loss can be very large even when the difference between body surface and surrounding fluid temperature is small. This is because the heat capacity of water is much greater than that of air, and the convective heat transfer coefficient of water is about 25 times greater than that of air.

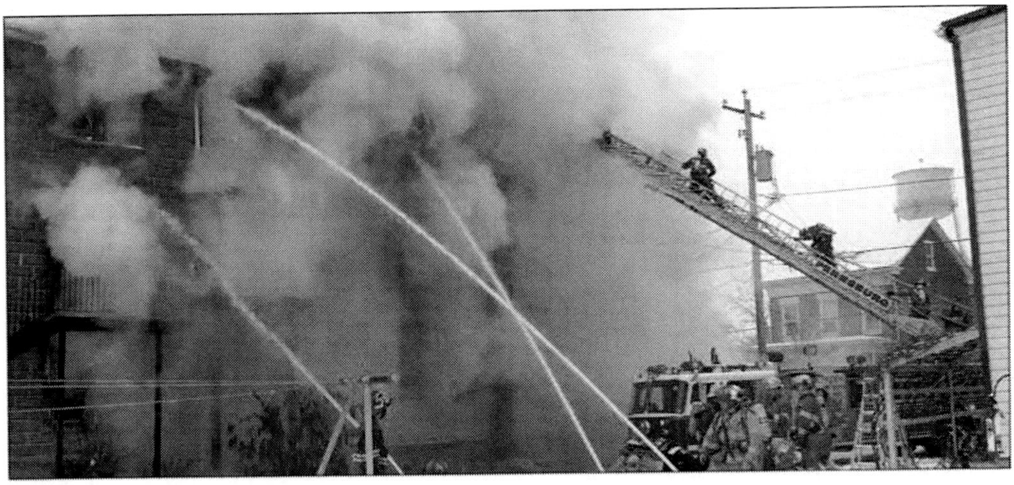

Figure 3.2. Courtesy of Bob Esposito.

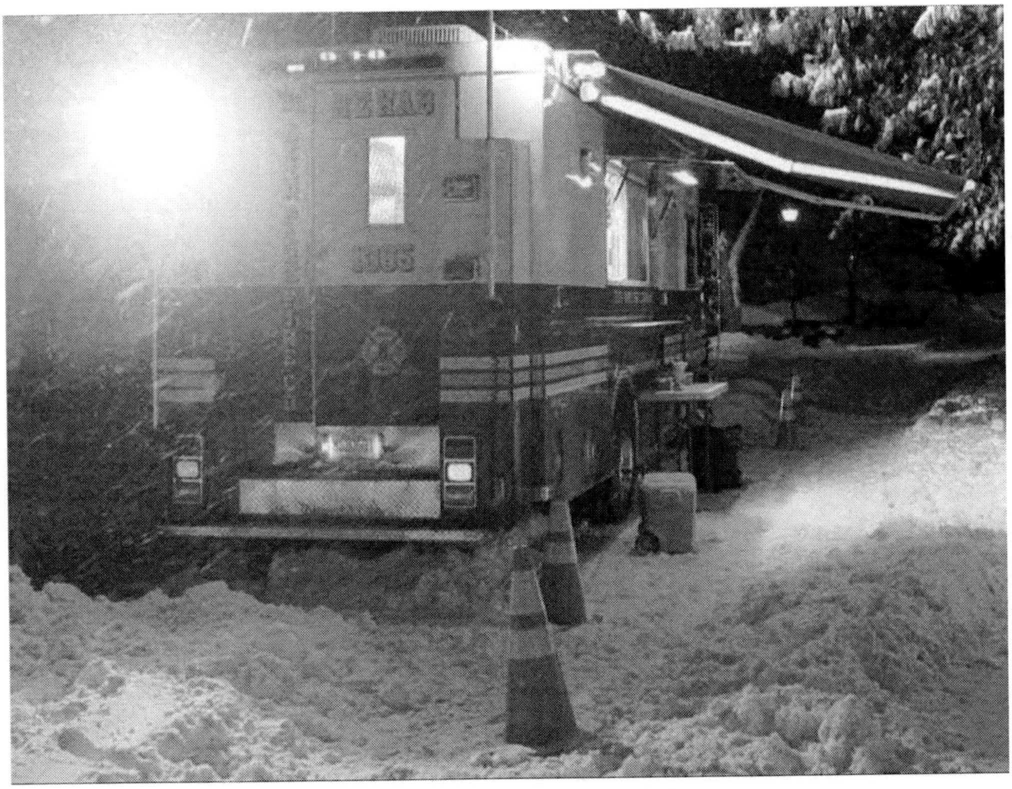

Figure 3.3. Courtesy of Cherry Hill, NJ Fire Department.

Radiative heat loss away from the body occurs when surrounding objects have lower surface temperatures than the body and are independent of air motion. However, radiation from the sun, ground, and surrounding objects can have a high radiative capacity and cause the body to gain heat even though the air temperature is below that of the body. For example, on a very sunny day a firefighter on a snowy surface may gain a significant amount of heat, despite low air temperatures. However, even when ambient air temperatures are relatively high, heat loss from exposed skin is greater under a clear, night sky than during daylight hours.

Conduction of heat occurs between two objects that are in direct contact and have different surface temperatures. Operating/Laying on cold ground/snow and touching metal objects or liquids are common ways this occurs during cold weather fire department operations. Heat conduction is greater during exposure when skin and clothing are wet than when the skin is dry. Wetness decreases the insulation of clothing and increases the contact area between skin and a surface.

Evaporative heat loss occurs when liquid turns to water vapor. Evaporative heat loss is associated with sweating and respiration. The rate of sweat evaporation depends upon air movement and the water vapor pressure gradient between the skin and the environment, so in still or moist air the sweat tends to collect on the skin. When firefighters perform strenuous exercise in heavy clothing, significant heat strain and sweating can occur. After exercise, the nonevaporated sweat will reduce clothing insulation capabilities and possibly form ice crystals. Breathing cold air can exacerbate respiratory water loss slightly during exercise, since cold air has lower water content than warmer air. Therefore, the most significant avenue of evaporative heat loss during exercise in cold conditions is the same as in warm conditions, which is sweating.

The key to effective operations on cold weather conditions is maintaining effective temperature regulation of the human body. Body temperature is normally regulated within a narrow range through two parallel processes: behavioral temperature regulation and physiological temperature regulation. Behavioral temperature regulation refers to conscious actions we take in order to minimize the impact of cold conditions on our bodies. This includes things such as wearing appropriate clothing, seeking shelter, and avoiding cold conditions. Physiological temperature regulation refers to the body's natural reaction to minimizing the impact on cold conditions. Two common physiological responses are reduced blood flow (vasoconstriction) to conserve the body's heat and shivering to produce additional heat.

Vasoconstriction begins when skin temperature falls below about 95 °F (35 °C) and becomes maximal when the skin temperature reaches 88 °F (31 °C) or less. If exposure to cold continues, the vasoconstriction will begin to occur in tissues beneath the skin, causing muscles to become cold and stiff. While the process of vasoconstriction helps to maintain the body core temperature, it does so at the expense of a decline in the peripheral tissue temperatures. Cold-induced vasoconstriction has pronounced effects on the hands, fingers, and feet, making them particularly susceptible to cold injury, pain, and loss of manual dexterity. The ears and nose are also highly susceptible to cold injury.

Cold exposure increases metabolic heat production in humans, which can help offset heat loss. Exposure to cold causes the skeletal-muscular system to contract. About 80 percent of the energy generated by this process is liberated in the form of heat. This process is initiated by one of two methods: voluntarily through increased physical activity or involuntarily by shivering. Shivering, which consists of involuntary, repeated, rhythmic muscle contractions, may start immediately or after several minutes of exposure to cold. Shivering typically begins in the torso muscles and spreads to the limbs. The intensity and extent of shivering will vary according to the amount of cold stress on the body.

Of the two metabolic methods for producing heat, physical movement will generate more heat than shivering. Running, for example, will generate twice the heat produced by shivering. However, shivering can be sustained longer than heavy or maximal exercise.

Individual Factors

Every individual responds to cold exposure in a slightly different manner. There are a variety of individual factors that influence the effect of cold exposure on a particular person. A summary of these is as follows:

- **Body size and fat**—People who have long and lean body types will lose heat faster than those who have short or stocky body types. The reason for this is that the principle means of heat loss in people exposed to cold is convective heat transfer at the skin surface. People with stocky, heavier body types have a relatively low body surface to mass ratio.

- **Gender**—Records kept by the U.S. Army show that women have a periphery cold injury rate that is twice that of males. Their research indicates that it is almost entirely attributable to women's generally greater body fat content and thicker subcutaneous fat layer than men of comparable age and weight. Thus, total heat loss in woman is greater due to the larger surface area for convective heat flux, and body temperature would tend to fall more rapidly for a given cold stress.

- **Race**—Again, records and research conducted by the Army shows that African-American soldiers were two to four times more likely to suffer a cold weather injury than their Caucasian counterparts. It is believed that this difference may be due to cold-weather experience, but more likely it is due to anthro pomorphic considerations (such as longer, thinner digits) and perhaps greater surface area-to-mass ratio.

- **Fitness and training**—The level of fitness in the individual has little impact on the physiological response to cold stress. The only significant advantage of a person with a high level of fitness dealing with cold stress is their greater amount of endurance, which will allow them to move for longer periods of time to keep warm.

- **Fatigue**—Physical fatigue will impair shivering and peripheral vasoconstriction during cold exposure **(Figure 3.4).** This will increase the person's risk for hypothermia.

- **Age**—Army research showed that people older than 45 years of age were less cold tolerant than younger people. This may be due to a decline in physical fitness or because of reduced vasoconstriction and heat conservation as compared to younger people.

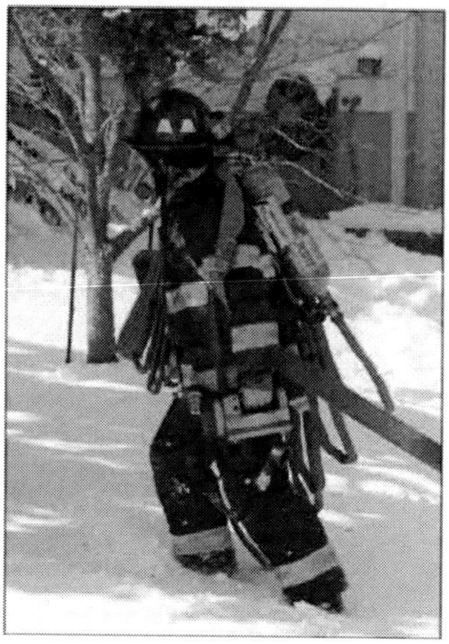

Figure 3.4. Courtesy of Dennis Wetherhold Jr., Allentown, PA.

- **Dehydration**—Dehydration can increase susceptibility to cold injury by decreasing the ability to sustain physical activity, particularly if accompanied by heat stress caused by working in heavy clothing, such as turnouts. Dehydration also can impair cognitive function and cause firefighters to use poor judgment.

- **Sustained operations**—Exertional fatigue, sleep deprivation, and poor nutrition (underfeeding) are common stressors during sustained operations and will impair the firefighter's ability to maintain thermal balance in the cold because of degradation of the metabolic heat production response, as well as impairment of the ability to sustain exercise performance.

- **Alcohol**—Although alcohol should not be an issue for emergency responders, its effects during cold exposure should be noted. Although alcohol may impart a sense of warmth, any peripheral vasodilation (which alcohol causes) will increase heat loss and the risk of hypothermia. It also impairs judgment and reduces the ability to feel the signs and symptoms of impending cold injury.

- **Nicotine**—Smoking or chewing tobacco can increase susceptibility to frostbite by increasing vasocon striction in peripheral body parts, such as the hands. Army research indicated that heavy (2 to 3 packs per day) smokers had a 30 percent higher incidence of peripheral cold injury.

Effects on Performance

When looking at the effects of cold on performance, there are three particular areas that must be considered: ability to work/exercise, manual dexterity, and cognition/thinking.

Exercise performance is not altered as long at the body core temperature drop is less than 0.9 °F and the muscle temperature remains above 97 °F (36 °C). However, for every 1.8 °F decrease in core or muscle temperature, maximal endurance exercise capability is lowered by about 5 percent, exercise endurance time is lowered by 20 percent, and maximal strength and power output is lowered by 5 percent.

Manual dexterity is important for many of the functions firefighters perform, particularly emergency medical functions. Pain sensations increase once the skin temperature is decreased to 68 °F (20 °C). Manual dexterity declines 10 to 20 percent after finger skin temperatures decrease below 60 °F (15.6 °C). Tactile sensitivity is reduced as skin temperature drops below 43 °F (6 °C) and further sharp decline in finger dexterity occurs at this point. It should also be noted that immersion of the hands and arms in 50 °F (10 °C) water for as short as 5 minutes can lower manual dexterity by 20 to 50 percent.

Cold strain can degrade mental performance on complex thinking tasks by 17 to 20 percent. The ability to remember new information is impaired when the body core temperature falls between 94 and 95 °F and short-term memory declines up to 20 percent with significant peripheral cooling absent of a decreased body core temperature. It also has been noted that a person's ability to provide and track rapid, accurate responses to questions or reactions that are required decreases by 13 percent at low ambient temperatures that cause skin temperatures to fall.

Predisposing Factors

When considering predisposing factors that may affect a firefighter's susceptibility to hypothermia, there are four categories of factors that must be considered:

- **Those that decrease the person's ability to produce heat.** These can include operational factors such as inactivity, fatigue, or excessive energy depletion. Physical problems affecting endocrine levels, such as hypopituitarism, hypoadrenalism, hypothyroidism, hypoglycemia, and diabetes also can reduce heat production within the body.

- **Those that increase a person's heat loss.** Firefighters work in environments that can easily cause increased heat loss. Wet clothing, immersion in water, excessive sweating, exposure to wind, and fatigue are all examples of things that can expedite heat loss. Skin conditions such as thermal burns, sunburn, and various forms of dermatitis also accentuate heat loss.

- **Those that impair the body's ability to thermoregulate.** Peripheral failures can be caused by trauma, neuropathies, and acute spinal cord transaction. A central failure of the body's ability to thermoregulate can be caused by a wide variety of factors, including nervous system lesions and trauma, stroke, hypothalamic dys function, Parkinson's Disease, multiple sclerosis, and drug and alcohol use. Psychotropic medications, in particular, increase the possibility of impaired thermoregulation.

- **Other miscellaneous clinical conditions, including infections, renal failure, and cancer.** We should not have firefighters operating on emergency scenes with these conditions.

The predisposing factors for frostbite and localized cold injuries can be categorized into five basic categories. These are summarized as follows:

- **Environmental factors**, including cold temperatures, wet skin, extended exposure duration, wind, and contact with metals, petroleum products, oils, and lubricants.

- **Mechanical factors**, including constrictive, inadequate and/or wet clothing, tight boots, and being in a cramped or prolonged stationary posture/position.

- **Physiological factors**, including hypothermia, prior cold injuries, trauma, erythrodermas, hypoxia, smoking, poor physical conditioning, and energy depletion.

- **Psychological factors**, including severe mental stress, poor training, and drug or alcohol use.

- **Medical factors**, including hypotension, atherosclerosis, anemia, sickle cell disease, diabetes, shock, and vasoconstrictors.

- Physical exams that are given to firefighters should seek to identify these predisposing factors ahead of time so they can be compensated for in field operations. SOPs must be established and enforced to ensure actual operations don't continue to place people in high risk situations for hypothermia or local cold injuries.

HYPOTHERMIA

Hypothermia can be defined as subnormal temperature within the internal body core. The condition can be caused by either exposure to cold environmental conditions without adequate protective clothing or by compromise of the body's physiological mechanisms by drugs, disease, or injury. A person suffering from hypothermia will exhibit poor coordination and often will stumble and slur speech. Mental dulling with impairment of judgment and ability to work may be prominent, even before other symptoms are manifested. The victim may not be aware of the degree of impairment and may resist treatment. Once severe shivering occurs the victim may not be able to rewarm without an outside heat source. For the firefighter, the danger of hypothermia exists when radiant heat loss from the face interferes with the body's heat conservation mechanisms allowing severe loss of internal core warmth. Hypothermia is associated with depression of normal circulation and vital signs, thus measurement of heart rate, pulse, and blood pressure may be difficult or impossible.

Accurate evaluation of the hypothermic victim can only be made by deep rectal temperature readings using a special low-temperature reading thermometer. However, careful observation of the patient can yield approximate results.

Table 3.2.

Wind Chill Chart

Temperature (°F)

Wind (mph) \ Calm	40	35	30	25	20	15	10	5	0	-5	-10	-15	-20	-25	-30	-35	-40	-45
5	36	31	25	19	13	7	1	-5	-11	-16	-22	-28	-34	-40	-46	-52	-57	-63
10	34	27	21	15	9	3	-4	-10	-16	-22	-28	-35	-41	-47	-53	-59	-66	-72
15	32	25	19	13	6	0	-7	-13	-19	-26	-32	-39	-45	-51	-58	-64	-71	-77
20	30	24	17	11	4	-2	-9	-15	-22	-29	-35	-42	-48	-55	-61	-68	-74	-81
25	29	23	16	9	3	-4	-11	-17	-24	-31	-37	-44	-51	-58	-64	-71	-78	-84
30	28	22	15	8	1	-5	-12	-19	-26	-33	-39	-46	-53	-60	-67	-73	-80	-87
35	28	21	14	7	0	-7	-14	-21	-27	-34	-41	-48	-55	-62	-69	-76	-82	-89
40	27	20	13	6	-1	-8	-15	-22	-29	-36	-43	-50	-57	-64	-71	-78	-84	-91
45	26	19	12	5	-2	-9	-16	-23	-30	-37	-44	-51	-58	-65	-72	-79	-86	-93
50	26	19	12	4	-3	-10	-17	-24	-31	-38	-45	-52	-60	-67	-74	-81	-88	-95
55	25	18	11	4	-3	-11	-18	-25	-32	-39	-46	-54	-61	-68	-75	-82	-89	-97
60	25	17	10	3	-4	-11	-19	-26	-33	-40	-48	-55	-62	-69	-76	-84	-91	-98

Frostbite Times: 30 minutes; 10 minutes; 5 minutes

$$\text{Wind Chill (°F)} = 35.74 + 0.6215T - 35.75(V^{0.16}) + 0.4275T(V^{0.16})$$

Where, T= Air Temperature (°F) V= Wind Speed (mph)

Effective 11/01/01

Table 3.3. Hypothermic Symptoms at various body Core Temperatures

Core Temperature	Symptoms
95 to 98.6 °F	Conscious, alert, but violent shivering.
90 to 95 °F	Conscious but mild to moderate loss of mental capacity; shivering usually present but may be impaired.
86 to 90 °F	Severe loss of mental capacity. Shivering gradually replaced by muscular rigidity. Cardiac arrest may occur. Pupils may be dilated.
80 to 86 °F	Impairment of respiration. Pulse rate and volume severely depressed. Pupils dilated and may be unresponsive to light. Cardiac arrest probable.
below 80 °F	Patients may appear dead with no discernable vital signs.

Recommended Treatment

Hypothermia that has progressed to the point that shivering has stopped is a true medical emergency. The patient should be evaluated with extreme care, since blood pressure and radial pulse may not be detectable due to decreased circulation in the extremities. In fact, the patient may even appear to be dead. However, successful resuscitations have been made even after extensive periods without notable vital signs. Therefore, all suspected hypothermia patients should be rewarmed at a hospital emergency department before death is assumed. In the emergency room, doctors typically operate by the philosophy that a hypothermic patient is not pronounced dead until they are "warm and dead."

In the field, the patient should be protected from further cold stress by removal to a warm place. Damp, frozen, or constricting clothing should be removed gently and replaced with blankets or other insulation. Particular care should be taken to insulate the head and neck with towels or other material. It is critical to note that cardiac arrest may be initiated by rough handling or attempts at field rewarming using external techniques such as electric blankets, hot packs, hot water bottles, or baths.

Available information suggests that the application of warm, humidified air by mouth-to-mouth breathing or special warmed air/oxygen respirators can be effective at stabilizing patients until rewarming can be implemented in a hospital emergency department. If the patient is trapped, such as in an apparatus accident or cave in, this technique often can be used with great success.

All patients with significant hypothermia should be afforded intravenous therapy. Intravenous solutions should be warmed before infusion by placing the bag next to a paramedic's body or in a warm water (98.6 °F (37 °C)) bath. IVs are often difficult or impossible to start in the hypothermia patient in the field due to poor circulation, therefore, transport should not be delayed significantly for this reason.

If the patient is in cardiac arrest, cardiopulmonary resuscitation (CPR) should be implemented in accordance with normal procedure. It must be remembered that shivering may mimic ventricular fibrillation on cardiac monitors. Since defibrillation and drug responses are usually ineffective at low body temperature, the hospital emergency department physician should be notified of the patient's history in regard to hypothermia before such therapy is initiated.

FROSTBITE

Frostbite is a soft-tissue injury resulting from exposure to environmental temperatures of less than 32 °F (0 °C). Injury results from freezing of cell and tissue fluids which mechanically and/or physically disrupt cellular function. General symptoms include sensation of coldness, followed by numbness. The skin turns red, then pale or waxy grey-white. Aching, tingling, and stinging may be experienced. Frostbite is divided into two categories although differentiation between them in the field may be impossible.

Superficial frostbite, sometimes referred to as frostnip, involves only the skin and/or tissue immediately beneath it. In the prethaw condition, the skin is waxy gray-white with yellow splotches possible. The skin is cold and resilient and may often be moved freely over joints and facial bones. After thawing, general swelling will occur and blisters may form after 24 hours. Throbbing, aching and burning pain may persist for several weeks. As swelling subsides, the skin usually peels, remaining red and tender. Cold sensitivity and dryness may continue for some time.

Deep frostbite involves not only the skin and subcutaneous tissue, but also deeper tissue down to the bone. It is manifested by a persistent lack of effective circulation with resultant ischemia and cyanosis. In the prethaw condition, skin is translucent, waxy, pallid and yellowish in color. The tissue is solid to touch and not movable over joints and bones. There is a marked lack of pain. After thawing, a throbbing, aching pain develops often followed by a period of sensation loss. Large blisters usually develop in about 72 hours. The area will generally be very swollen for a month or more. After about a month, the skin will peel leaving a thin, red, sensitive area of new skin. Itching and dryness may persist for many months. In extremely severe cases, blisters may form within the tissue along a line between tissue that will heal and tissue that is permanently damaged. The permanently damaged tissue can progress in one of two ways. The tissue may become dry, shriveled and black with little pain or swelling or the area may become infected, resulting in wet, swollen tissue and intense pain. Deep frostbite cases almost always require extensive medical care.

Recommended Treatment

The patient should be protected from further cold exposure by removal to warm place. Boots or clothing covering the affected area should be removed carefully and damp, frozen, or constricting clothing replaced with blankets or other insulation. In cases of minor superficial frostbite where only the outer layer of skin is affected, the area can be rewarmed by gently covering with a hand. Do not rub, massage, or apply ice or direct heat, such as from hot packs or from an open fire or apparatus exhaust. More serious cases of frostbite should not be thawed in the field, since thawing may be extremely painful and the possibility of refreezing exists. Such freeze-thaw-refreeze injuries are extremely serious. All cases of frostbite should be protected with a dry, sterile dressing and evaluated by a hospital emergency department. Again, smoking by the victim should not be allowed. If the injury is to feet or legs, patient should be handled as a stretcher patient to prevent further injury.

Immersion Injury

Immersion injury, also known as trench foot, is a tissue injury resulting from prolonged exposure to cold at temperatures that do not cause actual freezing. The condition results from compromise of circulation, especially in the extremities, by various means including local cooling, general body cooling, constriction by clothing such as gloves, socks, or boots or chronic circulatory disease such as arteriosclerosis. Even though freezing of tissue does not occur, this condition is almost impossible to distinguish from frostbite that has already been thawed. The condition presents itself in two distinct stages. Stage I, or ischemic stage, is due to a deficiency of circulating blood in the tissue. The area is cool, swollen, waxy, and mottled with blue to burgundy splotches. The skin is spongy to the touch and numb. Sensation often is lost and use of limbs is impaired by stiffness. Stage II, or hyperemic stage, is due to local relaxation of blood vessels. The area is red, warm, and swollen. Blister formation is common and constant; throbbing pain and burning are experienced also.

Trench foot is not likely to be found in firefighters who are involved in standard firefighting operations, regardless of the conditions. It is more likely to be encountered in personnel who are deployed to extended operations, such as major US&R operations that last for days at a time.

Recommended Treatment

Personnel should not use the affected area. Boots or clothing covering the injured area should be removed carefully and the area gently dried, elevated, and protected by a dry, sterile dressing. The area must not be rubbed, massaged, moistened, or exposed to ice or direct heat such as from hot packs or apparatus exhausts. Blisters should not be ruptured. Patients should be protected from further cold exposure by removal to a warm place and immediately replacing damp, frozen, or constricting clothing with blankets or other insulation. If the injury is to the feet or legs, patient should be handled as a stretcher patient to prevent further injury. Smoking should not be allowed. All immersion injury cases should be evaluated by a hospital emergency department.

CHILBLAINS

Chilblains are areas of skin, usually on the face or hands where circulation has been impaired for some time. The condition results from repeated or prolonged exposure to temperatures above freezing, especially when accompanied by high humidity. Initially the affected skin appears pale and blanched. Upon rewarm-ing, the area is red, swollen, hot, tender, and itchy. Skin may blister or ulcerate. One episode of chilblains can predispose occurrence during subsequent exposure to cold.

Recommended Treatment

The area should be rewarmed slowly by the bare hand or at room temperature. Do not rub, massage, or apply direct heat or ice. Itching may be relieved by application of a moisturizing ointment. In severe cases where blister formation occurs, the affected area should be protected with a dry, sterile dressing and evaluated by a physician, preferably a dermatologist.

Guidelines for Preventing Cold Stress Injuries

Most firefighting and rescue duties require firefighters to wear special protective clothing that also protects the wearer from the effects of cold temperatures. However, this does not mean the firefighters are immune from cold stress injuries. Various circumstances and conditions can place firefighters in a position of risk of cold stress injuries. The most common extinguishing agent that firefighters use is water. Firefighters will be exposed to water and steam during the course of their operations, even in very cold climatic conditions (Figure 3.5). Other special operations may cause firefighters to shed normal protective gear or actually operate in water. Incident Commanders (ICs) and other fire service personnel must always be cognizant of the possibility of cold injuries and ensure that tactical operations are always geared against this.

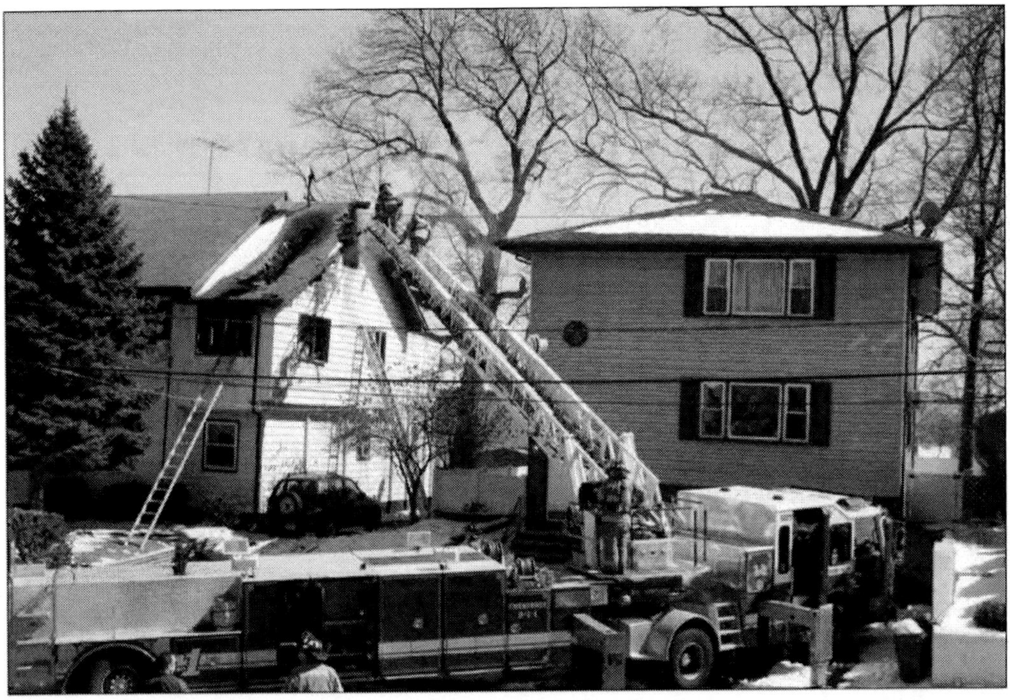

Figure 3.5. Courtesy of Ron Jeffers, Union City, NJ.

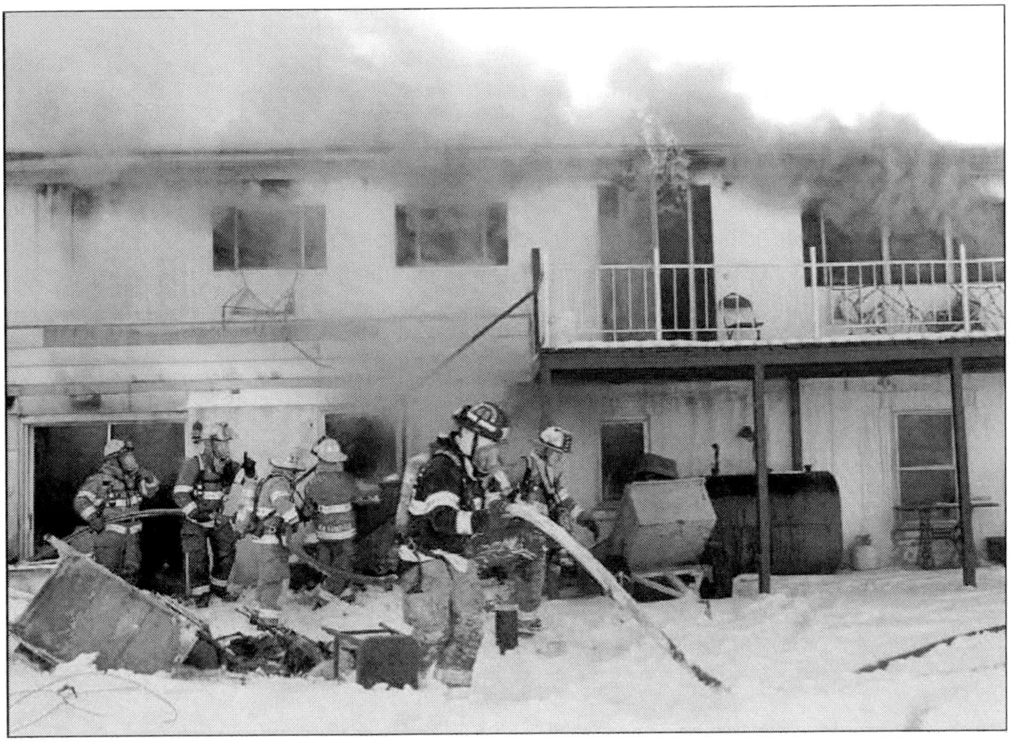

Figure 3.6. Courtesy of Bob Esposito.

Protective Clothing Effectiveness against Cold Stress

The first step toward prevention of cold injury lies in the issuance and maintenance of proper protective clothing as noted above. Insulation that is protected from wind and water stays dry and maintains its ability to protect the firefighter. Sometimes it is impossible to keep gloves, socks, and other clothing dry under extreme conditions. In particular, spare gloves and socks should be provided at the scene during cold conditions to allow changing when extended operations occur. Adequate provisions for drying clothing and equipment in a warm area at the fire station between alarms must be provided; hanging wet clothing in a poorly-heated apparatus room is not sufficient (**Figure 3.6**). In the most extreme conditions where frozen clothing must be thawed and dried, spare garments, including turnout clothing, should be provided to assure that dry clothing is available.

For clothing to effectively insulate the body, it must capture heat produced by body metabolism and prevent its loss to the environment. The insulating effect is provided by air trapped in spaces within and between layers of clothing. For clothing to maintain these spaces of trapped air effectively, the insulating layers must be protected from water and wind penetration. For example, in the standard three-layer turnout garment configuration of a fire-resistant outer shell, moisture barrier, and thermal barrier, the air trapped within the inner thermal liner and between the garment layers provides insulation, while the moisture barrier protects this insulation from water and wind penetration (**Figure 3.7**). This principle of garment construction is known as the "layer" or "synergis-tic ensemble" system, where several individual clothing layers are combined to provide a clothing ensemble that is a much more effective insulator than the sum of the layers taken individually. In essence, the air between the garment layers provides "free" insulation, as the trapped insulating air is weightless.

Additional insulating air spaces are also present between other garments, such as undergarments and station uniforms. Thus, a cold weather clothing ensemble consisting of cotton underwear, station/work uniform and turnout coat with thermal liner, vapor barrier, and outer shell, would have nine layers of air space and/ or insulation. This would yield an effective insulation thickness of slightly less than one inch. Some turnout clothing manufacturers further offer a winter lining, which as an additional layer inside the clothing provides further insulation.

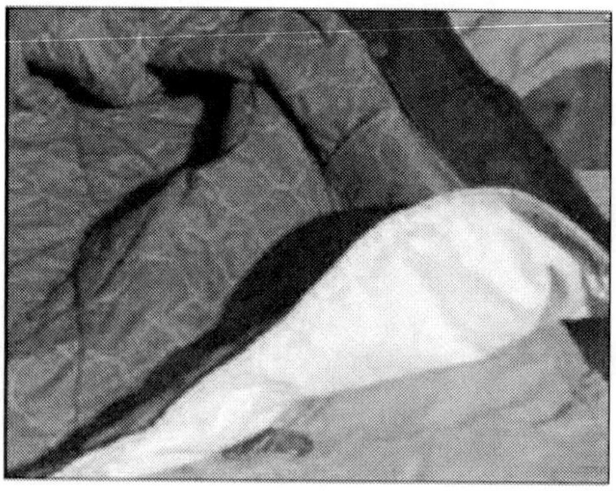

Figure 3.7.

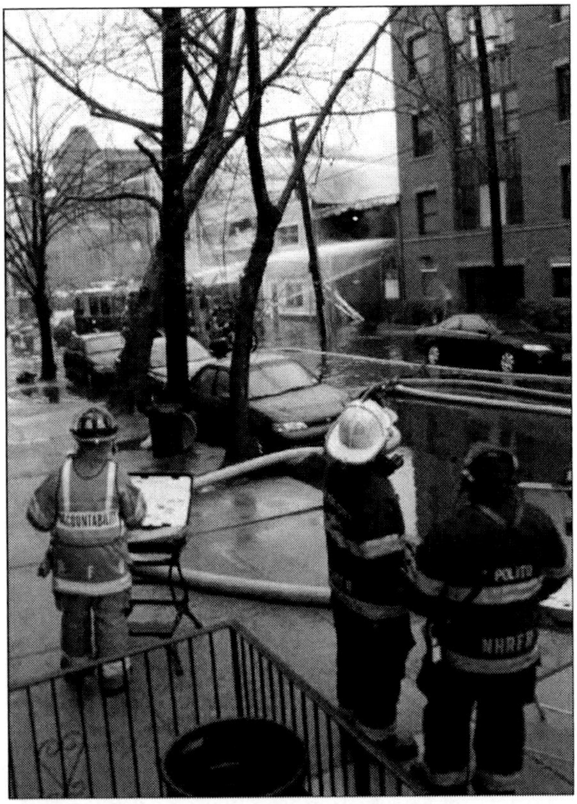

Figure 3.8. Courtesy of Ron Jeffers, Union City, NJ.

The amount of insulation thickness that is required to protect the wearer from cold temperatures depends on both the temperature being protected against and the amount of work the wearer will be doing. This presents a problem to both protective clothing manufacturers and wearers. Firefighters can operate in a variety or temperatures and at an equally diverse level of workloads. A firefighter properly insulated for light work will sometimes be in danger of overheating when heavy work is per formed, even though the motion of activity "pumps" air through the insulating garments and reduces the insulation value by about one- half. In addition, garments can be ventilated during nonfire exposure by opening the coat and collar closures to allow additional air circulation. Therefore, it is probably wise to provide insulation adequate for light work levels, accepting that some overheating will occur during periods of strenuous activity and that chilling will occur during periods of inactivity. Personnel who are relatively inactive, such as pump operators, aerial device operators, and supervisors are difficult to insulate properly and may require more frequent rewarming (**Figure 3.8**).

Another critical problem that must be considered in cold weather applications is the effect of perspiration. The body, even when inactive, emits several pints of perspiration from the skin each day. Under periods of heavy work, especially when overheated, far greater amounts of perspiration are emitted. Some of this moisture is removed from the clothing by the ventilation effect noted above. However, much of the perspiration is absorbed by the clothing next to the skin, then transferred to the outer clothing by a process known as "wicking." If no barrier material is encountered, the moisture can evaporate from the outer clothing layer. If a non-breathable barrier material is encountered, the moisture condenses on the barrier layer and within the underlying clothing layers. Turnout clothing manufactured to National Fire Protection Association (NFPA) 1971, *Standard on Protective Ensembles for Structural Fire Fighting and Proximity Fire Fighting* requires only breathable moisture barriers that limit the effect of condensation and permit the free escape of moisture buildup inside the garment under the majority of work conditions.

Moisture that is trapped in clothing has several effects. First, the insulation value of the clothing layers is impaired due to matting of the fabrics and filling of the insulating air spaces with water. After the clothing has absorbed a certain amount of moisture, it can hold no more and perspiration will accumulate on the skin itself. Since water transfers heat 25 times faster than air, a chilling effect occurs, especially after exercise. Second, if high heat conditions are encountered, this trapped moisture may be converted to steam, causing burns. Advances in breathable protective clothing liners, such as those using breathable moisture barriers, have reduced the effect of moisture building up on the firefighter's skin.

Since up to half of the body's heat can be lost from the head and neck, it is critical that firefighters be adequately protected. As with the torso, extra insulation to these areas will allow the body to send extra heat to the extremities, keeping hands and feet warm. Unfortunately, most standard helmet liners do not provide a high level of cold, wind, and water protection. The ear covers now required for NFPA 1971-compliant helmets offer greater protection in combination with turned up collars and a protective hood. Yet many of the fabrics used generally allow wind and water penetration which will compromise the insulating layer, if present **(Figure 3.9).** Only a few protective hoods and helmet ear covers use moisture barriers to offer some protection from wind or water penetration **(Figure 3.10).**

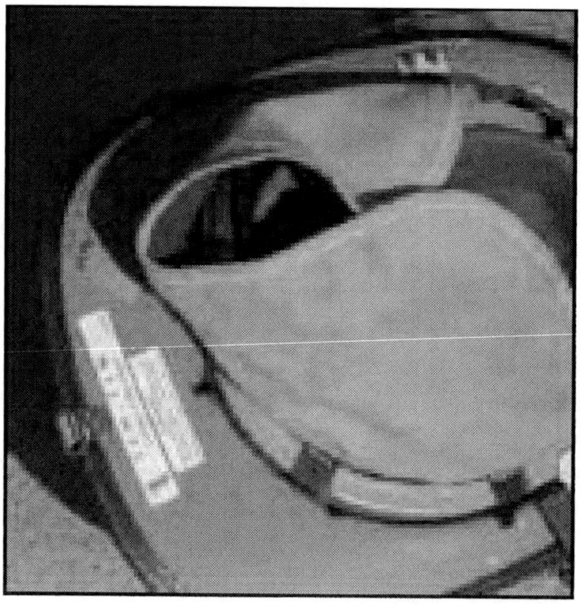

Figure 3.9.

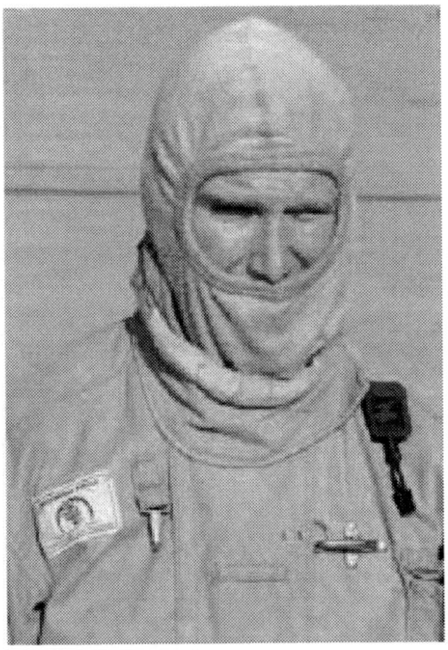

Figure 3.10. Courtesy of IFSTA/ Fire Protection Publications.

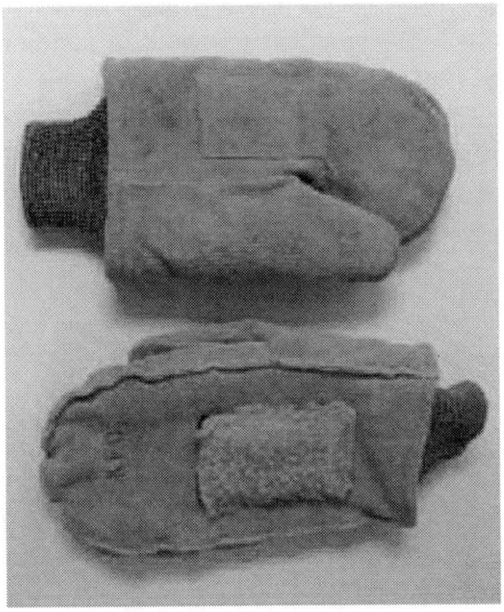

Figure 3.11.

The hands are probably the most difficult part of the body to protect from cold. Unfortunately, the requirements of insulation and dexterity are almost completely in opposition. Current NFPA 1971 glove criteria require the use of a moisture barrier, which does provide water and wind-resistance protection to the hands. Unfortunately, some departments use gloves that do not use an adequate moisture barrier, which may still offer adequate protection from heat and flame while allowing good dexterity and fit, but provide little protection from water penetration.

While an ideal cold weather firefighter's glove is not available, gloves that meet NFPA requirements will provide some degree of cold protection. As described in Chapter 2, these gloves employ outer leather or combined fabric shells, a moisture barrier, and lining material. There is currently no requirement for glove moisture barrier breathability, but some gloves are available with a breathable moisture barrier, which permits the escape of perspiration inside gloves. Fire departments that operate in severely cold climates use mittens that are designed for firefighting to maximize warmth of all the fingers **(Figure 3.11).**

It must be noted that when any glove or mitten liner becomes dampened from perspiration or external moisture, insulation value is lost and local cold injury can result. If the glove has interchangeable liners, they should be switched out for dry liners. If they do not, the firefighter should change to dry gloves.

Like the hands, the feet are difficult to insulate effectively while maintaining ease of movement. Standard rubber fire boots provide protection from wind, water, and snow, but provide little insulation, even when lined with a thin layer of insulating felt. However, when worn with a thick insulating sock, boots of this type will provide adequate insulation for the feet to tolerate limited exposure under cold-wet conditions, where temperatures do not fall below 14 °F. Modern, leather firefighting boots, that typically use breathable moisture barrier liners, offer far superior protection in cold weather conditions.

When addressing protective clothing and its impact on preventing cold injuries, the impact of breathing apparatus should also be considered. Self-contained breathing apparatus (SCBA) and SCBA cylinders must be protected from cold also, since frostbite can occur if skin contact to severely cooled facepieces is allowed. In addition, the National Institute of Occupational Safety and Health (NIOSH) has issued bulletins stating that SCBA may not operate effectively in below freezing conditions. To prevent freezing of regulators, special care should be taken to ensure that proper moisture removal from breathing air supplies is maintained. In addition, nose cups should be used on all SCBA used in cold conditions in order to prevent fogging; antifog preparations have been shown to be almost useless in field conditions.

Avoiding Hypothermia

A firefighter's body core temperature during cold exposure reflects a balance between heat production (physical activity, shivering, etc.) and heat loss. Increasing heat production and decreasing heat loss will reduce the risk for hypothermia, which is defined as a core temperature less than 95 °F.The environmental conditions (whether cold-dry or cold-wet) will determine the risk for hypothermia. Convective heat loss is about 25 times greater in water than air. Wet clothing (from rain or sweat) and immersion increase heat loss substantially, increasing the likelihood of hypothermia.

Firefighters can avoid falling victim to hypothermia by following two important concepts when dressing for activities in the cold: layering and staying dry. Firefighter protective clothing is designed to protect against hypothermia by reducing heat loss to the environment. Insulation is determined by how much air is effectively trapped by the clothing, both the personal protective clothing and the clothing worn beneath it. Multiple layers of clothing allows air to be trapped and serve as insulation. This also allows the individual to adjust clothing layers according to the environmental conditions and activity level. Layers can be removed as the ambient temperature or physical activity levels increase, thereby reducing sweating and moisture buildup within clothing. Of course, in the case of personal protective clothing, only so much can be removed before it presents a hazard to the wearer. Thus, we must find other ways to reduce the threat posed by moisture buildup inside the protective clothing as a result of sweating.

To assist in removing moisture caused by sweating, the innermost layer of personal protective clothing in contact with the skin must have wicking properties that allow water vapor to be transmitted to the outer layers for evaporation. When clothing becomes wet, the insulation provided is degraded, and conductive heat losses increase substantially. Care must be taken when wearing personal protective clothing, because even those equipped with breathable moisture barriers have a limited vapor transfer rate that cannot keep up with sweat produced by high activity levels.

Most people who work outside in cold weather conditions have the ability to adjust the amount of clothing they wear based on the temperature and the level of work activity they will be performing. Firefighters are not as flexible in their ability to do this. A certain minimum amount of protective clothing and equipment is always required for safety purposes and the amount of energy expended can vary widely. It is important that firefighters operating in cold climates dress in layers beneath their personal protective equipment (PPE) and then make adjustments based on conditions. Certainly any clothing that becomes wet should be removed and/or replaced as required.

An important planning consideration is not only knowing how much clothing is needed during activity in the cold, but also recognizing that as soon as physical activity stops, body heat loss will be significant. Exercise increases peripheral blood flow, resulting in greater heat transfer to the environment. Sweating that may occur with heavy exercise, even in cold conditions, also will increase heat loss when activity stops. This highlights the problem of needing less clothing during a movement, but then needing more layers after being forced to remain stationary in a foxhole or defensive position. Other clothing items always need to be available to be put on if firefighters cease physical activity, but must remain in the cold environment.

Firefighters should be encouraged to keep wearing their helmets and hoods, or other suitable head protection, when operating for extended periods in cold weather. Heat loss from the bare head can be up to 50 percent of the total loss in 25 °F (3.9 °C) air when firefighters are clothed adequately elsewhere.

It goes without saying that firefighters typically do their work in extremely dirty environments. All clothing, including PPE, becomes less effective if it becomes dirty. Dirt compresses the insulation in the fleece and clogs the pores in breathable fabrics. This is just another reason that firefighters should keep their turnout clothing as clean as possible.

Working in standing water, rain, or overspray from hoselines substantially increases a firefighter's susceptibility to hypothermia because water has a high thermal conductivity. For example, a person could sit in 50 °F air for 3 to 4 hours and not experience a fall in core temperature, whereas immersion in 50 °F water could cause a person to become hypothermic in 1 to 2 hours (**Figure 3.12**).

Firefighters must be aware of potential changes in weather and working conditions that can increase susceptibility to hypothermia. For example, going from 70 °F (21 °C) with sunshine to 55 °F (12.8 °C) air with heavy rain causes dramatically different conditions for people operating in that climate. Incident command personnel must recognize these types of changes in climate and adjust operations as necessary.

Water immersion causes profound physiological changes and challenges to body temperature homeostasis. Core temperature cooling during immersion depends on both the water temperature and the immersion depth. Cold water temperatures have higher radiative, convective, and conductive heat losses compared to warm water temperatures. Deeper immersion covers a greater amount of the body surface area and significantly increases body temperature cooling rates and risk for hypothermia. Fast-moving streams increase convective heat loss and cause body temperatures to cool faster than still bodies of water.

Table 3.4 shows the allowable exposure time during immersion at various water temperatures and immersion depths as developed by the U.S. Army. Certainly this information would be applicable firefighting and rescue operations that exposure firefighters to standing water. These exposure times reflect the time it takes the body core temperature to fall to 95.9 °F (35.5 °C).The immersion time limits in the table based on average Army soldiers, which would be comparable to well-conditioned firefighters. Leaders must recognize that some personnel will cool faster than the time limits predicted by the table. Firefighters who have low body fat and a high surface area-to-mass ratio are more susceptible to faster cooling rates. Also, firefighters who have not eaten in a while (particularly over 24 hours) are more susceptible, as are those who are fatigued because of physical exhaustion or sustained operations. Time limits when immersed to the neck are very short to avoid the possibility of drowning.

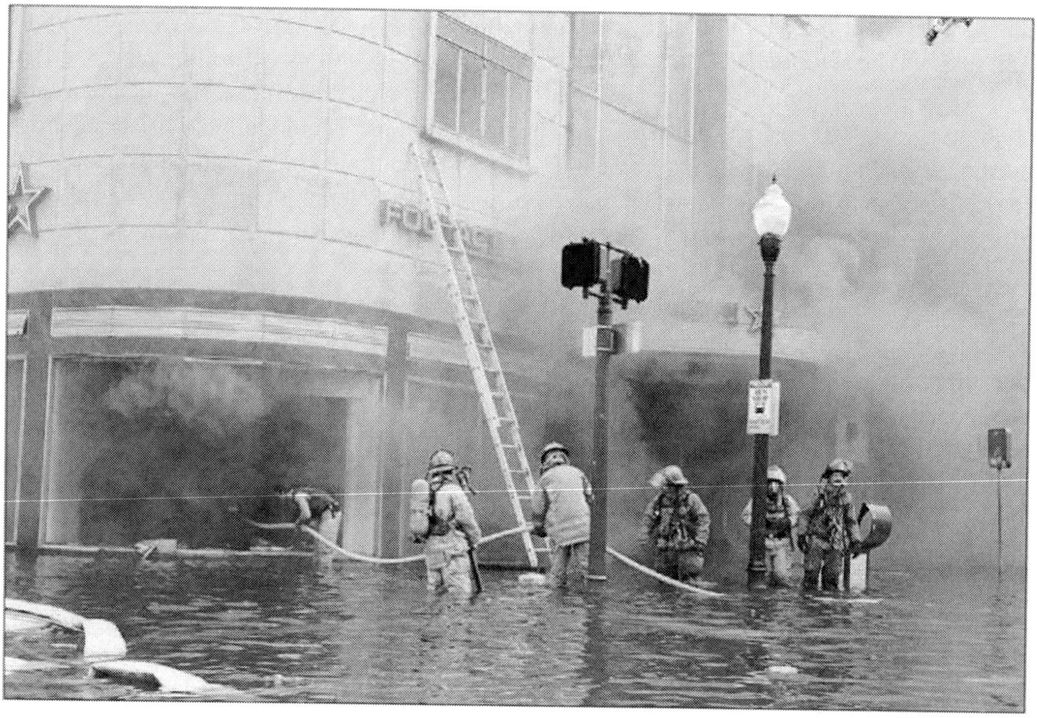

Figure 3.12. Courtesy of Chris Mickal, New Orleans Fire Department.

Table 3.4. Immersion Time limits at Different Water Temperatures and Immersion Depths

Water Temperature	Ankle-deep	Knee-deep	Waist-deep	Neck-deep
50 to 54 °F	7 hours; if raining, 3.5 hours	5 hours; if raining, 2.5 hours	1.5 hours; if raining, 1 hour	5 minutes
55 to 59 °F	8 hours; if raining, 4 hours	7 hours; if raining, 3.5 hours	2 hours; if raining, 1.5 hours	5 minutes
60 to 64 °F	9 hours; if raining, 4.5 hours	8 hours; if raining, 4 hours	3.5 hours; if raining, 2.5 hours	10 minutes
65 to 69 °F	12 hours; if raining, 6 hours	12 hours; if raining, 6 hours	6 hours; if raining, 5 hours	10 minutes
>70 °F	No limit	No limit	No limit	30 minutes

Certainly, the most effective way for ensuring firefighters do not fall victim to hypothermia is to minimize the amount of time that they are exposed to the cold conditions. Firefighters should be rotated from operational positions to rehab areas that allow them to rewarm and dry off. The amount of time required to do this will depend on the conditions. More detailed information on rotating personnel and the appropriate locations to rewarm them will be detailed in Chapters 4 and 5 of this document.

In summary, firefighters need to remember the acronym, COLD, for operating in cold weather and avoiding hypothermia:

- Keep it Clean—The dirtier clothing is, the less it will protect against cold weather.
- Avoid Overheating—Firefighters who overheat and sweat excessively ultimately will be more susceptible to hypothermia.
- Wear it Loose and in Layers—Air insulation between the layers of clothing is the most effective insulation. It also allows for adjusting the amount of clothing if conditions warrant it.
- Keep it Dry—Water causes cooling 25 times faster than dry air. Replace wet clothing when extended operations are required in cold weather.

Avoiding Frostbite

Frostbite injuries are far more likely to affect firefighters than generalized hypothermia for fire departments that operate in cold weather conditions. Inadequate planning or training and lack of experience contribute to a higher probability of frostbite injuries. However, frostbite can be avoided by simple, yet effective, countermeasures.

ICs and officers should follow a systematic risk assessment of weather conditions before settling on specific cold weather operations. The goal should be to identify potential hazards and plan accordingly. At high cold-injury risk levels, the likelihood of cold weather injury may outweigh the benefit of certain means to carry out the required emergency scene functions. While some acclimatization to cold weather conditions is beneficial, it does not significantly increase the firefighter's ability to avoid frostbite. It merely provides him/ her the information he/she needs to avoid such injuries or recognize them in their early stages.

The only way to determine the relative risk of frostbite is to monitor the air temperature and wind speed. Air temperature is the most important determinant for the risk of frostbite. As the air temperature falls below freezing, the risk of frostbite increases. However, wind speed also has a role. Wind increases convective heat loss by disturbing the boundary layer of air that rests against the skin and causes the skin to cool at a faster rate than if no wind was present. However, wind cannot cool skin, or any tissue, below the ambient air temperature. Therefore, frostbite cannot occur if the air temperature is above 32 °F.

Physical activity is an effective countermeasure for increasing skin temperature when wind is not present; however, when exposed to wind, physical activity does not alter the temperature of exposed or covered skin. For example, at 14 °F with no wind, moderate activity can increase finger temperature from 63 to 80 °F. However, the addition of an 11 - mph wind reduces finger temperatures below 59 °F, a critical temperature where decreases in manual dexterity begin to appear.

ICs and officers must evaluate the relative risk of frostbite by using the wind chill Temperature (WCT) index **(Table 3.2).** WCT integrates wind speed and air temperature to provide an estimate of the cooling power of the environment. It standardizes the cooling power of the environment to an equivalent air temperature for calm conditions. **Table 3.3** gives the general guidance that is to be followed for the different time-to-frostbite risk zones in most personnel. **Table 3.4** provides frostbite risk zones based upon the period of time in which exposed cheek skin will freeze in more susceptible persons in the population, assuming they are using precautions (gloves, proper clothing). Cheek skin was chosen because this area of the body typically is not protected, and studies have observed that this area, along with the nose, is one of the coldest areas of the face. Wet skin exposed to the wind will cool even faster.

Table 3.5. Wind Chill Danger Zones in Susceptible Personnel

Wind Speed (mph)	**Air Temperature (°F)**											
	10	5	0	–5	–10	–15	–20	–25	–30	–35	–40	–45
5	>120	>120	>120	>120	31	22	17	14	12	11	9	8
10	>120	>120	>120	28	19	15	12	10	9	7	7	6
15	>120	>120	33	20	15	12	9	8	7	6	5	4
20	>120	>120	23	16	12	9	8	8	6	5	4	4
25	>120	42	19	13	10	8	7	6	5	4	4	3
30	>120	28	16	12	9	7	6	5	4	4	3	3
35	>120	23	14	10	8	6	5	4	4	3	3	2
40	>120	20	13	9	7	6	5	4	3	3	2	2
45	>120	18	12	8	7	5	4	4	3	3	2	2
50	>120	16	11	8	6	5	4	3	3	2	2	2

Note: Wet skin could significantly decrease the time for frostbite to occur.
White—Low risk, freezing is possible, but unlikely.
Light Gold—High risk, freezing could occur in 10 to 30 minutes.
Dark Gold—Severe risk, freezing could occur in 5 to 10 minutes.
Medium Gold—Extreme risk, freezing could occur in less than 5 minutes.

The following frostbite preventive measures can be taken depending on the risk level present at the emergency scene:

Low-Risk Level

- encourage members to check on each other;
- wear appropriate clothing and wind protection (true for all risk levels);
- cover exposed flesh, if possible; and
- avoid sweating.

High-Risk Level

- require members to check on each other every 20 to 30 minutes;
- always work in groups of at least two, regardless of the circumstances;
- require exposed skin to be covered;
- provide warm shelter for rehab operations; and
- stay active, but avoid sweating.

Severe-Risk level

- Same as high-risk level, except require members to check on each other every 10 minutes.

Extreme-Risk level

- may consider modifying tactical operations based on conditions; and
- other requirements the same as severe-/high-risk levels.

While much of the above information was based on cheek skin temperatures, keep in mind that exposed fingers will freeze at a WCT that is about 10 °F warmer than the cheek freezing points.This is because there is less blood flow in the fingers compared to the face during cold exposure. Therefore, when the WCT is below -9 °F (-22.8 °C), there is an increased risk of finger frostbite and firefighters must take appropriate precautions, such as always wearing dry gloves and changing gloves when they become wet. The risk for frostbite is less at a WCT above -9 °F, but appropriate actions to reduce the risk must still be taken.

Low skin or body core temperatures increase susceptibility to peripheral frostbite because they reduce or abolish the firefighter's ability to recognize impending danger. When firefighters begin to feel numbness (occurs at a skin temperature around 45 °F (7.2 °C)), they need to increase their physical activity levels to raise their core temperature and increase blood flow to the extremities. As skin temperature falls below 45 °F, further cooling to freezing levels will not be perceived by the firefighter.

Fingers and other open skin areas can cool rapidly when touching cold materials, especially metal and liquids. Extreme caution must be taken if it is necessary to touch cold objects with bare hands at temperatures below freezing as contact frostbite can occur. Gloves always should be used to create a barrier between the hand and material, and can reduce performance decrements associated with hand cooling even at temperatures above freezing.

Cold injury surveillance (tracking, observation, and rehabbing) of firefighters is one of the most effective means to prevent frostbite. Firefighters that operate in cold conditions must be taught to check on their partners on a regular basis by looking for blanched skin on the fingers, ears, cheeks, nose, and toes. Members operating rehab areas also should be alert for these signs. Leaders also must ensure that firefighters are comfortable about reporting any potential problem and must understand that there will be no negative consequences from reporting. Many cold injuries occur because a firefighter is afraid to appear "weak" by mentioning to the chain of command that something is wrong (for example, fingers are numb). In such instances, a cold injury develops because appropriate preventive measures that could resolve the problem are not taken.

AVOIDING NONFREEZING COLD INJURIES

Firefighters are susceptible to a variety of nonfreezing injuries when working in cold conditions. Nonfreezing cold injuries occur most commonly when conditions are cold and wet (air temperatures between 32 and 55 °F), the hands and feet cannot be kept warm and dry, and firefighters are relatively immobile, which isn't all that common. The feet are the most common area of nonfreezing cold injuries. In the military this type of injury is referred to as trench foot. Operating for extended periods of time and in cramped conditions, such as during extended US&R operations, may lead to these types of injuries. If these areas are cold and damp, trench foot can become a serious problem, whether the dampness is caused by the environment or from sweat accumulation in the socks.

Prevention of trench foot can be achieved by encouraging firefighters to remain active and increase blood flow to the feet, rotating personnel out of cold-wet environments, and keeping feet dry by continually changing socks. Changing socks two to three times throughout the day is mandatory in cold-wet environments. Vapor barrier boots do not allow sweat from the foot to evaporate. Boots should be taken off after each incident (or at least daily on extended missions), wiped out, and allowed to dry.

When operating for extended periods of time in daylight snowy conditions, fire service personnel also should be alert for the possibility of snow blindness and/or sunburn. Snow blindness and sunburn are caused by exposure of unprotected eyes and skin to ultraviolet (UV) radiation. The threat of snow blindness and sunburn depends on the intensity of sunlight, not the air temperature. Snow, ice, and lightly colored objects reflect the sun's rays, increasing the risk for injury.

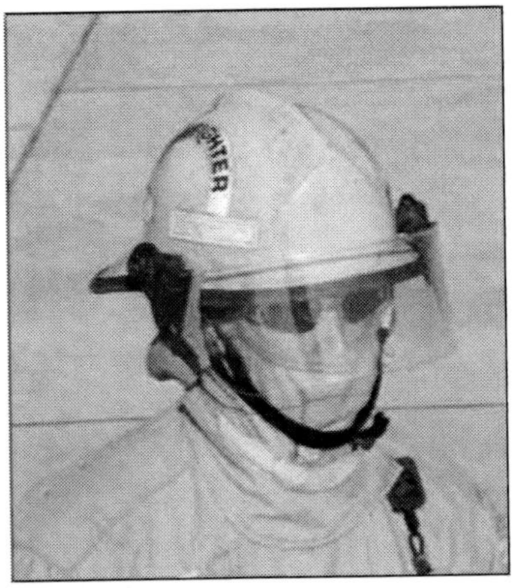

Figure 3.13. Courtesy of IFSTA/Fire Protection Publications.

Snow blindness results when solar radiation "sunburns" unprotected eyes. Eyes may feel painful, gritty, and there may be tearing, blurred vision, and headache. The use of protective eyewear or goggles that block more than 90 percent of UV radiation will help to prevent snow blindness (**Figure 3.13**).

Sunburn to exposed skin increases heat loss during cold exposure, increasing susceptibility to hypothermia. It also leads to uncomfortable/painful feelings that decrease firefighter performance. Sunburn can be prevented by using a sunscreen that contains at least a 15 sun protection factor (SPF). For cold weather, an alcohol-free sunscreen lotion that blocks both ultraviolet A and ultraviolet B rays is most desirable.

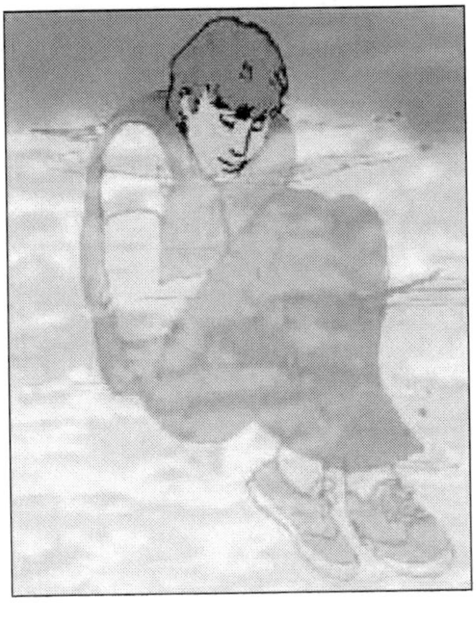

Figure 3.14.

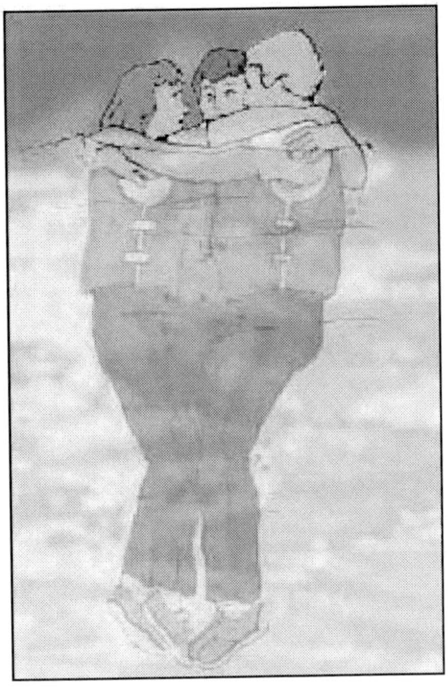

Figure 3.15.

Special Precautions for Cold Water Immersion Situations

On rare occasions, firefighters may find themselves accidentally cast into standing cold water. In some of these cases they will not be able to self-rescue and will need to assume as safe as possible in a position before being reached by rescuers. U.S. Coast Guard research has shown that swimming, treading water and drown-proofing are not effective in prolonging survival in cold water. This research suggests that firefighters who are wearing flotation devices should instead use the Heat Escape Lessening Position (H.E.L.P.) and the Huddle Position **(Figures 3.14 and 3.15)** when exposed to cold water. The object of these techniques is to keep the head and neck out of the water and lessen heat loss from the upper and lower torso. U.S. Navy research suggests that rescue divers who are exposed to more than one cold water dive per shift, even when apparently rewarmed, may be in danger of developing circulatory collapse with resultant death due to hypothermia upon subsequent exposure. Thus, firefighters who must dive into cold water during rescue operations should make sure that extra manpower is available when extended operations occur.

In: Rehab, Protection and Safety Measures or Firefighters … ISBN: 978-1-60741-566-4
Editor: Andreo Rios

Chapter 4

ESTABLISHING AND OPERATING A REHAB AREA

Ensuring that firefighters are in good physical condition, properly hydrated, and well-fed prior to responding to an incident are important in helping to ensure their safety during operations. However, even physically fit firefighters can suffer the consequences of overexertion and exposure to harsh environmental conditions during the course of emergency operations and extended physical/practical training activities. Most of the illnesses and injuries discussed to this point in the document can be avoided by establishing and operating a proper emergency incident rehabilitation, or rehab, area.

This chapter will provide detailed information on establishing and equipping a rehab area. The chapter begins by highlighting how to determine when it is necessary to establish rehab operations at an incident or training activity. It is important that rehab operations operate under the umbrella of the Incident Command System (ICS) structure being used at the scene, so suggestions on how to do that are covered also. The latter portions of the chapter discuss selecting, organizing, and equipping rehab operations for duty.

CRITERIA FOR ESTABLISHING REHAB OPERATIONS

One important fact must be realized before getting too far into the discussion on criteria for when rehab operations should be established at an incident. Unlike so many other areas of the fire service that are highly regulated by codes and standards, there is no law or standard that sets out specific criteria for when to establish rehab operations. The closest to any requirement in the code world can be found in National Fire Protection Association (NFPA) 1584, *Recommended Practice on the Rehabilitation of Members Operating at Incident Scene Operations and Training Exercises* (2003 ed.). Objective 4.2.4 of that document states that "procedures should be in place to ensure that rehab operations commence whenever emergency operations pose the risk of pushing personnel beyond a safe level of physical or mental endurance." Little concrete direction can be derived from that statement and much is left to the judgment of incident command personnel.

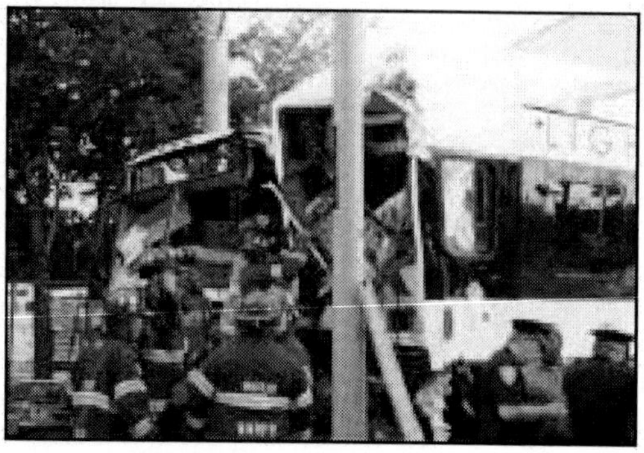

Figure 4.1. Courtesy of Chris Mickal, New Orleans Fire Department.

The truth of the matter is that determining when to establish rehab operations at an incident remains more of an art than it is a science. Many fire departments place specific benchmarks in their Standard Operating Procedures (SOPs) identifying when a rehab area should be established. However, even these benchmarks may require adjustments depending on conditions. For example, suppose a fire department's SOPs state that a formal rehab area will be established when an incident goes to a second alarm. Depending on the incident and the conditions, the Incident Commander (IC) may rightfully need to deviate from this I policy in certain situations. A one-alarm fire on an extremely hot and humid day might necessitate the establishment of a formal rehab operation at this smaller incident. One the other hand, a second alarm response to a multicasualty motor vehicle collision with entrapment may not require rehab operations at all (**Figure 4.1**).

In reality, regardless of departmental SOPs, the IC must consider a variety of factors when determining the need to establish rehab operations. These factors, when considered as a whole, will make the need for a rehab operation apparent. One fact is clear: ICs should not play "catch-up" when deciding the need for a rehab area. That is, do not wait for people to starting dropping over from exhaustion before putting rehab operations in motion. At this point you are acting too late. Rather, the establishment of rehab should be a routine, proactive measure to prevent personnel from getting to the point of injury or illness at an incident.

The IC will use a variety of information sources, combined with their personal experience, departmental SOPs, and a little old-fashioned common sense in determining the need for rehab operations at an incident. The incident factors that enter into this decision basically boil down to two general considerations: the type of incident and the climatic conditions during the incident.These considerations, combined with feedback from personnel operating at the scene, will aid the IC in determining when rehab is needed. The section below provides a little more insight into the factors influencing the need for rehab at common types of incidents and in various weather conditions.

Structure Fires

Municipal fire departments most commonly equate the need for incident rehab operations with structural firefighting operations (Figure 4.2). For the purpose of this section we are referring to structural firefighting using the historical definition provided by the NFPA, which is "the activities of rescue, fire suppression, and property conservation involving buildings, enclosed structures, vehicles, vessels, aircraft, or like properties that are involved in a fire or emergency situation."

As alluded to previously, some fire departments set criteria for establishing rehab operations in their SOPs based on the size of the incident, the number of resources assigned to the incident, and/or other conditions, such as the weather at the time of the incident. These SOPs, combined with the IC's judgment, as used to decide when a rehab area will be established.

NFPA 1584 does not provide a hard and fast benchmark on when rehab operations should be established at these types of incidents. It does however give some direction on when firefighters operating at these incidents should enter rehab. Using this information the IC can make sure that a rehab area is set up when firefighters meet the criteria for seeking rehab services. NFPA 1584 provides the following two guidelines for company or crew rehabilitation in terms of work-to-rest ratio and/or self-contained breathing apparatus (SCBA) usage:

Guideline # 1: The company or crew must self-rehab (rest with hydration) for at least 10 minutes following the depletion of one 30-minute SCBA cylinder or after 20 minutes of intense work without wearing an SCBA. The Company Officer (CO) or crew leader must ensure that all assigned members are fit to return to duty before resuming operations.

Guideline #2: The company or crew must enter a formal rehab area, drink appropriate fluids, be medically evaluated, and rest for a minimum of 20 minutes after any of the following:

- depletion of two 30-minute SCBA cylinders;
- depletion of one 45- or 60-minute SCBA cylinder;
- whenever encapsulating chemical protective clothing is worn; and
- following 40 minutes of intense work without an SCBA.

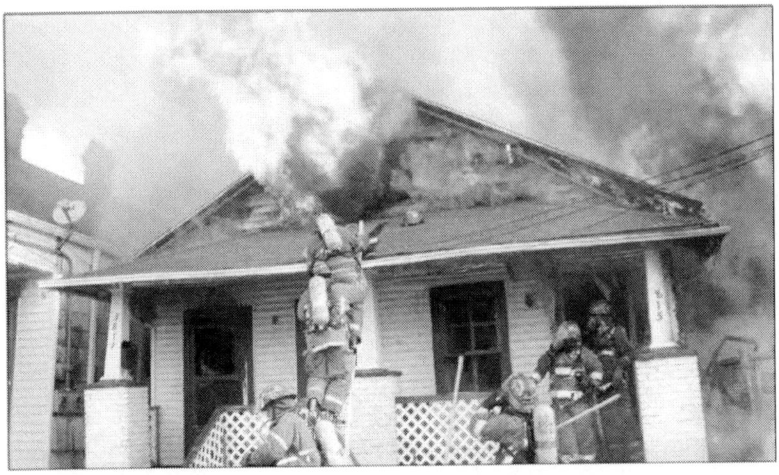

Figure 4.2. Courtesy of Chris Mickal, New Orleans Fire Department.

Let's look at these requirements in the context of a "typical" fire department response to a working structure fire. In this scenario the fire department uses standard 30-minute SCBA cylinders.

- Following an initial fire attack, the hose team is forced to leave the hazard area because the low air- pressure alarm in one of the members' SCBA is sounding. The team reports back to their vehicle or a ser vice vehicle to replace SCBA cylinders, drink some water or other appropriate fluid, and rest for at least 10 minutes. Once the CO is certain that all members are ready to resume operation, he or she advises the IC that the team is ready for another assignment.
- The team receives another assignment and continues operations until one of the members' low air- pressure alarm sounds again.
- The team retreats from the hazard area the second time and this time reports to the rehab area that has been established.
- At the rehab area, all members must undergo a medical evaluation, receive fluid replenishment, and rest for at least 20 minutes before being allowed to return to service again.

According to NFPA 1584, if members enter the rehab area prior to going through two 30-minute SCBA cylinders (or any other of the criteria listed above in Guideline #2) they still must be medically evaluated and drink fluids. However, their rest period may be lowered to only 10 minutes before they are allowed to return to duty, if they are fit to do so.

When looking at the requirements and the scenario described above, one should note that the NFPA requirements predominantly focus on changing SCBAs as a benchmark for rehab needs. The reason for this is because it is much easier to track SCBA changes than it is to keep track of time during the course of an incident. The NFPA requirements do require time-tracking when SCBAs are not in use, but in the vast majority of cases it will be the SCBA usage that guides rehabbing of individual firefighters. Given that realization, the IC is provided with some insight into the need for establishing rehab operations at standard structural fire operations. If it will be a relatively quickly handled incident where members will only require one SCBA during the course of the incident, a formal rehab area may not be required. This is, of course, assuming that suitable beverages are available. If it appears that more than one SCBA cylinder will be required of members or they will be engaged in more than 20 minutes of very hard work without an SCBA, early preparations for establishing a rehab area should be made.

There are a couple of special considerations that ICs must keep in mind relative to this issue. First, even though the fire may be knocked down quickly, in some cases extensive overhaul may be required. Oftentimes the work is harder during overhaul than during the fire attack. Long overhaul operations may require a rehab area to be set up on what was otherwise an insignificant fire.

Secondly, the IC may be able to adjust the size of the rehab operation accordingly based on the changing size of the incident. The rehab area must be capable of accommodating all of the firefighters operating at the incident. However, as the incident winds down, the number of firefighters remaining at the incident typically decreases accordingly. In these cases the scope of the rehab operation may be adjusted down as well. The IC just needs to make sure that the remaining resources in the rehab unit are still capable of performing all the required duties.

Procedures for scaling down and terminating rehab operations are detailed in Chapter 6 of this document.

Highrise Building Fires

Fires in highrise buildings, typically defined as buildings that exceed 75 feet in height, present additional challenges above and beyond those presented in other structural firefighting situations (**Figure 4.3**). While high-rise structures pose many of the same hazards to firefighters as low-rise structures, there are two additional challenges with fires in highrises that determine the need for rehab operations at these incidents.

The first challenge is the large amount of energy firefighters must expend simply to reach the location of the fire. Safety concerns may not permit firefighters to take elevators to the fire floor or even a floor close to it. This means that fully bunked-out firefighters must carry all the firefighting equipment they need to the fire. In extremely tall structures the firefighters may require rehab before they even reach the fire floor and begin operations.

Many fire departments use a rule-of-thumb that it will require three companies to perform every task in a highrise fire that would require one company in a low-rise fire. This is due to the tremendous amount of energy expended simply reaching the work area. For example, if we wish to place a single handline in service in a one-story building, one company will be required to perform the task. The same task in a highrise will require three companies being used as follows:

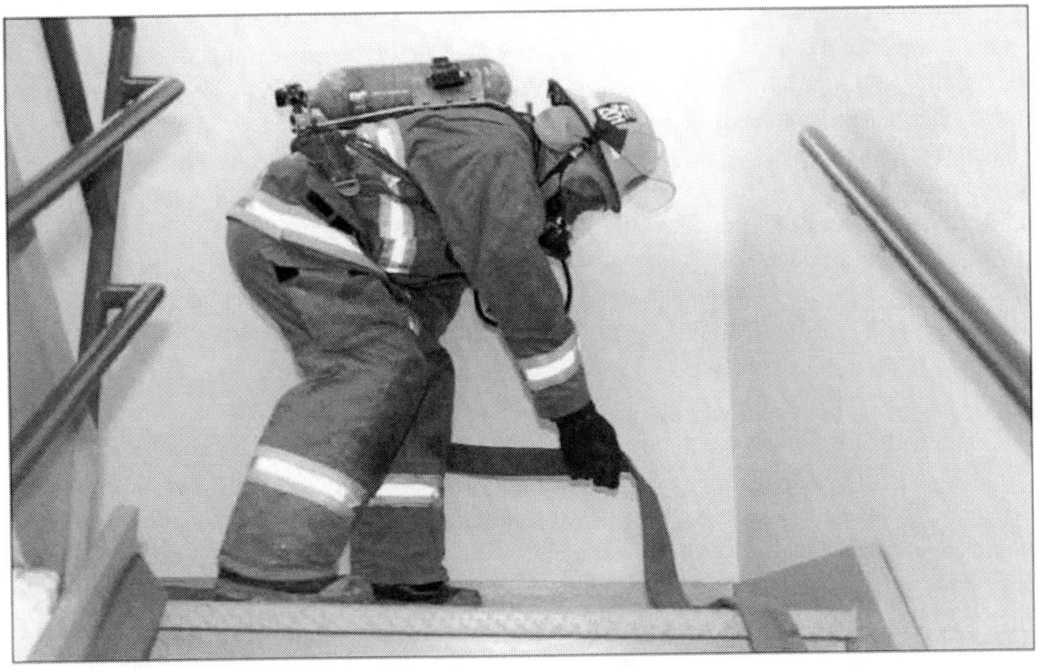

Figure 4.3. Courtesy of Rick Montemorra, Mesa, AZ Fire Department.

- Company 1 will operate the handline in the fire area.
- Company 2 will be on standby outside the door leading to the fire floor where the handline is being operated.
- Company 3 will be at the Staging Area that typically is located two floors below the fire floor. This company will be resting, replacing SCBA cylinders, and preparing to move up into the standby position.

Thus, this high expenditure of energy coupled with the large number of personnel operating on the scene will place both importance and strain on incident rehab operations. Details of how to compensate for this strain are discussed later in this chapter.

The second challenge posed by highrise fire operations is the fact that once the location of the fire is reached, firefighters often will face extreme high-temperature conditions because the difficulty often encountered in effectively ventilating these structures during fire incidents. This will place additional wear and tear on the firefighters that is often above what they would encounter in a properly-vented, low-rise building fire.

Formal rehab area operations must be established any time a working fire is being attacked in a highrise structure. The rehab area should be setup as soon as possible as a large number of fatigued firefighters will add up early in the incident. Most departments that frequently encounter highrise fires use a tiered rehab system on these incidents. In a tiered rehab operation some basic rehab functions are performed at a forward location in the fire building near the fire floor, while other, more extensive rehab is being performed at a location farther from the fire.

One source of confusion that seems to be more prevalent at highrise fires than other types of fires is the difference between Staging Areas and rehab areas. Companies that are in the Staging Area are assumed to be ready for duty and simply awaiting an assignment. Minor rehab functions, such as fluid replenishment and basic medical monitoring may be performed in Staging, but the companies should be ready to deploy when needed. Companies that are assigned to the formal rehab area are out-of-service and not ready for an immediate assignment. They should not be relocated to the Staging Area or given another assignment until they have been rehydrated, rested the appropriate amount of time, and have otherwise been deemed fit for duty.

Wildland Fires

Wildland fires, which are fires that involve natural-cover fuels such as grasses, weeds, crops, shrubs, and trees, range widely in size and pose a variety of challenges to firefighters depending on the size and circumstances of the fire **(Figure 4.4)** .These fires may range in size from just a few square yards to over a half-million acres. They may be in relatively easily accessible agricultural lands or in virtually inaccessible natural terrain. Extinguishing these fires may take only a few minutes or the fights can last for weeks on end. Organizations that handle these fires must have plans to rehab personnel at significant wildland fires that are compatible with the scope and length of the operation they are faced with.

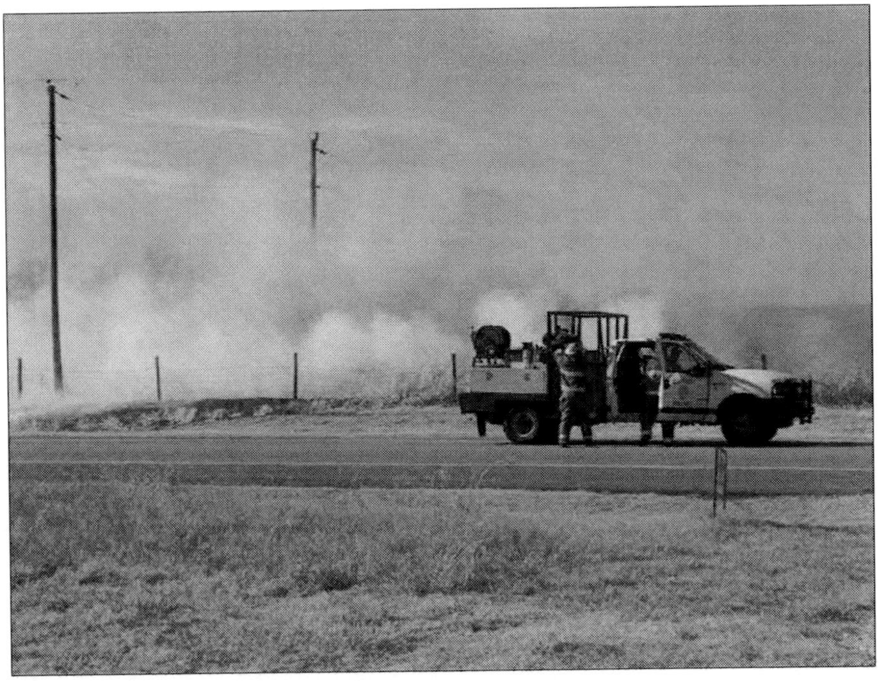

Figure 4.4.

When dealing with relatively small wildland fires that can be handled during the course of a single day, rehab operations and requirements for individual firefighters can be addressed in much the same manner as those described above for structure fires. A rehab area of an appropriate size to handle the number of personnel who will need it should be established. Personnel typically will be rotated into the rehab area based on the difficultly of the work they have been performing and the time they have been at it. The amount of time a firefighter can operate on these fires will vary depending on the nature of the tasks they are performing and the weather conditions of the incident. Firefighters who are performing heavy manual labor, such as hand cutting fire lines and who are operating in warmer weather conditions will require shorter work times and more frequent rehabbing. Firefighters who are operating in more temperate conditions or who are doing simpler tasks, such as operating a nozzle while riding an apparatus that is performing a pump and roll attack, will be able to operate for greater periods of time between breaks and rehab.

Firefighters who operate at large-scale at wildland fires typically work 12- to 24-hour shifts on the fire line. Firefighters may have to walk long distances over rugged or hilly terrain simply to reach the fire/work area. As in highrise firefighting, they may be tired and in need of rest and rehab before they even begin the actual fire attack. Once they reach the work area, they may be exposed to high atmospheric temperatures, high humidity, and sometimes high elevations. High elevations have less oxygen available for breathing (as well as combustion) and cause firefighters to tire more rapidly.

It should be noted that formalized, long-term, wildland firefighting operations typically involve State and Federal response agencies that use the ICS in a fairly rigid manner. As will be detailed later in this chapter, the term "rehab" is not a term that typically is used within ICS in the same way it is by structural firefighters. In ICS, rehabbing firefighters is a function of the Medical Unit within the Logistics Section of ICS. Wildland personnel typically use the term "rehab" to describe the process of reforesting and improving the land following devastation by fire. Responders who are not used to operating within the wildland fire arena need to be aware of this difference in terminology.

Major wildland firefighting operations may require multiple rehab areas scattered around the incident. These areas must be capable of providing resting firefighters with protection from the elements, fluids for drinking, and medical evaluation, at a minimum. Firefighters working distant from the rehab areas need to practice self-preservation techniques. This includes monitoring their own and their crew members' conditions, taking short breaks from time to time, and keeping hydrated. NFPA 1500, *Standard on Fire Department Occupational Safety and Health Program* requires wildland firefighters to be provided with 2 liters or quarts of water and for a system to replenish this water to be in place at all incidents. NFPA 1584 states that responders should be limited to 12-hour shifts on the emergency scene followed by a multihour break before they are allowed to return to service.

In summary, ICs should consider the following when determining the need to establish rehab operations at a wildfire event:

- Estimate the size of the fire and the amount of time that will be needed to extinguish it completely. As specified in NFPA 1584, the IC must establish a rehab operation when the fire will involve heavy manual labor for more than 40 minutes.
- Consider the weather conditions at the time of the fire. The hotter and more humid the weather is, the greater the need for early rehab operations.
- Know the elevation above sea level at which the fire is located. Fires that occur at high altitudes are more demanding on firefighters.
- How the fire will be attacked is important. The heavier the manual labor that will be performed, the greater the need for rehab operations.

Hazardous Materials Incidents

Because of the unknown and/or threatening nature of the products involved in a hazardous materials (hazmat) incident, personnel working in proximity to the hazardous materials must wear special chemical protective equipment in order to prevent falling victim. The process of donning this equipment and then performing incident-required tasks while wearing it is labor-intensive and stress-producing on the wearer. In order to meet the guidelines established in NFPA 1584, rehab operations should be established on every incident where the donning of chemical protective equipment will be required. Wearers of the equipment should be decontaminated properly after leaving the incident hot zone and then remove the equipment before reporting to the rehab area **(Figure 4.5)** .The rehab area must be ready to go by the time the first entry personnel have been deconned and have removed their equipment. The rehab area itself should be located upwind from the incident and in the cold zone.

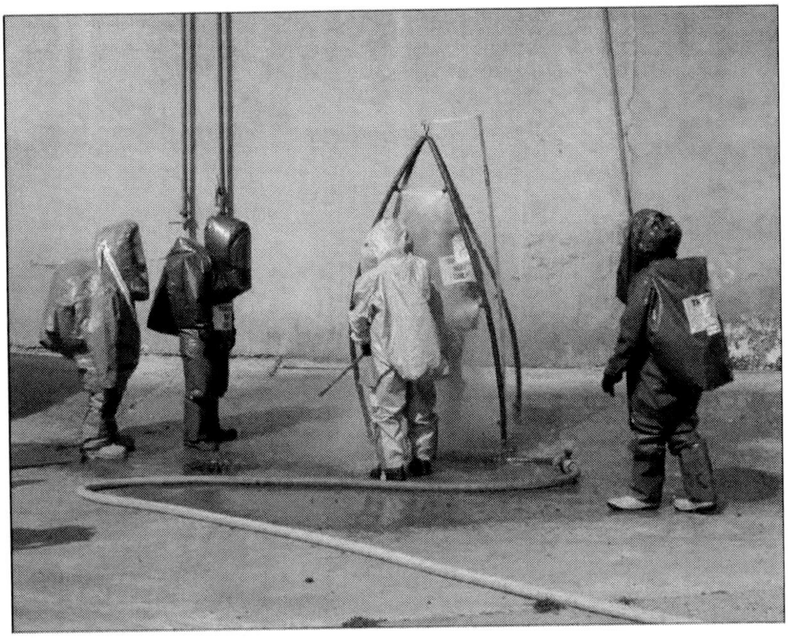

Figure 4.5. Courtesy of IFSTA/Fire Protection Publications.

Hazmat incidents that do not require the special protective clothing, such as an overturned, leaking gasoline tanker, still may require firefighters to wear standard personal protective equipment (PPE) for extended periods. Rehab areas should be set up on these incidents so that the guidelines for work-to-rest ratios outlined in NFPA 1584 can be followed also.

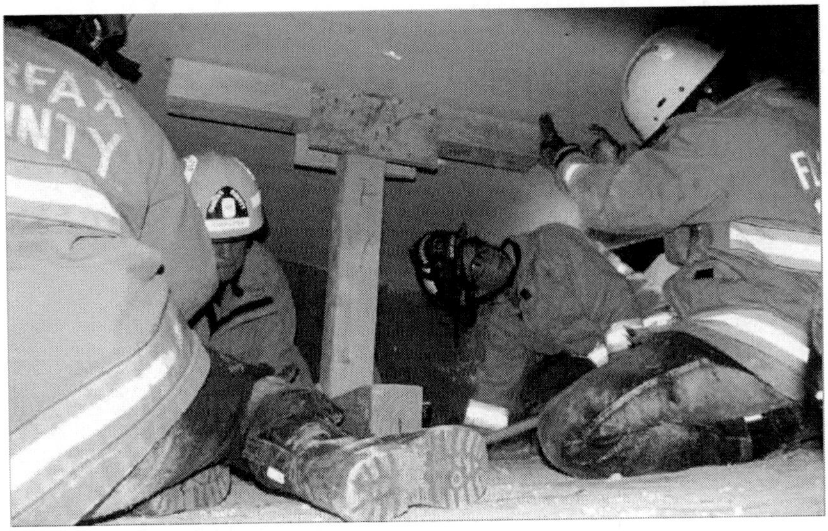

Figure 4.6. Courtesy of IFSTA/Fire Protection Publications.

Urban Search and Rescue Incidents

Urban search and rescue (US&R) incidents can range from small localized incidents, such as a trench cave-in rescue, to wide-scale, long-term incidents like the response to a major earthquake or hurricane (**Figure 4.6**). The need for rehab operations and the manner in which those services will be provided is very much analogous to that described above for wildland fire incidents. Localized incidents that will only last from a few hours to a day or so will be rather simple to provide rehab services for. Large-scale incidents that spread over a vast area will be more challenging and will require more self-observation of personnel who are working together for extended periods of time. In general, follow the guidelines described above in the wildland fire incident section.

Warm Weather Criteria

Regardless of the type of incident, warm weather will greatly affect the need for rehab operations. Simply, the warmer and more humid the weather, the greater the level of stress it will impart on personnel operating on the scene. This was described in detail in Chapter 2 of this book. To review, the amount of heat stress that firefighters are exposed to is actually a combination of three important elements:

- ambient temperature;
- relative humidity; and
- direct sunlight.

Ambient air temperature and relative humidity can be factored together to create what is often referred to as the heat stress index, heat index, or humiture. In arid climates the thermal impact on the body might actually be slightly less than that of the ambient temperature. For example, note on **Table 4.1** that when the ambient temperature is 94 °F and the relative humidity is 10 percent, the heat stress index is 89 °F (31.7 °C). More common is the effect of this combination in humid environments. In these cases the impact on the body will exceed that of the ambient temperature alone. For example, again referring to Table 4.1, when the ambient temperature is 94 °F as above, but the relative humidity is 60 percent, the heat stress index is 111 °F (43.9 °C).

To determine the total thermal stress on firefighters, two factors in addition to the heat stress index may be required. First, keep in mind that the sun shining on the surfaces of objects produces radiated heat. If the firefighters are working in direct sunlight, factor in an additional 10 °F to the heat stress index reading. If the firefighters are wearing heavy protective clothing, add an additional 10 °F to the heat stress index. Thus, if the firefighters were working in 94 °F heat with 60-percent humidity and they were wearing full turnout gear in the sunlight, the total thermal impact on their bodies would be a very dangerous 13 1 °F (55°C). **Table 4.2** provides some guidelines on danger levels relative to various thermal stresses on firefighters.

Table 4.1. Heat Stress Index

				Relative Humidity					
Temperature °F	**10 percent**	**20 percent**	**30 percent**	**40 percent**	**50 percent**	**60 percent**	**70 percent**	**80 percent**	**90 percent**
104	98	104	110	120	132				
102	97	101	108	117	125				
100	95	99	105	110	120	132			
98	93	97	101	106	110	125			
96	91	95	98	104	108	120	128		
94	89	93	95	100	105	111	122		
92	87	90	92	96	100	106	115	122	
90	85	88	90	92	96	100	106	114	122
88	82	86	87	89	93	95	100	106	115
86	80	84	85	87	90	92	96	100	109
84	78	81	83	85	86	89	91	95	99
82	77	79	80	81	84	86	89	91	95
80	75	77	78	79	81	83	85	86	89
78	72	75	77	78	79	80	81	83	85
76	70	72	75	76	77	77	77	78	79
74	68	70	73	74	75	75	75	76	77

Note: Add 10 °F when protective clothing is worn and add 10 °F when in direct sunlight.

NFPA 1584 does not provide any specific benchmark temperatures at which rehab operations should be established. In a previous publication on rehab released by the U.S. Fire Administration (USFA) (FA-114), they recommended that rehab operations be initiated whenever the heat stress index exceeds 90 °F.

Table 4.2. Injuries Associated with Heat Stress Index Conditions

Humiture,°F	**Danger Category**	**Injury Threat**
Below 60	None	Little or no danger under normal circumstances
80 to 90	Caution	Fatigue possible if exposure is prolonged and there is physical activity
90 to 105	Extreme caution	Heat cramps and heat exhaustion possible if exposure is prolonged and there is physical activity
105 to 130	Danger	Heat cramps and heat exhaustion likely and heat stroke possible if exposure is prolonged and there is physical activity
Above 130	Extreme danger	Heat stroke imminent

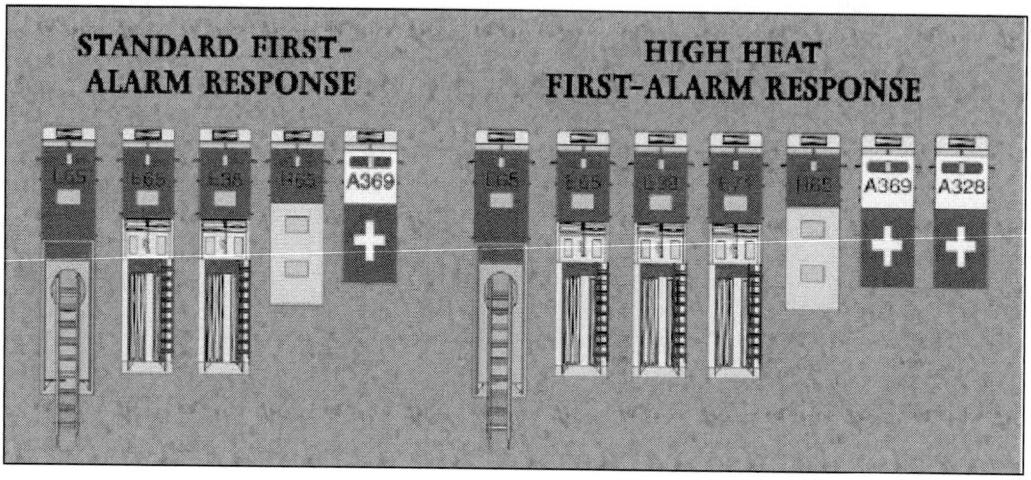

Figure 4.7.

Each fire department needs to establish high temperature benchmarks for initiating rehab operations based on their experience and what their firefighters are acclimated to. Departments in regions of the country that experience frequent hot weather conditions may have a higher heat threshold than those areas were high temperatures are less frequent. For example, an 85 °F day in Maine may require additional rehab operations to be considered, when the same 85 °F day in southern Arizona would not be considered a serious concern.

There are additional actions that some fire departments choose to implement during heat conditions that exceed the predetermined benchmark for their department. These actions typically involve increasing resources assigned to an incident to compensate for personnel tiring faster due to the heat. The following are some examples of these measures:

- Automatically dispatch specialized rehab equipment that would otherwise only respond via special call by the Incident Commander (IC).
- Dispatch one or more extra engine or truck companies on first-alarm assignments **(Figure 4.7).**
- Dispatch additional ambulances or emergency medical services (EMS) responder units to all working incidents.
- Require firefighters to report to rehab after expending one 30-minute SCBA cylinder rather than two cylinders.

Refer back to Chapter 2 of this book for additional information on high heat stress conditions.

Cold Weather Criteria

While most people automatically equate the need for rehab operations with warm, humid weather, fire departments that operate in cold weather climates also must develop plans to rehab personnel who are working in the cold **(Figure 4.8).** While personal protective clothing will offer a significant level of protection against cold weather, it does not make firefighters immune from the effects of cold. Firefighters who are sweating heavily underneath their gear or who become wet during the performance of their duties will have an increased chance of cold injury Because many operations require firefighters to work outside for extended periods of time, localized cold injuries to exposed areas, such as the face and ears, may also result.

Another often overlooked factor in cold weather is the fact that the human body burns more calories when temperatures are cold than when they are warm. This is because extra energy is required to maintain the body's normal core temperature in colder temperatures. Thus, firefighters are likely to become hungry faster in cold weather than in warm weather.

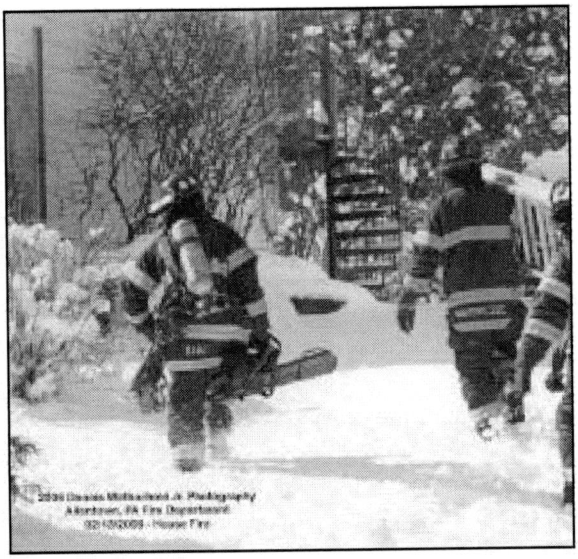

Figure 4.8.

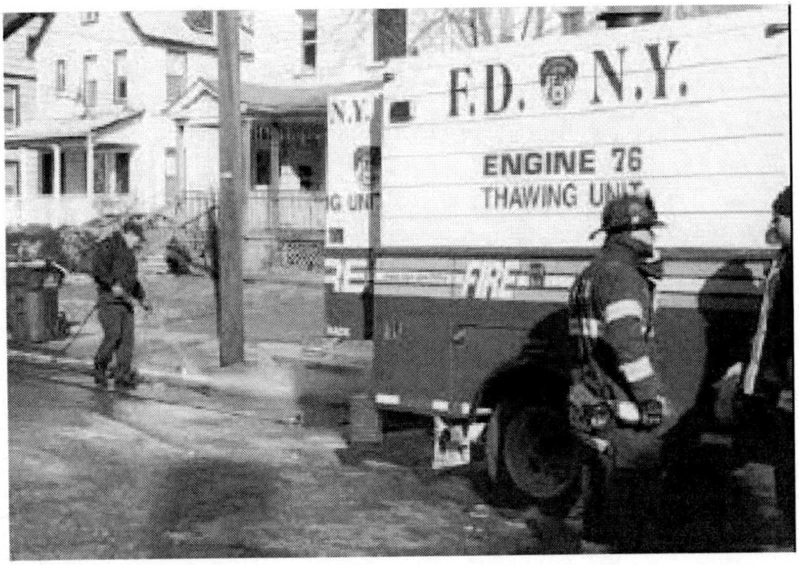

Figure 4.9. Courtesy of Ron Jeffers, Union City, NJ.

Just as described above for hot weather conditions, there are no standards-driven benchmarks at which rehab operations should be established for cold weather operations. In most cases it will be necessary for individual fire departments to determine at what wind chill index level rehab operations should be initiated or expanded.This determination is based on the normal weather conditions in the jurisdiction and the level of experience personnel have with cold-weather operations. The only documented recommendations that have been released previously were in the previous USFA report (FA-114) on emergency incident rehab operations. That document recommended initiating rehab operations whenever the wind chill factor dropped to 10 °F or lower based on the Siple and Passel chart.

Some of the same tactical adjustments that were described for hot weather operations can be applied to cold weather scenarios also. This includes more frequent rotation of personnel and adding additional personnel or companies to responses. Keep in mind that postincident operations also can be complicated by extremely cold weather. Hoses, ladders, and other equipment may become frozen in place. This would require firefighters to expend considerable effort in freeing, retrieving, and stowing the equipment **(Figure 4.9).** This will increase the need for rehab services long after the incident is controlled.

Other Situations Requiring Rehab Operations

The section above highlighted the most common incident and weather-driven situations that impact the need for rehab operations at an incident. Certainly, the need for rehab services is not limited to the situations described above. There are a wide variety of other situations that could require rehabbing of personnel.

Fire department personnel often are called in to support law enforcement agencies during extended operations. This can include crime scene investigation, criminal standoff situations, civil unrest situations, and clandestine drug lab scenes to name a few. In these situations both the law enforcement and fire service personnel could be operating in stressful positions for extended periods of time. Fire departments should develop rehab plans for these types of incidents.

Fire departments are also called to assist in open area search operations. These incidents typically involve looking for disoriented young, old, or injured people who have wondered off and are in need of being found and assisted. In some cases these searches may involve finding otherwise healthy outdoor enthusiasts who have become lost in unfamiliar areas. These situations may require firefighters to perform long searches, sometimes over difficult terrain. This can be very tiring for the personnel involved in the search. Provisions must be made to give these personnel a break and meet their fluid and nutritional needs. In extremely large area searches, multiple rehab areas may be required.

The following are examples of other types of duties that may require firefighters to be deployed for extended periods of time. Fire departments who get involved in these types of situations should have commensurate rehab procedures in place to aid personnel who are working them. Because most of these events are known well in advance, there is no reason why fire departments should not have good rehab plans in place when these events take place:

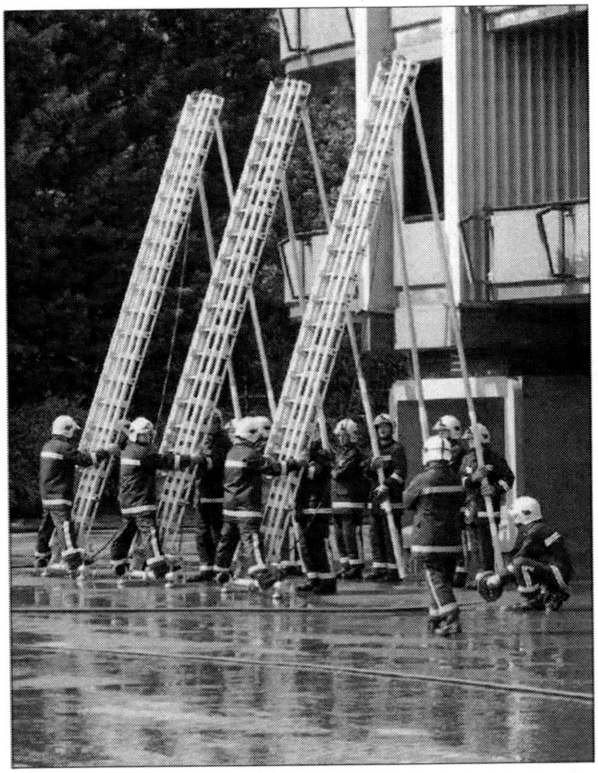

Figure 4.10.

- Fairs, carnivals, or other festivals;
- auto races;
- parades;
- concerts;
- major sporting events;
- political rallies or conventions; and
- large-scale religious ceremonies.

Lastly, fire department should not overlook the importance of good rehab operations during training exercises. Training exercises often involve strenuous work that continues for extended periods of time, often a full day **(Figure 4.10)**. Firefighters in recruit academies can work at these levels for multiple days on end. The same precautions taken for overexertion and responder fitness should be used at a training activity as they would be used at an emergency incident. All training classes or exercises should be designed so that rehab will be available to the participants for appropriate amounts of time at regular intervals.

Fire departments that train at a fixed training facility should have suitable areas for rehabbing personnel planned out and ready to go (**Figure 4.11**). When possible the rehab set-up and procedures used in training should mirror those that are used in the field.This will serve as a proper training on field rehab procedures and make the process more familiar and comfortable when faced with the same conditions at real-life incidents.

REHAB'S PLACE IN THE INCIDENT COMMAND SYSTEM

In order for any emergency incident, regardless of its size, to be handled in the utmost safe and efficient manner it is essential that an incident management system be used to organize and manage the responders assigned to the incident. All components of the incident operations must fit into the operational framework of the incident management system used for that incident.

Though some individual fire departments and regional agencies developed a localized incident management system dating back 100 years or more, it wasn't until the early 1970s that widespread use of model incident management systems began to be common around the U.S. In the early 1970s two different model incident management systems were developed and began widespread use throughout the U.S.The ICS was first developed by Fire Resources of California Organized for Potential Emergencies (FIRESCOPE), a consortium of local, State, and Federal agencies, that had been tasked with some of the first large-scale urban/wildland interface fires in southern California. Those agencies soon adapted that system for everyday use in standard fire department operations. ICS eventually was adopted for teaching the National Fire Academy (NFA) and became the standard system used anytime a Federal response to an incident was required. Many other jurisdictions around the U.S. also adopted ICS for their everyday operations.

At relatively the same time that ICS was being developed and growing in popularity, members of the Phoenix, Arizona Fire Department developed a somewhat different incident management system that they called the Fireground Command System (FGC). This system also gained wide popularity in departments throughout the U.S. through the publishing and teaching efforts of many of the Phoenix Fire Department members.

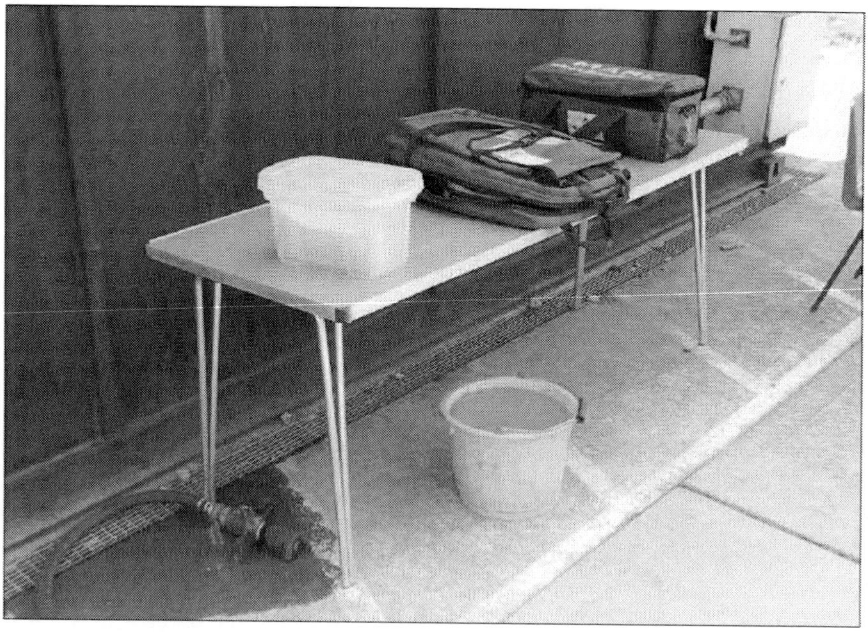

Figure 4.11.

Without going into detail, there were enough differences between these two systems that it caused problems when agencies used to either one of them were forced to work with agencies that used the other one at incidents. In the early 1990s the National Fire Service Incident Management System Consortium was formed by all of the involved organizations using or supporting both of these systems for the purpose of resolving these differences and merging them into one agreeable system. The resulting National Fire Service Incident Management System (IMS) was approved in 1994. Though FIRESCOPE, the Fireground Command folks, and the Federal response agencies all still kept their own identities, each of them adopted the recommendations of the IMS Consortium and a more uniform consistency was achieved.

In the flurry of homeland security activities following the terrorist attacks of September 11, 2001, President George W. Bush issued a number of Homeland Security Presidential Directives (HSPD) aimed at improving our nation's response to future terrorist incidents, as well as other nonterrorist, large-scale disasters. The two directives that most impacted incident management were HSPD-5 and HSPD-8. HSPD-5 identified steps for improved coordination in response to incidents. As part of that effort it mandates the development of a National Incident Management System (NIMS) for responding to emergencies. HSPD-8 described the way Federal departments and agencies would prepare for such a response, including prevention activities during the early stages of a terrorism incident.

Within the total NIMS documentation that was developed, was a mandated ICS system that was required to be used on all responses involving Federal entities. It was also strongly suggested that this system be used in all local responses. The components and design of the ICS system mandated in NIMS were virtually identical to the IMS system that emerged as a result of the National Fire Service Incident Management System Consortium's work to merge the original ICS and FGC. Only a few minor terminology changes and the addition of an Intelligence component separated the NIMS ICS from the system used previously. Though some jurisdictions have been resistant to change from the incident management systems they were using, it is strongly recommended that all U.S. response agencies adopt NIMS ICS as soon as practical.

Rehab's Position in a Fully-Expanded Incident Command System

Because the scope of this manual is limited to discussing emergency incident rehabilitation operations, this document will not provide an extensive overview of the ICS. In short, formal incident command must be established at every incident. Only those portions of the model ICS structure that are actually needed at an incident should be activated and staffed. The responsibilities for any portion of the ICS structure that are not activated remain the responsibility of the IC.

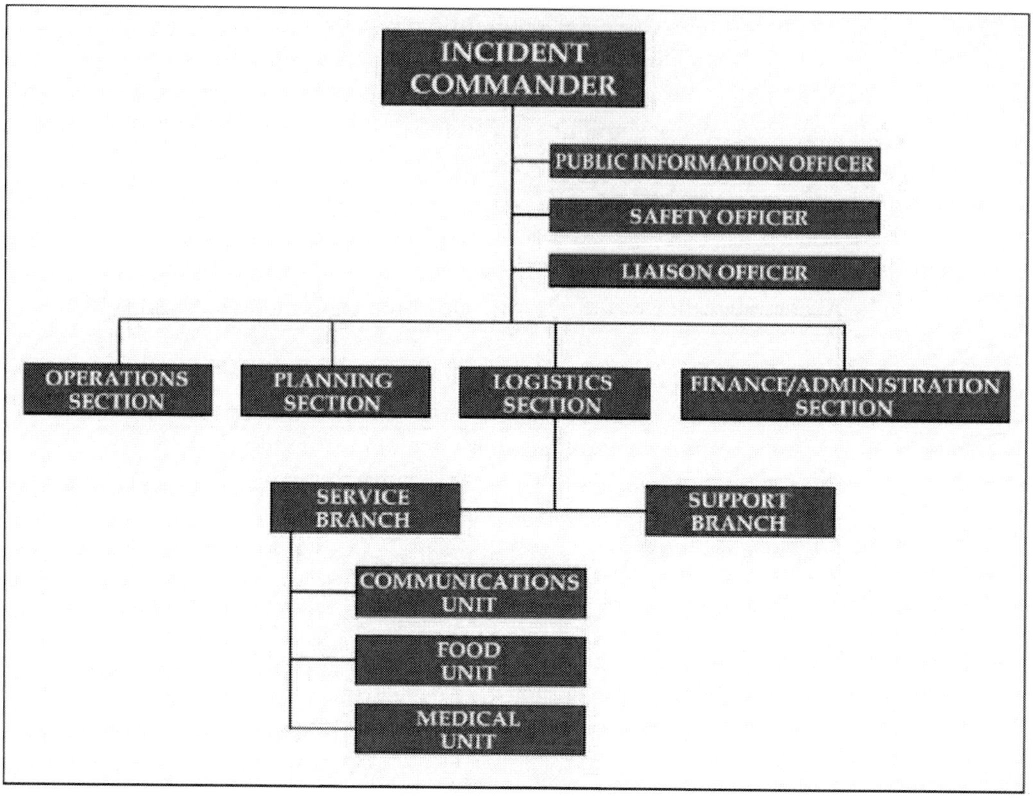

Figure 4.12.

According to NIMS ICS, when fully implemented the ICS structure will include five major sections: Command, Operations, Planning, Logistics, and Finance/Administration. The Logistics Section is further divided into two Branches: the Service Branch and the Support Branch. The Service Branch is comprised of three designated Units: the Communications Unit, the Food Unit, and the Medical Unit **(Figure 4.12).**The Medical Unit is not responsible for victims of the incident, rather for emergency personnel assigned to work at the incident. The Medical Unit develops the medical plan and provides first aid and light medical treatment for personnel assigned to the incident. It also develops the emergency medical transportation plan (ground and/or air) and prepares medical reports. It is within the Medical Unit that the responsibility for emergency incident rehab operations fall.

The Rehab Group is just one portion of the overall Medical Unit. In cases when there are no significant responder medical issues, rehab may be the only portion of the Medical Unit that is activated. In other cases, it will be necessary to integrate rehab functions into the other medical functions of the Medical Unit. Typically, this occurs only with very large scale incidents.

Only the largest of incidents will ever require the full implementation of the ICS structure. In some cases fire officers will go their entire careers without working within an incident structure that is developed to the point of formally operating the Medical Unit within the Service Branch of the Logistics Section. Because of this fact, the following section examines rehab's placement in incidents encountered more commonly.

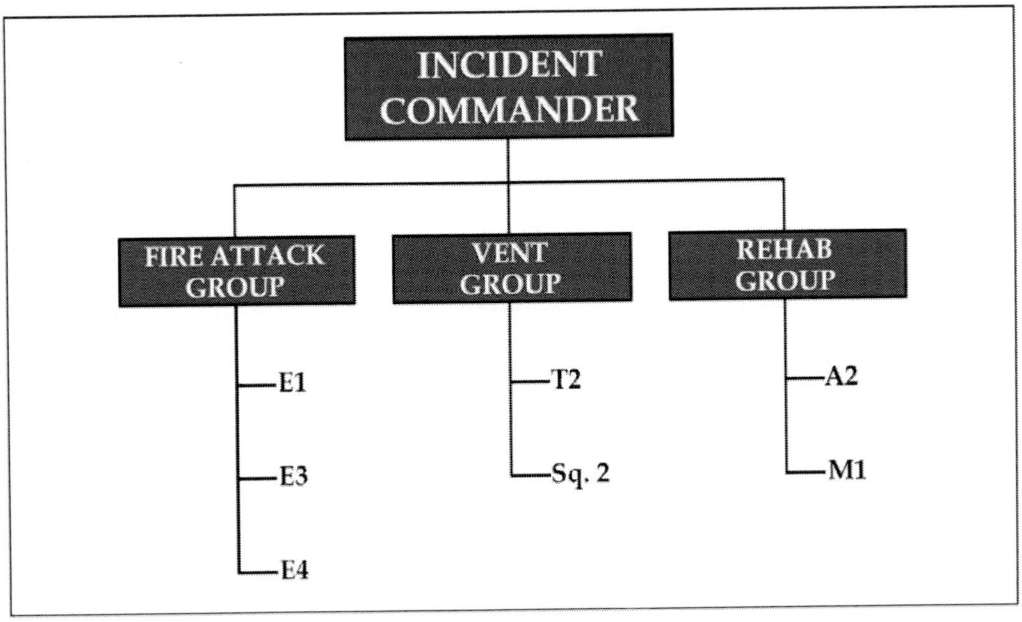

Figure 4.13.

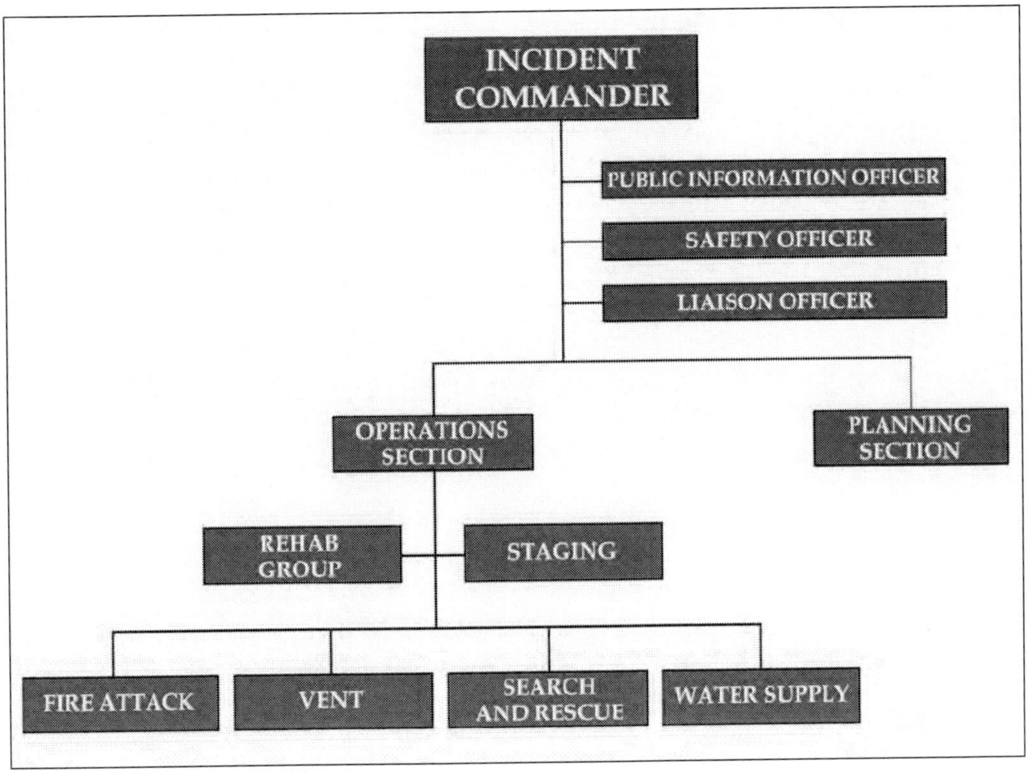

Figure 4.14.

Rehab's Position in Routine, Daily Incidents

As mentioned above, the IC is responsible for all portions of the IMS structure that are not specifically activated at a given incident. In the vast majority of daily incidents, the ICS structure will not be expanded beyond having tactical level management units, such as Divisions, Groups, and/or Branches, report directly to the IC. In these situations a Rehab Group will be established under the direction of a Rehab Group Supervisor **(Figure 4.13).** If the incident is divided into Branches or if sections other than Logistics are implemented, the Rehab Group typically continues to report to the IC.

In some cases where the Operations Section has been activated at an incident, the IC may choose to place the Rehab Group under the direction of the Operations Section Chief. In this respect this places Rehab in the same position as Staging (**Figure 4.14**). Technically, this is an incorrect usage of ICS, however some jurisdictions feel that placing both Rehab and Staging under the same reporting structure works more efficiently.

Regardless of whether the rehab operation is in a small or large incident operation, there will be command positions within the Rehab Group that need to be filled.These positions will each be responsible for overseeing a part of the rehab function. These positions will be detailed more fully later in this document.

Performing Rehab Within the Personnel Accountability System

Fire and emergency scenes are very dynamic places. Depending on the size of the incident, there can be a large number of emergency responders operating on the scene. Though all of these responders should be operating in teams of at least two and within ICS, even if they are it is often difficult to account for every responder's exact whereabouts at any given time during incident operations. Personnel accountability on the emergency scene has been a struggle for ICs for as long as firefighters have been fighting fires. Although Federal Express (FedEx®) and United Parcel Service (UPS™) are capable of tracking the exact location of a package you ship anywhere in the world at any given moment, most ICs cannot do the same for firefighters on their emergency scene. Fire service accountability systems have not kept pace with accountability and tracking systems in other parts of the work world. This is despite the fact that lost or disoriented firefighters account for a significant percentage of traumatic fireground deaths.

A series of firefighter deaths attributed to becoming lost or disoriented in structure fires in the early 1980s led several U.S. fire departments to develop personnel accountability systems for emergency scene operations. The use of a personnel accountability system in emergency incident operations also has been mandated by NFPA 1500 since its first edition in 1987. NFPA 1500 does not detail a specific type of accountability system to be used. It simply requires fire departments to establish written SOPs for a personnel accountability system that is in accordance with NFPA 1561, *Standard on Emergency Services Incident Management Systems*. NFPA 1561 also does not give very specific details on the type of system to be used.

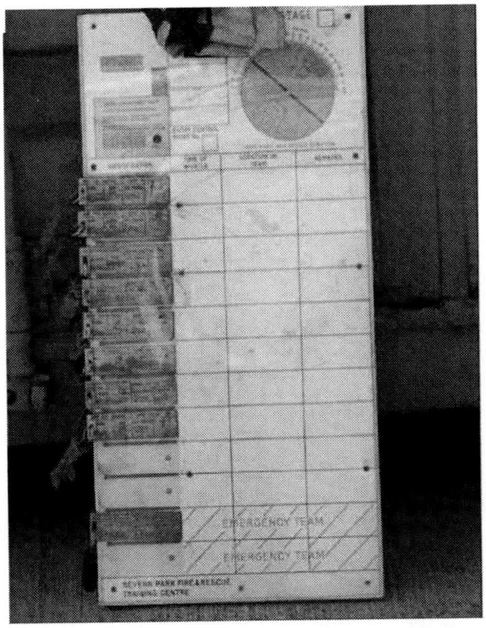

Figure 4.15.

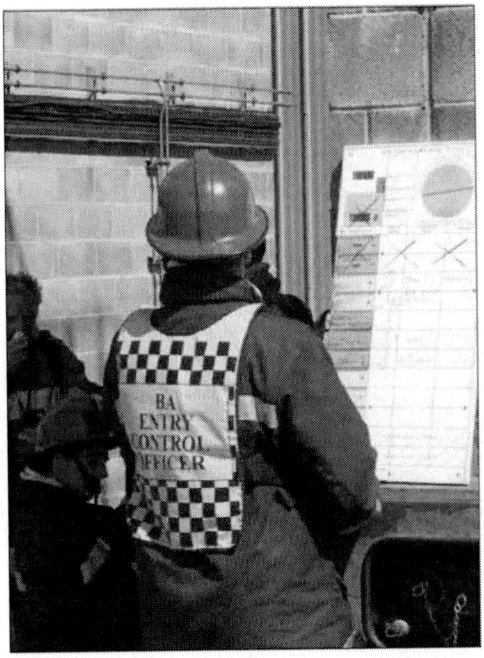

Figure 4.16.

It is not the purpose of this document to detail the various personnel accountability systems that are in use around the U.S. fire service. Suffice to say that the current status of accountability systems in the fire service is comparable to the situation surrounding incident management systems in the 1970s. Many different departments and agencies have developed systems for use in their jurisdictions, but there is little consistency among the systems used throughout the country. Some common systems that are used in the North American fire service include the Seattle PASSPORT System, the Phoenix Fireground Accountability System, and the Prince George's County, Maryland, Personnel Accountability Tag (PAT) System. More modern technologies, such as bar coding systems, have also entered use in some jurisdictions. We are in the infant stages of exploring the use of global positioning system (GPS) technologies for tracking the whereabouts of firefighters as well.

Regardless of which system is used, most of them work in much the same manner. The system uses some type of tag, token, or marker that identifies a member and that is turned in when the member rides in position on a company or reports for duty at the scene of an emergency **(Figure 4.15).** No accountability system will work unless every single member follows the system's procedures every time. In addition to locating some type of marker at the riding position on the apparatus, most systems have a procedure for collection and accounting of these markers at the point of entry to the hazard area **(Figure 4.16).** The markers must be organized in a way that instantly identifies where firefighters are working and which are in and which are out of the hazard area. Local procedures will dictate whether regular command system officers or a designated accountability officer monitors the markers and whereabouts of personnel for a portion of the emergency scene. All personnel should pick up their accountability markers when they leave an area or change assignments and take them to the new location to which they are moving.

When personnel are reassigned from forward operating positions and sent to rehab, the members must pick up their markers and present them to the Rehab Group Supervisor or rehab accountability officer when they reach the rehab area. The Rehab Group Supervisor then places the markers on an accountability board or chart and records the entry of those personnel on a check-in/check-out log sheet. By doing this the exact attendance in rehab at any given time will be known. This is important in the event that a serious problem, such as an explosion or structural collapse, occurs on the emergency scene. Knowing that personnel are in rehab will negate the need to search for them in a rubble pile.

Once the personnel are ready to leave rehab and be reassigned to the incident, the IC or Staging Manager is notified of their availability. When the group receives its next assignment, its members retrieve their markers from the Rehab Group Supervisor and take them along to their next assignment. The Rehab Group Supervisor notes on the log sheet the time that these personnel are checking out. When the personnel and their company are returned to service they place the markers on their apparatus.

If one member of a crew or company who is in rehab is deemed unfit to return to service, the Rehab Group Supervisor should not return the markers to any members of that company or crew until they are all ready to go. If that member will not be fit for the remainder of the incident, or they are transported to a medical facility, that person's marker should be removed from the rest of the group's. The marker of the out-of-service person is then forwarded to the IC. The rest of the crew, if sufficient in number, then may be reassigned.

Rehab Area Functions

Before getting into selecting a site for rehab operations and outlining the resources that will be required to operate it, it is important to outline the essential functions that will be performed there. All of the considerations that go into selecting, equipping, and staffing a rehab area are based on providing these essential functions.

According to NFPA 1584, rehab operations should, at a minimum, have the ability to meet the following five emergency incident rehabilitation needs:

1. Medical evaluation and treatment.
2. Food and fluid replenishment.
3. Relief from climatic conditions.
4. Rest and recovery.
5. Member accountability.

When designing an SOP to meet these requirements of NFPA 1584, it may be difficult to develop a coherent procedure strictly following the five needs exactly as they are described above. The authors of a book titled *Emergency Incident Rehabilitation* (Brady/Prentice-Hall) took these five needs and broke them down into seven basic functions that must be performed at any rehab operation. These seven functions can be more easily integrated into a logical SOP for carrying out rehab operations at an incident scene. The seven basic rehab functions are

1. **Physical assessment**—Every firefighter must be given a basic physical assessment when they first enter the rehab area. This includes both a visual assessment and monitoring of basic vital signs (**Figure 4.17**). A firefighter who shows signs of present or potential illness or injury should be sent to the Medical Evaluation and Treatment portion of the rehab area for more intensive treatment. Firefighters who are simply tired, thirsty, and or hungry can also be sent to the appropriate location to address those needs.

2. **Revitalization**—The basic intent of this function is to provide rest, rehydration, and nutritional support for responders who have been actively participating in incident operations. Other than the initial assessment that is given to every responder who enters rehab, this Figure 4.17 is probably the most common function performed during most City, NJ. rehab operations. The purpose of this function is to make sure that personnel rest long enough to regain their energy and allow their vital signs and body core temperatures to stabilize, replace fluids lost during exerting periods of work, and meet nutritional needs they may have (**Figure 4.18**).The goal is to send the person back into action or back to the station in relatively the same condition in which they arrived at the incident.

3. **Medical evaluation and treatment**—Firefighters whose initial assessment reveals present or pending injury or illness must receive more thorough evaluation and treatment in order to minimize the chance of their condition worsening (**Figure 4.19**). Firefighters displaying these signs must receive immediate atten tion. They should not be directed to the revitalization area first before getting treated.

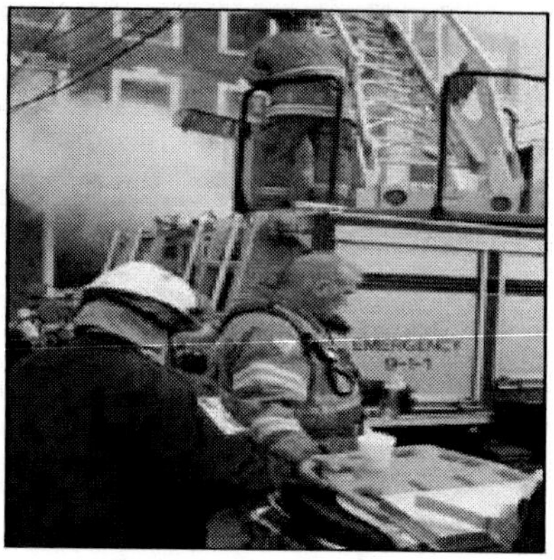

Figure 4.17. Courtesy of Ron Jeffers, Union City, NJ.

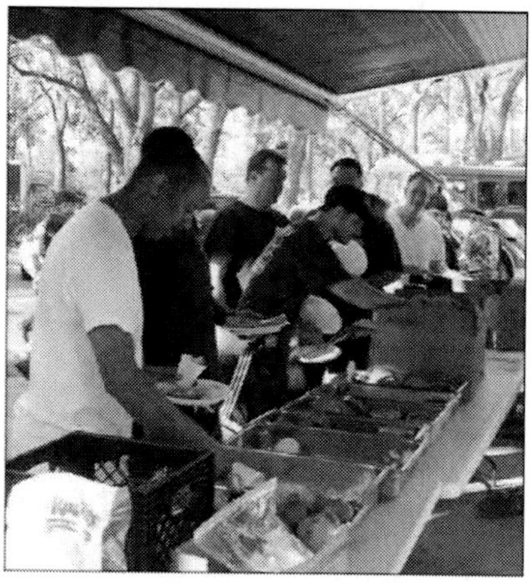

Figure 4.18. Courtesy of Chris Mickal, New Orleans Fire Department.

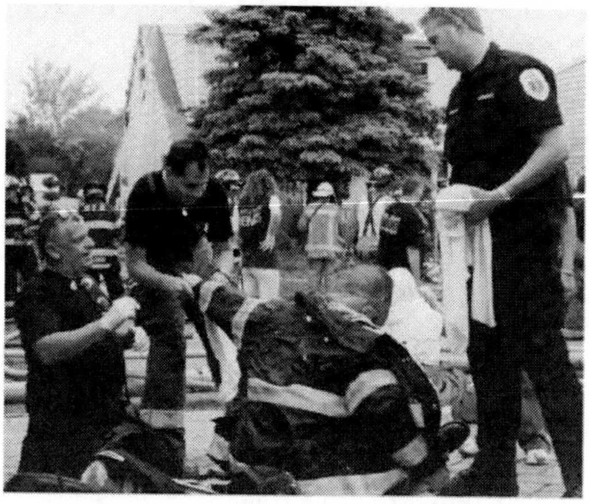

Figure 4.19. Courtesy of Ron Jeffers, Union City, NJ.

4. **Continual monitoring of physical condition**—Firefighters who are in either the revitalization area or the treat ment area should both receive continual evaluation

during their stay in the rehab area. Firefighters who do not have easily treatable conditions or who do not show signs of recovering will require a greater level of medical attention, usually following transport to a medical facility.

5. **Transportation for those requiring treatment at a hospital**—Rehab SOPs must establish responsibilities and plans that address how firefighters who need more intensive medical care will be transported to a hospital. The plan also may designate specific hospitals to which the firefighters may be transported, depending on the type of care they are in need of. The number of ambulances needed to stand by at the rehab area will be dependent on the number of people operating at the incident. There should always be at least one available. It is not recommended that vehicles other than ambulances be used to transport members to a hospital. In some cases, conditions that seem extremely minor can change quickly during the transport. If the person is not in a properly equipped and staffed ambulance, proper medical treatment could be delayed.

6. **Initial critical incident stress assessment and support**—Incidents that require large rehab operations often involve situations that can be emotionally stressful to firefighters. These include situations involving civilian and/or firefighter injuries and deaths. In recent years the emergency services have realized the impor tance of implementing aggressive critical incident stress management (CISM) programs in maintaining the overall wellness of their members. Most departments that have well-developed CISM plans choose to implement them as part of the rehab operation.

7. **Reassignment**—Each department will have their own procedures on how to handle firefighters who been restored to acceptable physical and emotional condition and are ready to be either reassigned to the incident or sent back to their quarters. This procedure must not violate the integrity of the member accountability system and be orderly in nature.

With these seven vital functions outlined, we can turn our attention to addressing how to select a good area for rehab functions to be performed and determining the resources that will be required to equip and staff the area.

Choosing the Location of a Rehab Area

Other than determining the need to start rehab operations, the next most important question that must be answered is where to locate the rehab area. The goal is to choose a site that will comfortably hold all of the personnel who will need to be rehabbed or who will provide those services and that will be strategically located to support the incident operations. It is hoped that the initial site selection will result in a rehab area that can be operated from that location for the duration of the incident. Although occasionally necessary due to changing incident conditions, moving the rehab area during the course of an incident is extremely challenging and can be confusing to personnel operating on the scene.

Fire department SOPs should outline the responsibility for choosing the rehab area location. In some cases it is the SOPs themselves that dictate this location. This is particularly true for departments who rely on special rehab apparatus and portable shelter for operating rehab areas. In these cases the SOPs generally provide very specific details on where the rehab area should be set up in relation to other incident functions. Commonly SOPs dictate that the rehab area be set up relatively close to the Incident Command Post (ICP). These SOPs should always be followed, as personnel who are operating at the scene and are assigned to report to rehab will be heading to the location specified in the SOPs.

Other jurisdictions leave selection of the location of the rehab area up to either the IC or the person assigned to command the rehab operation. Depending on the degree to which ICS has been activated, this person could be called the Rehab Group Supervisor or Medical Unit Leader. Regardless of which one of these people takes on the task, they will all be evaluating the same factors in making this decision. These factors include the possibility of positioning close to the portion of the scene where the most intensive work is being performed, the availability of a location upwind of any hazardous gases or smoke, and the potential size and duration of the incident and the number of responders who may require rehabbing. If this is the procedure used by a particular jurisdiction, there must be a parallel procedure for notifying all personnel on the scene as to the location of the rehab area so they know where to report once they have been assigned to do so.

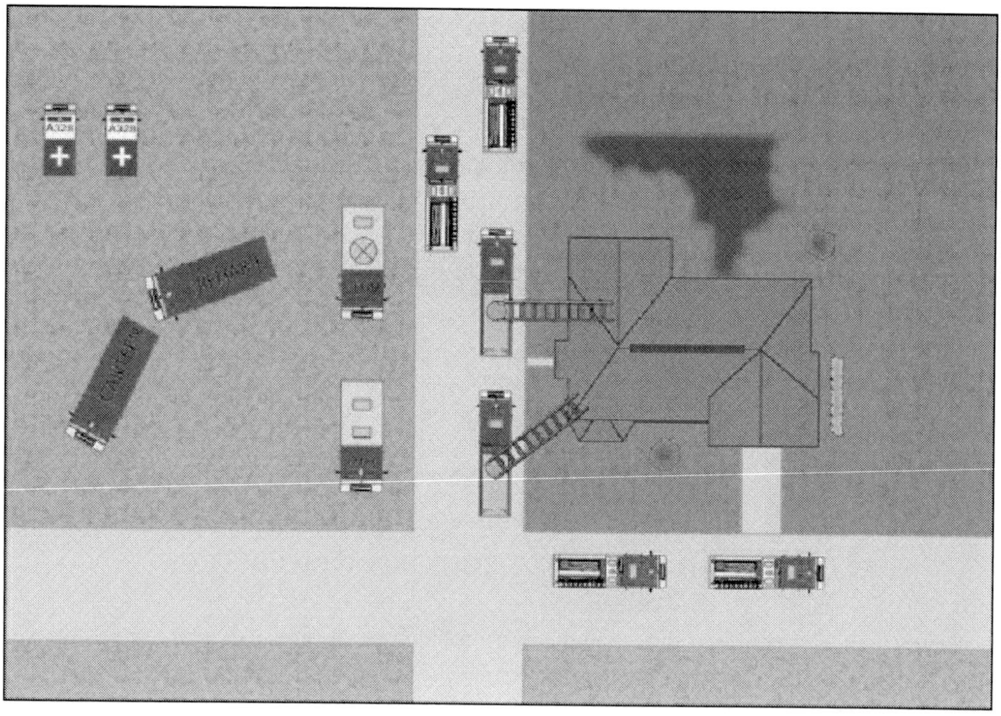

Figure 4.20.

Regardless of who decides on where the rehab area should be located, they will be faced with two general schools of thought on where the best location might be. Some jurisdictions choose to locate rehab as close to the incident Command Post as possible. Others prefer a location that is more remote from the Command Post and incident operations, yet reasonably accessible to firefighters who need to go there. Both options have their advantages and disadvantages.

Jurisdictions that like to locate their rehab operation close to the Command Post (CP) usually do so in order to facilitate the ICs ability to keep track of how many people are in rehab and who is becoming available for reassignment. Departments that operate rehab apparatus, as well as SCBA replenishing and other support apparatus, also like this arrangement as it allows them to group these vehicles in one location and share resources and equipment **(Figure 4.20).** For example, an air/power/light unit that is replenishing SCBA cylinders also can provide electrical power to the CP vehicle. The downside of this concept is that because ICs have a view of firefighters who are resting (as they should be) in the rehab area, they often are tempted to order them back into service before the firefighters are really ready to do so. As well, the firefighters themselves are less likely to temporarily "detach" themselves from the demands of the incident and may be prone to offering to return to service too quickly. This can jeopardize their health and well-being.

The primary reason that some jurisdictions choose to use a more remote rehab location is the belief that the further the responders are from the incident, the more easily they will be able to rest and relax. A more distant site is also advantageous on large-scale rehab operations at large incidents. In these situations the rehab area will require lots of resources and space. It may not be practical to operate such an extensive rehab operation in close proximity to the incident work area. The movement of supplies and injured personnel requiring transportation to a medical facility could be impaired if too close to the incident operations. On the other hand, the downside of this strategy is the obvious distance between the work area and the rehab scene. Expecting already tired personnel to hike a long distance to rehab is also not desirable. If the rehab area is more than a short, reasonable walk from the work area, some form of transportation should be required.

Rehab Site Selection Criteria

The most basic criteria for selecting a good rehab area is making sure the chosen location maximizes the firefighter's ability to get proper rest and revitalization, as well as medical attention as required. For fire departments that choose to locate rehab in close proximity to the ICP, there is little discretion in evaluating site criteria. The rehab area will be relegated to a pretty standard location based on the position of the CP. There may be a little leeway in using some available features, such as buildings or shady trees close by, to support the rehab area, but that will be about the extent of it.

In jurisdictions that provide flexibility for locating the rehab area, there are a number of factors that the person making the decision must take into account when selecting the rehab area location. The "big three" considerations that will need to be taken into account are

1. **The estimated number of responders who will need to be rehabbed.** At small incidents with a limited number of fire fighters on the scene, typically less than five or six personnel will be in rehab at any given time. This will not require a substantial

amount of space or equipment to accomplish. As the size of the incident and the number of firefighters grow, so will the need for space in the rehab area.

2. **The climatic conditions at the time of the incident.** If the weather is mild and dry, it may not be necessary to select a location that shelters the responders, other than to get them out of direct sunlight. Excessively hot, cold, or wet weather will require a site that shelters the firefighters from the elements.

3. **The duration of the incident.** Rehab at short duration incidents (less than 6 to 8 hours) may be handled adequately using apparatus and portable equipment. If the incident is going to last for the better part of a day or longer, it may be better to locate rehab in an available building. If a building is chosen, make sure it is suitable for proper rehab operations and that displacing occupants of the building for a period of time will not affect them adversely in the name of firefighter safety.

NFPA 1584 does provide some recommendation on desirable site characteristics for rehab operations. The following is a summary of characteristics and considerations that must be evaluated in addition to the "big three" described above:

- Locate the rehab area in the incident's "cold zone" so that personnel in the area can remove protec tive equipment and truly relax and recharge. In general, the rehab area should be outside, uphill, and upwind of the hazard area.
- Be reasonable in the distance from the work area to the rehab area. You don't want to be so close that the rehab area is in the way of incident operations. On the other hand, it should not be so remote that firefighters are tired by the time they get back to the work area.
- Choose a site that protects responders appropriately from the weather conditions. Look for a shaded, cool area in hot weather and a warm, dry, wind-protected area during cold-weather operations **(Figure 4.21**). Always try to stay out of precipitation.
- Make sure the site is large enough to comfortably fit all those peo ple who will be rehabbing or operating the site. Cramped rehab areas work against the goals trying to be accomplished there.
- The site should be free of vehicle exhaust. If running vehicles are a part of the rehab operation, they should be positioned so that their exhausts discharge downwind of rehabbing personnel.
- Excessive, loud noise can have a negative impact on people's ability to relax and recharge. Look for as quiet a location as possible.
- Make sure that you are able to restrict media access to the rehab area. Dealing with media works against trying to rest and relax. Tired or otherwise stressed personnel often do not make the best spokespersons.
- Apparatus capable of replacing and/or refilling expended SCBA cylinders should be collocated at the rehab area (**Figure 4.22**).
- The rehab area must be easily accessible, in both directions, for ambulances that may be needed to transport injured firefighters to a medical facility.

- Rehab operations require substantial amounts of drinking water. On smaller, shorter incidents these needs usually can be easily met with drinking water that is brought to the scene on apparatus. For long-term incidents it helps to have a rehab area located in a loca tion where a drinking water supply source is available.
- It is helpful if restroom facilities are a part of the rehab area or are in close proximity to it. Some departments have apparatus equipped with portable restrooms (**Figure 4.23**). On long-term incidents, portable restrooms may be brought to the scene. Provisions must be made to service these restrooms over the duration of the incident.
- Make sure the rehab area is remote from gruesome sights. Relaxing fire-fighters should not have to view disturbing incident conditions.

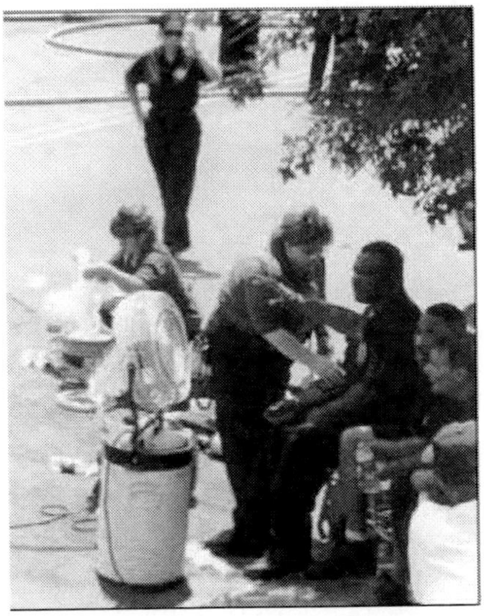

Figure 4.21. Courtesy of Ron Jeffers, Union City, NJ.

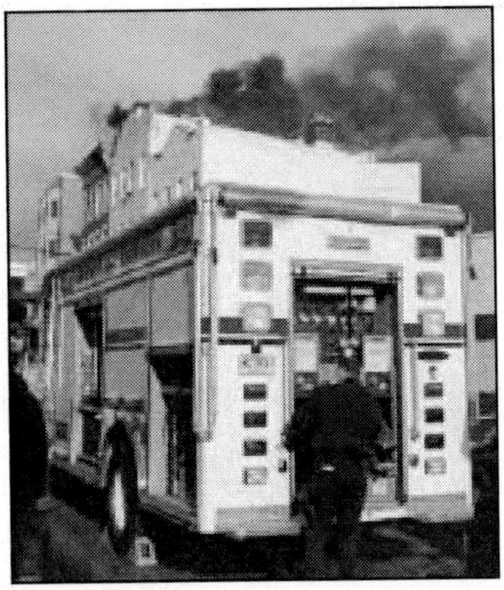

Figure 4.22. Courtesy of Ron Jeffers, Union City, NJ.

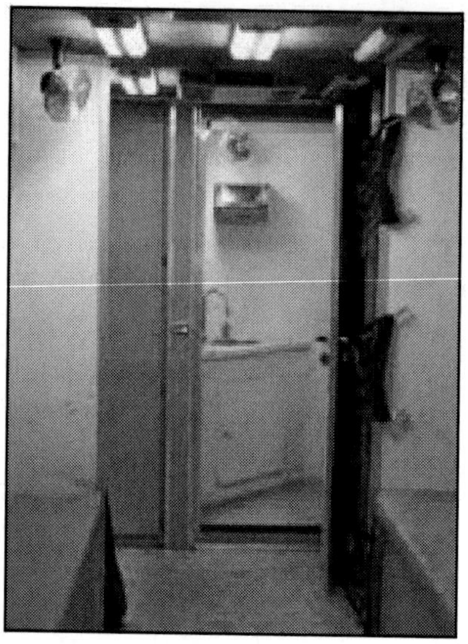

Figure 4.23. Courtesy of Phoenix, AZ Fire Department.

Fire departments should have SOPs for naming rehab areas and announcing their locations to the personnel on the scene. Departments that locate rehab close to the CP probably don't need to make any significant announcements. Most personnel know where Command is located. This becomes more important in departments that are more flexible in locating the rehab area. A general broadcast noting the location of rehab should be made over a fireground radio frequency. As well, companies being assigned to report to rehab should be reminded of its location.

Some incidents, particularly larger ones, may require more than one rehab area. In these situations the fire department should have an SOP for providing names for each site. NFPA 1584 recommends that each rehab area be identified by its geographic location at the incident site. For example, they might be named North Rehab Group and South Rehab Group or 6th Street Rehab Group and 9th Street Rehab Group. Proper accountability system recording of personnel entering rehab becomes even more important when there are two or more rehab areas. In the event of the need for a rapid accounting of personnel, both rehab areas will have to be checked.

Rehab Area Facilities

How a rehab area will be established and operated highly depends on the type of facility that will house the operation. Depending on the situation and the resources available to the fire department, rehab areas may be located in fixed facilities, apparatus, or portable structures or open areas. This section highlights considerations that apply to each of these options. The necessary equipment and supplies needed to run a rehab operation in any of these locations is covered in the next section of this chapter.

Fixed Facilities

In some situations ICs will have the option of establishing rehab in a building or fixed structure. Typically this will occur on a case-by-case basis and be dependent on the availability of a suitable structure in proximity to the incident. The use of fixed facilities is especially helpful on long-term incidents and in wet or otherwise extreme climatic conditions. Buildings with large, open spaces immediately adjacent to entrance/exit doors make the best rehab areas. Examples of these structures include cafeterias, gymnasiums, warehouses, mall areas, hangers, and large lobbies. Open structures such as parking garages, pavilions, and the undersides of stadiums or grandstands also can be used to provide relief from direct sunlight and inclement weather.

When considering looking for a structure in which to locate rehab operations, the following considerations should be taken into account:

- Look for a structure that is reasonably close to the incident scene and is easily accessible to the firefight ers who will report there.
- Try to locate the rehab area on the ground level, if possible. It is not desirable to have firefighters using stairs during rehab operations.
- Make sure the portion of the facility that will be used for rehab is large enough to comfortably contain all the people and resources that will be located there. People tripping over each other is not conducive to effective rehab operations.
- Facilities that have running water and restroom facilities are highly desirable. On long-term incidents it is a bonus to have suitable kitchen facilities as well.
- Facilities that are climate-controlled are helpful in extremely cold or hot conditions.
- Try not to select structures whose use for fire department operations will negatively affect the operations or finances of the buildings' occupants.
- Avoid structures in which the equipment worn and used by firefighters may cause damage to the facility. This includes structures that have expensive carpeting, furniture, and other features not conducive to being used by dirty, wet firefighters.
- Make sure that access to the rehab area can be controlled and that civilians, media, and other nonessential personnel cannot easily access the rehab area unchecked.

In situations where the fire department does take over a structure for rehab operations, every attempt should be made to ensure that the structure is left in relatively the same condition it was in at the onset of the operation. All trash and supplies should be cleaned up from the area. If the area has been otherwise soiled, arrangements must be made to clean it up. The owner or occupant of the building should be provided information on who to contact in the event that damages will have to be repaired.

Apparatus-Based Rehab Operations

The vast majority of rehab operations that are established at regular day-to-day incidents will not use fixed facilities and structures. More commonly, rehab areas will be established in open areas using emergency vehicles as the backbone of the operation. Vehicles will be positioned in a manner that allows their features to be most effectively used for the task at hand. This section looks at the various types of vehicles that may be useful in rehab operations and describes how they may best be used.

Pumpers and Aerial Apparatus

Though they are the most common apparatus at most emergency incidents, most fire department pumpers (engine companies) and aerial apparatus have limited usefulness for rehab operations. Climate-controlled cabs do allow firefighters to get out of extreme environments and into a more climatically-comfortable setting **(Figure 4.24).** However, these cabs are not very spacious and are not suitable for proper medical evaluation and monitoring of personnel. Except in very small incidents, with few responders rehabbing at the same time, apparatus cabs should not be used for this purpose.

Pumpers and aerial apparatus' roles in rehab apparatus generally will be limited to transporting personnel who will perform the rehab operation and any medical equipment they may require. In hot weather conditions, pumpers and aerial apparatus equipped with pumps and water tanks may use small hoselines to assist in cooling firefighters down when they enter the rehab area **(Figure 4.25).**

Rescue and Squad Apparatus

Depending on their design, rescue and squad apparatus have many of the same limitations as those described above for pumpers and aerials when it comes to being of assistance at rehab operations. Some rescue vehicles have larger seating areas in the rear portions of their apparatus bodies and may be a little more suitable for rehabbing small numbers of responders than are apparatus cabs (**Figure 4.26**). However, they still are not ideal for treating firefighters who require medical attention.

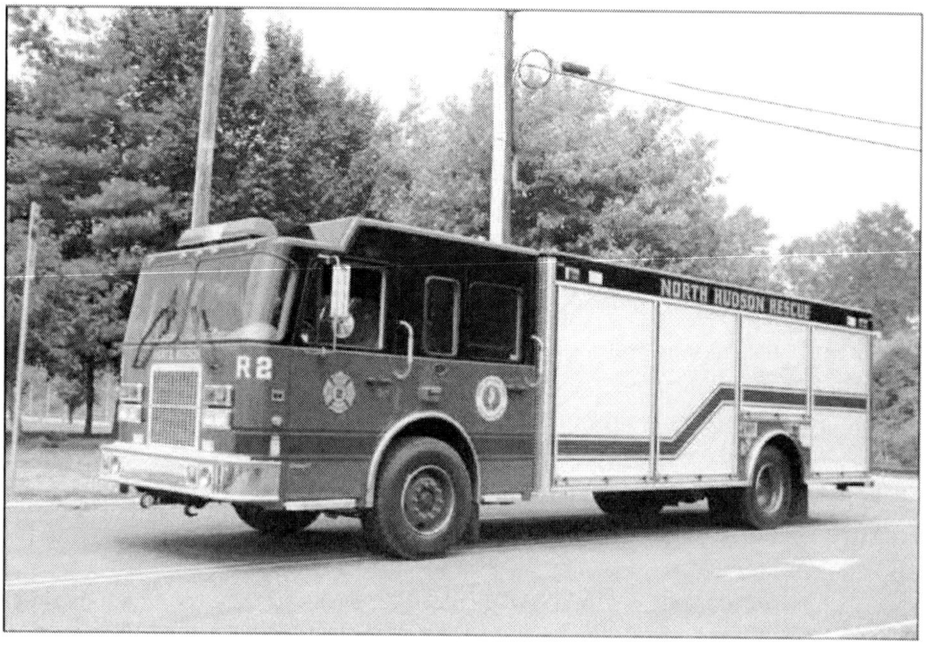

Figure 4.24. Courtesy of Ron Jeffers, Union City, NJ.

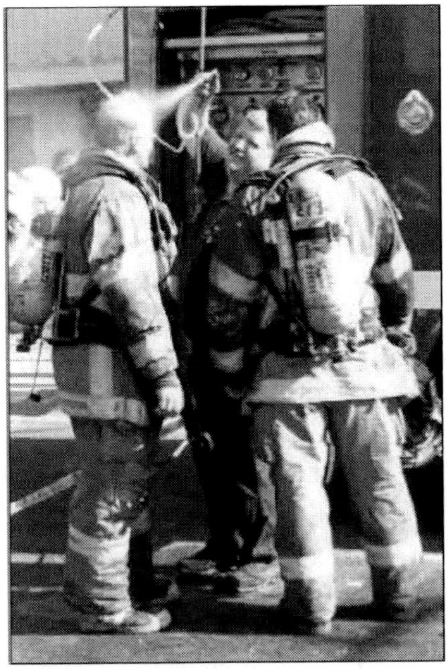

Figure 4.25. Courtesy of Phoenix, AZ Fire Department.

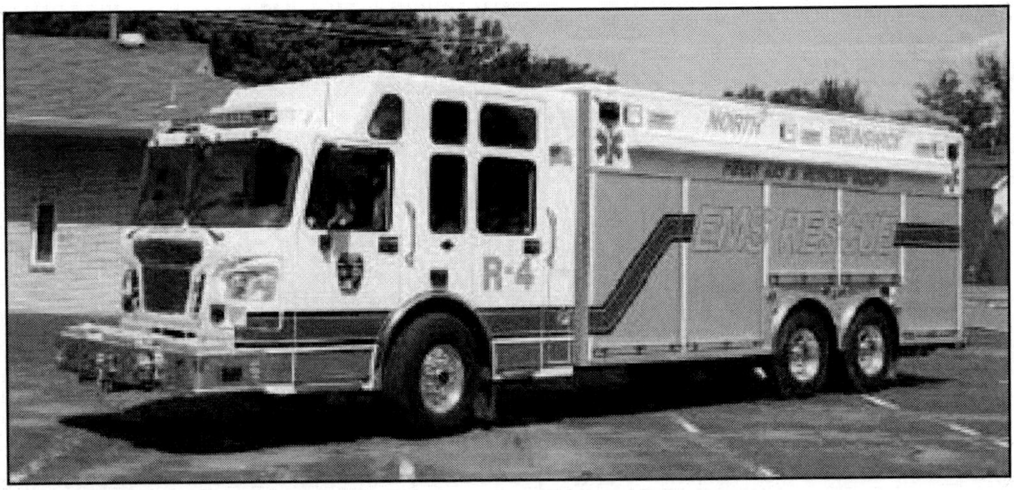

Figure 4.26. Courtesy of Ron Jeffers, Union City, NJ.

Many fire departments choose to equip rescue apparatus with quantities of supplies that can be used to initiate and operate an incident rehab area. This often is done because of the large amount of compartment space on these vehicles and the additional medical training the members of these companies often have. Rescue vehicles may be equipped with beverage containers, medical equipment, fans, awnings, and other equipment usable in establishing a rehab area (**Figure 4.27**). Many rescue vehicles also carry spare SCBA cylinders or SCBA cylinder refill equipment, such as cascade systems or breathing air compressors, on board. The ability to service SCBA equipment is an important function of an overall rehab area.

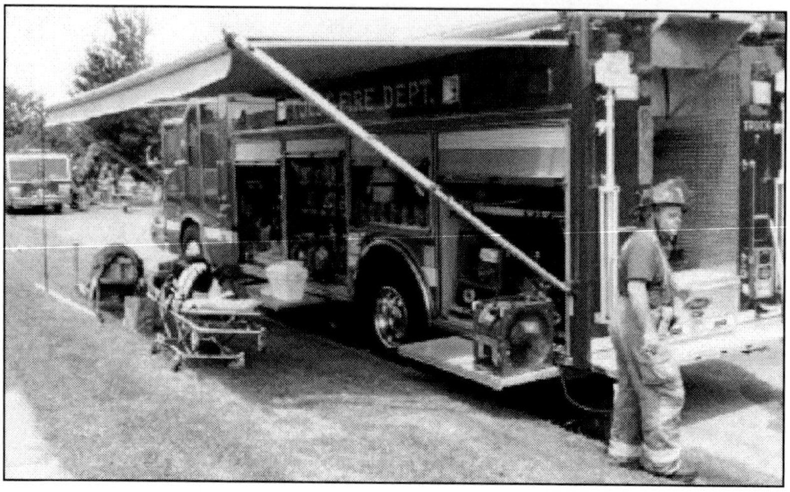

Figure 4.27.

Emergency Medical Services Vehicles

EMS vehicles can be divided into two basic categories: those that transport victims and those that don't.Transport vehicles, more commonly known as ambulances, are designed to treat patients within their rear compartments and then transport them to a suitable medical facility (**Figure 4.28**). NFPA 1584 recommends that at least one ambulance be assigned to the rehab area in the event that a firefighter needs expedient transportation to a medical facility for more aggressive treatment. Ambulances that are assigned to rehab areas may perform a variety of functions, including those that are described below.

- The ambulance crew may be assigned to support and staff the rehab operation.
- The ambulance may be used to transport injured firefighters to a medical facility.
- The ambulance EMS supplies may be needed in the rehab area.
- The patient compartment may be used for shelter during inclement weather or for evaluating and treating firefighters who have suspected injuries or illnesses.

If ambulances are used in the rehab operation, they should be parked in a manner that allows them to load their patient (s) and leave for a hospital in a quick manner if necessary. An open route from the rehab area to a roadway leading to the hospital must be maintained at all times.

Nontransport EMS vehicles are used by emergency medical technicians (EMTs), paramedics, or EMS supervisors to respond quickly to scenes and to begin treatment of victims until an ambulance can arrive and provide transport to a hospital **(Figure 4.29).** These vehicles may carry a variety of equipment that could be useful in the rehab area. In some jurisdictions, it is common to appoint an EMS supervisor or responder unit paramedic as the Rehab Group Supervisor or Medical Unit Leader. When this occurs that person likely will want to work out of their vehicle in a Command/ support role.

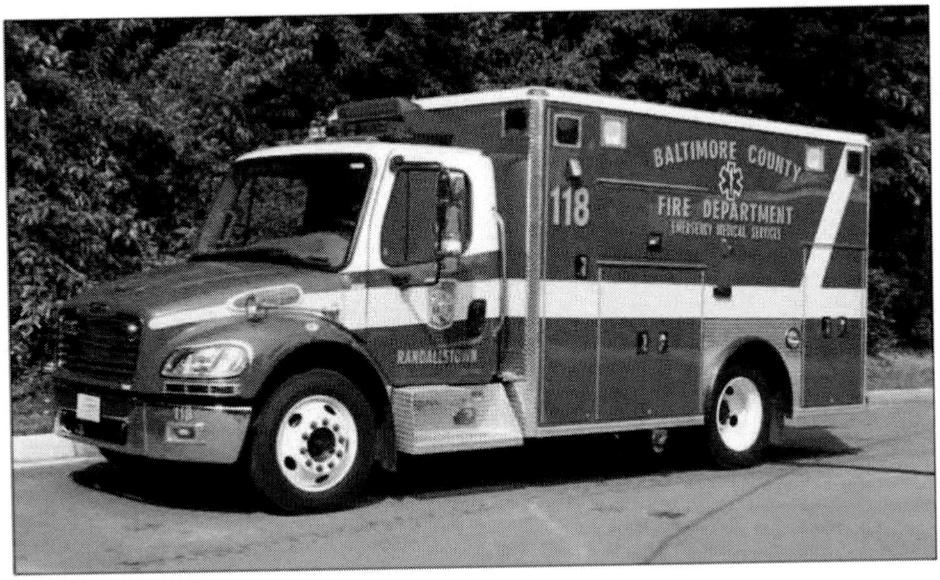

Figure 4.28. Courtesy of Ron Jeffers, Union City, NJ.

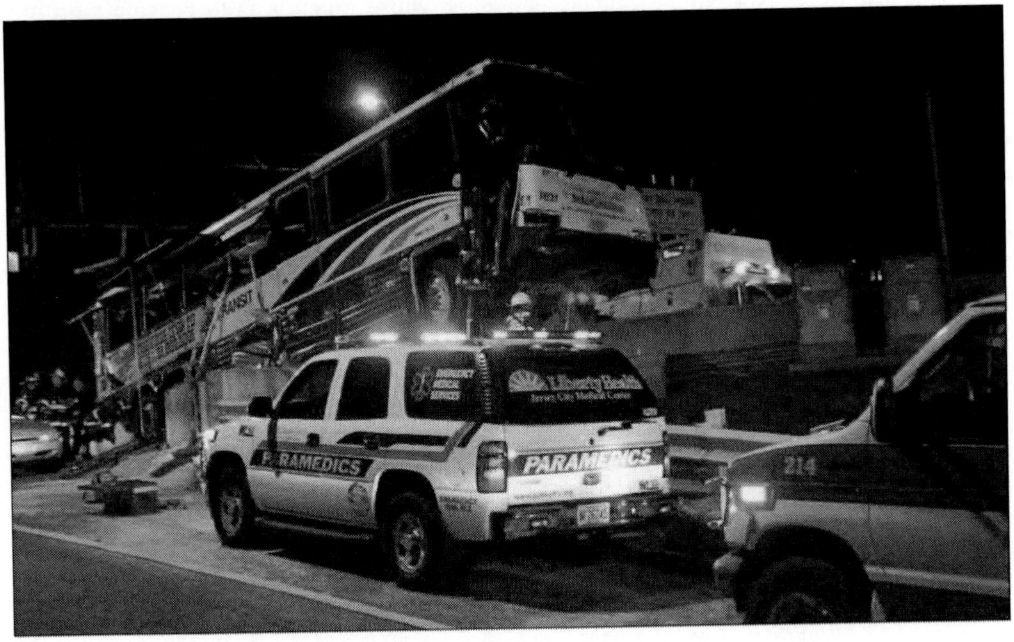

Figure 4.29. Courtesy of Ron Jeffers, Union City, NJ.

Air/Power/Light Units

Many fire departments operate special vehicles to provide electrical power, floodlighting, and/or resupply SCBA equipment on the emergency scene **(Figure 4.30).** Depending on local preferences, these vehicles may be referred to as air/power/light units, utility vehicles, or squads. These vehicles typically have large-capacity electrical generators that are driven either by an auxiliary engine or a power takeoff source from the apparatus' main engine and/or transmission. The apparatus also is equipped with large banks of elevating floodlights and various types of portable floodlights for lighting nighttime incident scenes. This ability to supply power and lighting can be very useful for operating an effective rehab area. Much of the equipment that is required to operate the rehab area requires a power source.

Air/Power/Light units also typically carry a large number of SCBA air cylinders for replacement of expended units at the scene, as well as a cascade system or breathing air compressor for refilling SCBA and cascade cylinders. As mentioned above in the rescue vehicle section, these vehicles are necessary at the rehab area because most personnel entering the rehab area will need to have their SCBAs serviced. Regardless of whether firefighters in rehab receive another onscene assignment or are told to return to quarters, their SCBAs should be refilled before they leave rehab. Jurisdictions that routinely send mobile air-supply units to structure fires and hazmat incidents commonly carry some rehab supplies on the unit **(Figure 4.31).** So that they meet the intent of the NFPA 1584 requirement that fluids to be available wherever spare SCBA cylinders are located, mobile air-supply units may carry items such as water jugs and cups or coolers full of bottled drinks for fluid replenishment.

Canteen Units

Canteen units are specially-designed apparatus whose function is to provide nutritional support to firefighters and other personnel working at extended operations **(Figure 4.32).** Depending on local traditions and preference, the canteen units may be operated by the fire department itself, or by a variety of other service organizations. Examples of these types of organizations include fire buff organizations, professional service organizations such as the Red Cross or Salvation Army, fire department Ladies'Auxiliaries, community service clubs (Lions, Elks, etc.), and other similar organizations.

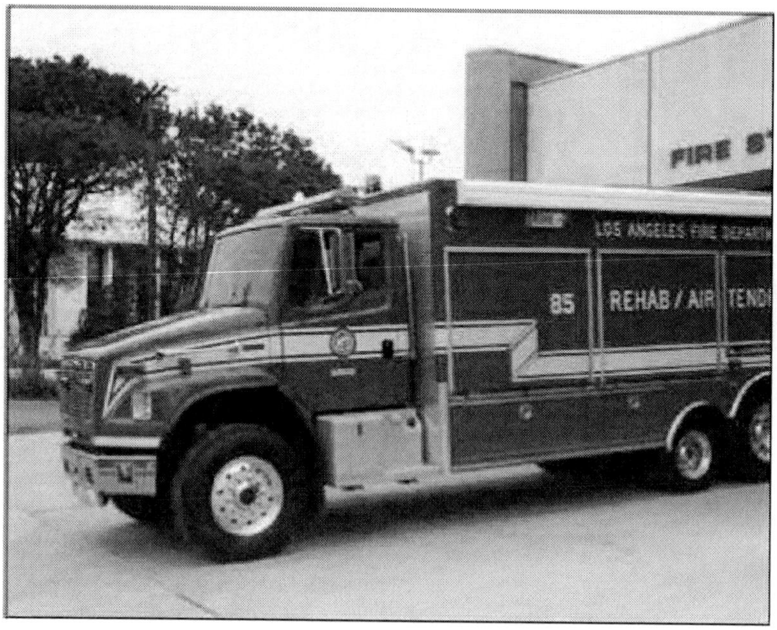

Figure 4.30.

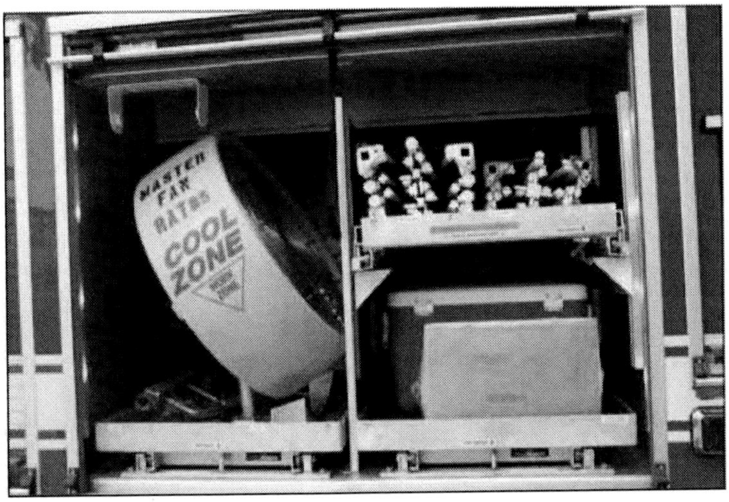

Figure 4.31.

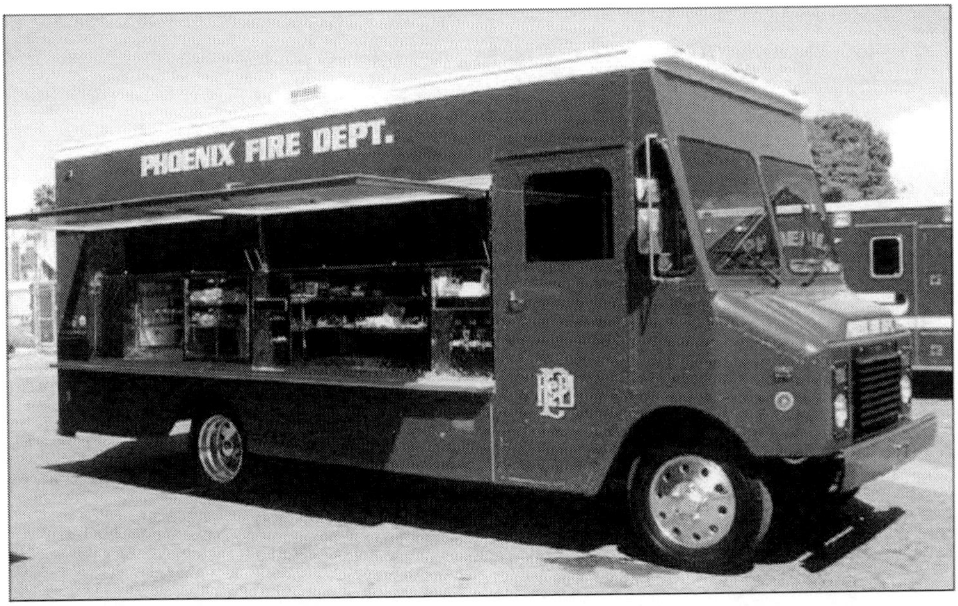

Figure 4.32.

The types of equipment carried on a canteen unit may vary depending on the level of nutritional support the organization intends to provide. Simple canteen units are set up to provide drinks and prepackaged foods that do not require heating or other preparation. More elaborate canteen units are intended to prepare hot meals and major nutritional support at the scene. These units are true mobile kitchens that include ranges, cooking griddles, conventional and/or microwave ovens, freezers/refrigerators, sinks and water tanks, large hot- and cold-drink dispensing equipment, and trash receptacles. These apparatus require onboard electric generators for independent operation, though most also are equipped with ground-shore connections that allow external power sources to be used on extended operations.

Organizations that operate these units should ensure that they meet applicable health department and sanitary regulations when these units are in service. Failure to do so could result in making responders ill during the course of an incident. Operators of these units should have policies and procedures on what types of food and drinks should be served. This should be coordinated with those officials who oversee health and safety requirements for the fire department or other organizations that are served by the canteen unit. The goal is to ensure that only foods and beverages that are best suited for providing appropriate nutritional support for firefighters and other responders is provided during the course of operations. More information on appropriate nutritional support is found in the next chapter of this document.

Buses

In the absence of permanent facilities or dedicated rehab vehicles to support rehab operations during extreme weather conditions, many fire departments choose to use buses to shelter firefighters who are rehab-bing. Of all the possible types of vehicles that could be used for this purpose, buses tend to be the most ideal. This is particularly true of urban transit or airport-type buses. These vehicles have open floor plans and their interiors are not particularly susceptible to being damaged by dirty, wet firefighters. Rehab personnel can easily move around in these vehicles to evaluate firefighters and monitor their conditions. Most of these buses are equipped with heating and air conditioning systems that allow the interior climate to offset adverse exterior weather conditions and allow firefighters to doff their equipment for maximum rest and recovery.

In some cases local agencies will donate buses they have been removed from service for permanent assignment. This allows the fire department to make any modifications they wish to the bus **(Figure 4.33).** This also makes the fire department responsible for getting the bus to the incident. In other jurisdictions the fire department works out a prearranged agreement with the agency providing bus service to have buses dispatched to emergency scenes when they are required. These agreements should be written so that the fire department is assured that there is some way to get a bus to the scene in a reasonable period of time, any time it may be needed.

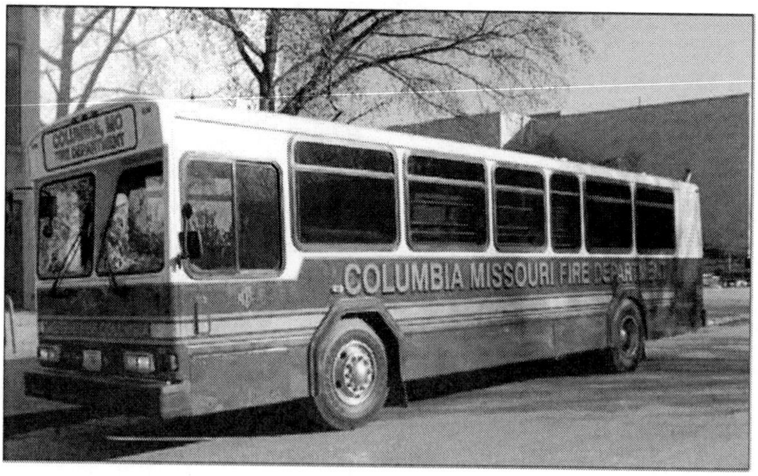

Figure 4.33.

Rehab Vehicles

The increased emphasis on firefighter safety and the recognized benefits of improved rehab services at emergency scenes has led many fire departments to develop dedicated rehab units for response to incident scenes in recent years. Typically the sole purpose of these units, and the personnel assigned to them, is to respond to incidents where rehab operations may be required and then provide that service. In many cases these vehicles will not have everything on them needed to provide an effective rehab operation; however, they will carry the items that are needed and generally not carried on other standard response units.

Depending on the desires and resources of the particular fire department, the rehab unit can fall into one of two basic designs: those that are designed to carry rehab equipment and those that are designed to provide rehab functions within the apparatus themselves. In many cases the vehicles are designed to do both of these. Rehab vehicles that are intended only to transport rehab equipment tend to be smaller vehicles and often are vehicles that previously served another function, such as a retired ambulance or service vehicle **(Figure 4.34).**

Vehicles that are designed to carry out rehab functions often are custom-designed and built for that purpose. These vehicles may have a variety of features, including enclosed seating areas, medical evaluation and treatment areas, toilets, refreshment dispensing areas, exterior awnings, misting systems, and other helpful features **(Figure 4.35).** Onboard electrical supply is important for powering the unit, but they also should be capable of taking onshore power for extended operations.

The type and amount of equipment carried on these vehicles will depend on local preferences. Any equipment carried on these units should be easily deployable and storable. It needs to be durable because of the situations in which it will be used. The vehicle also should be equipped with trash containers to ensure that all expendable supplies are collected properly for disposal in an appropriate manner.

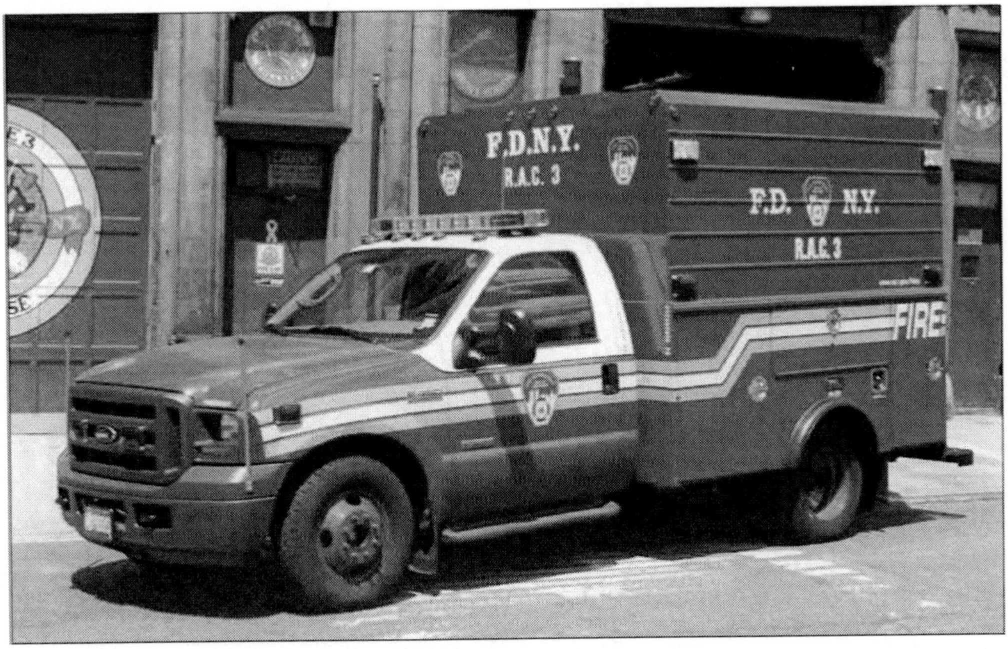

Figure 4.34. Courtesy of Ron Jeffers, Union City, NJ.

Portable Equipment Used For Rehab Operations

In order to provide effective rehab operations at an incident scene, a variety of portable equipment will be required. There is no "ideal" or model list of rehab equipment that should be available to use. The types and amount of equipment used by a particular department will vary depending on the resources available to that department and the level of rehab services they will provide. This section gives a brief description of the various types of equipment that may be used for rehab operations. Note that this section does not cover emergency medical equipment that may be used as part of the effort. Again, that will depend on the level of care provided by the EMS provider assigned to assist in the rehab operation.

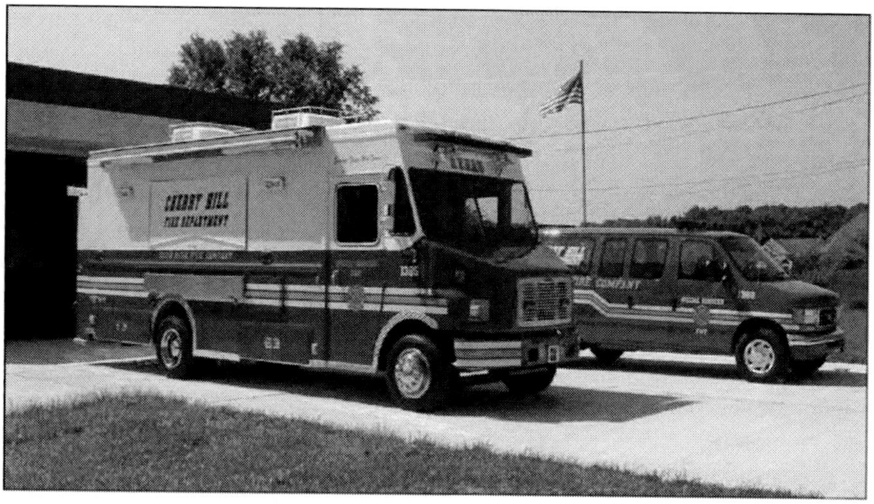

Figure 4.35. Courtesy of Cherry Hill, NJ Fire Department.

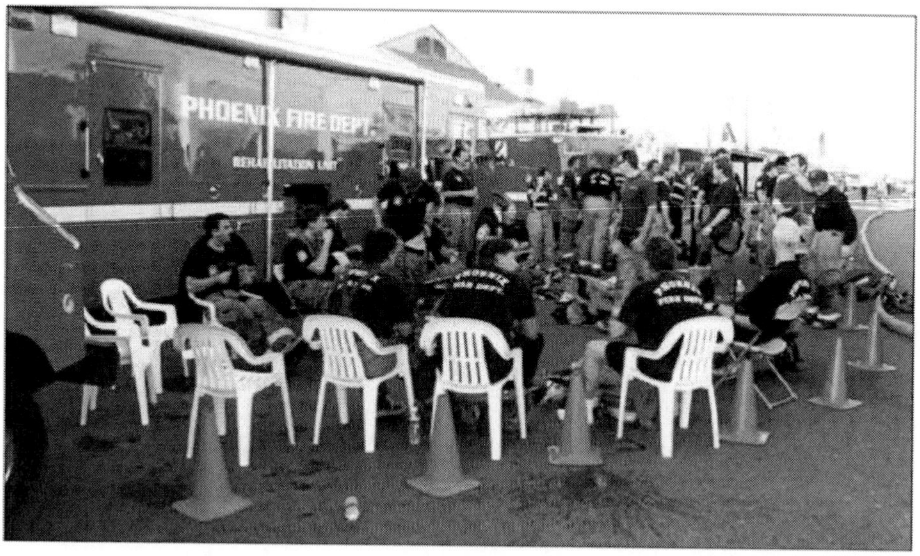

Figure 4.36. Courtesy of Phoenix, AZ Fire Department.

Rehab Area Marking Equipment

In order for a rehab operation to be completely successful, the area must be easily located and defined. In some cases the location of the rehab area will be denoted by a designation or the location of specific apparatus used to provide rehab services. In other cases the department may choose to have a formal procedure for marking or cordoning the rehab area.This may be done by using signs, banners, traffic cones, vinyl boundary marker tape, rope, or other similar items **(Figure 4.36).** Some agencies use a different color of boundary tape for the rehab area than is used elsewhere on the scene. Apparatus that are used commonly to provide rehab services should be equipped with this marking equipment.

Blankets/Tarps

Blankets and tarps can be used for a number of purposes during rehab operations. In the absence of hard or otherwise clean surfaces, tarps and blankets can be placed on the ground to make a more suitable place for personnel to sit or for equipment to be placed on. In a pinch they can be used to construct simple shelters from the sun or wind. Blankets may be useful for aiding personnel in warming themselves during cold weather operations. These blankets and tarps do not have to be anything special or fancy. Standard fire service tarps and military-type wool blankets work well for rehab operations and are commonly carried on a variety of fire apparatus.

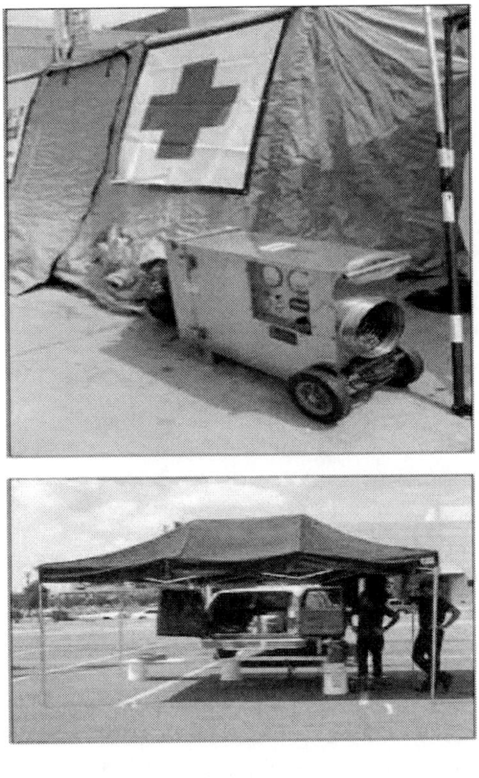

Figure 4.37. a & b.

Portable Shelters

In the absence of a permanent structure to be used for rehab operations, many fire departments choose to use some type of portable shelter to house part or all of the rehab function. How much of the rehab function that is housed in the portable structure is dependent on the wishes of the department and the size of the structure. Some portable structures, such as pop-up pavilions, air-inflated structures, and foldout awnings on the sides of apparatus can be deployed in a matter of minutes and are practical for almost any incident requiring rehab operations **(Figures 4.37 a and b)**. Other portable structures, such as tents and similar types of portable buildings may be practical on long-term, larger incidents.

All of these portable structures provide some level of protection from the elements. Some of them, such as air-inflated structures and tents can even be equipped with air conditioning or heating equipment when necessary. During heavy snow falls, these structures may not be able to handle the weight of snow on top of them without collapsing. In windy conditions they may need to be secured to the ground to prevent being toppled or otherwise blown away.

Portable Heaters

As mentioned above, portable heaters may be needed for rehab operations in jurisdictions that operate in colder climates. In addition to those mentioned above for portable shelters, many jurisdictions place heating equipment in open rehab areas. This allows personnel to sit or stand near them and warm up while resting. It may also be helpful in assisting clothing and PPE in drying. The two most common types of portable heaters used in rehab areas are electric and liquefied petroleum gas (LPG)-fired models. Portable electric heaters similar to those used in home or work settings can be used. They will require some source of electricity for power. In general, portable electric heaters do not put out as much heat (British Thermal Units (BTUs)) as LPG-fired units, which is one of their primary disadvantages.

LPG-fired portable heaters, often referred to as bullet heaters or salamanders, are commonly used in the construction industry (**Figure 4.38**). These devices are fueled by small (typically 5 gallon) LPG cylinders that are connected to the heaters by flexible hoses. Emergency responders must be aware that gas-fired units produce carbon monoxide as they burn and they must only be used in extremely well vented areas. If they are used within a confined space, carbon monoxide monitoring equipment should be used to ensure that the atmosphere remains safe for those who are operating in it. of which type of heater is used, they should be kept a safe distance from combustible objects and inspected regularly to ensure that they are in safe working condition.

Misting/Cooling Devices

Agencies that are located in jurisdictions subject to warm or hot weather may carry cooling or misting equipment to assist in rehab operations. This type of equipment is divided into two general types: air conditioning equipment and misting equipment. Portable air conditioners operate in much the same manner as fixed air conditioning equipment in structures or automobiles. They generally are not effective in open air settings and are only used to cool enclosed, portable structures. They require an independent source of power for operation.

Misting equipment is only effective in jurisdictions that have hot, arid climates. When finely-atomized water mists hit hot, arid air, the resulting evaporative process cools the surrounding air by up to 30 °F (20 °C) in perfect conditions. The evaporative cooling effect increasingly loses its effectiveness as the relative humidity of the atmospheric air increases. For this reason, misting equipment is not particularly effective in environments that have moderate to high relative humidity.

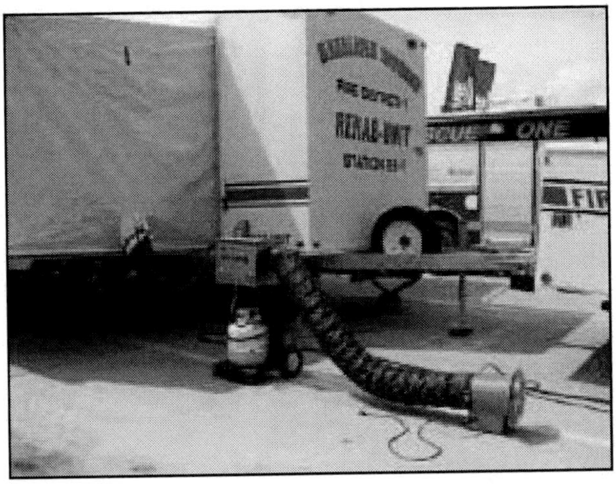

Figure 4.38.

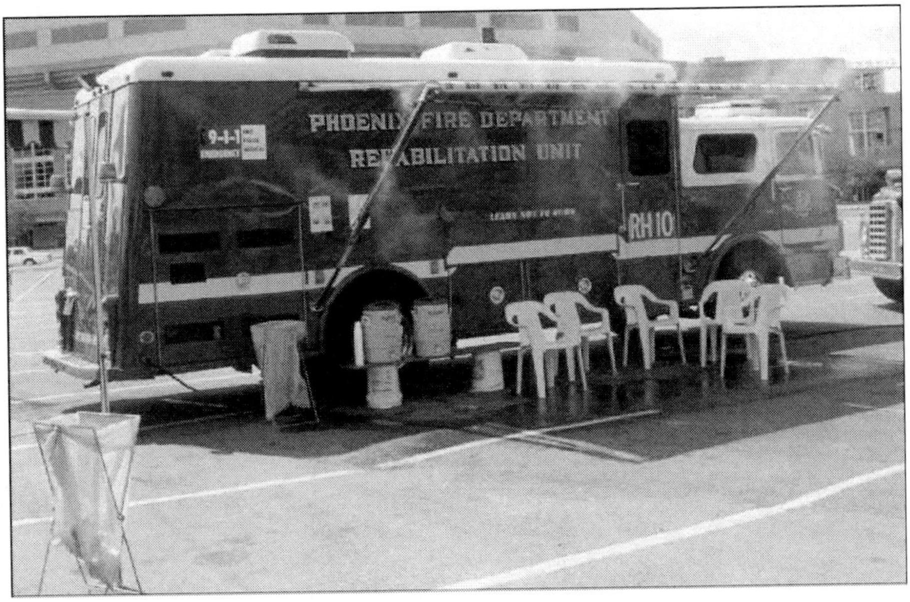

Figure 4.39.

There are a number of types of misting equipment that can be used in rehab settings. Several of these require an external source of water supply. One is a tent-awning or pavilion-type structure whose structural members are piping systems with spray nozzles located around the perimeter of the device **(Figure 4.39).** When the system is charged with water, a very fine spray mist is discharged from the openings. These structures can be raised very quickly and located anywhere where there is a water supply source nearby. Another common device is a mechanical blower that has a water injection line run within it. A spray nozzle within the unit introduces a water mist into the discharge side of the blower. This device cools both by movement of the air by the fan and by evaporation of the water.

Any device requiring an external water supply source should only be attached to a source that has clean water. Otherwise the risk of spraying contaminated water on the people using the equipment is real. If the cooling equipment cannot be attached to a municipal or similar water supply, it can be supplied with water by a fire department pumper, assuming the pumper filled its tank at a potable water source.These devices flow a very low volume of water (in some cases 5 gpm or less), so a pumper operating off its tank can supply the device for a substantial period of time.

Another device that is seeing increasing use in rehab operations is a smaller mechanical blower that is designed to be attached to the top of an insulated drink dispensing container **(Figure 4.40)**. These containers may hold anywhere from 5 to 20 gallons of ice water. The chilled water is dispersed through the blowing action of the fan. The drink containers will need to be refilled on a frequent basis. Although ice water is not required, it does maximize the cooling effect of this equipment. An external electrical source will also be required to power the blower.

Fans and Blowers

Portable fans or blowers are used commonly in rehab operations for assisting in cooling responders who are resting there.The air moving across the resting responders will help their bodies more effectively dissipate the heat they are generating internally.

Though gasoline-powered blowers are probably now the most commonly used mechanical blowers for ventilation operations, these devices should not be used for cooling firefighters in a rehab area. The exhaust from their gasoline engines is dispersed in the air stream and is counterproductive to the rehab effort. Only electrically powered fans should be used for rehab area cooling.

Many fire departments have repurposed old electric smoke ejectors for use as cooling devices in rehab operations (Figure 4.41). They move a relatively large amount of air and they are rugged. When available, it is desirable to fit the smoke ejector with a flexible duct that allows the unit to be placed a short distance away from the point where the air is actually discharged. This reduces the noise level in the area where firefighters are resting.

Standard household box fans also work for this purpose. They do not move quite as much air as a smoke ejector and do not stand up to rugged use over a long period of time. However, they are considerably less expensive than a smoke ejector should you need to purchase them.

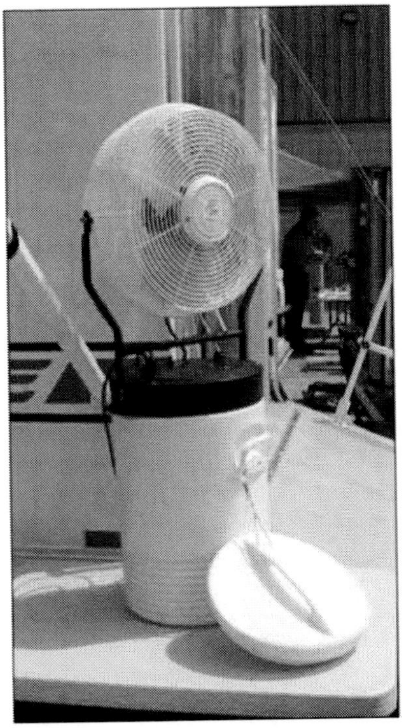

Figure 4.40.

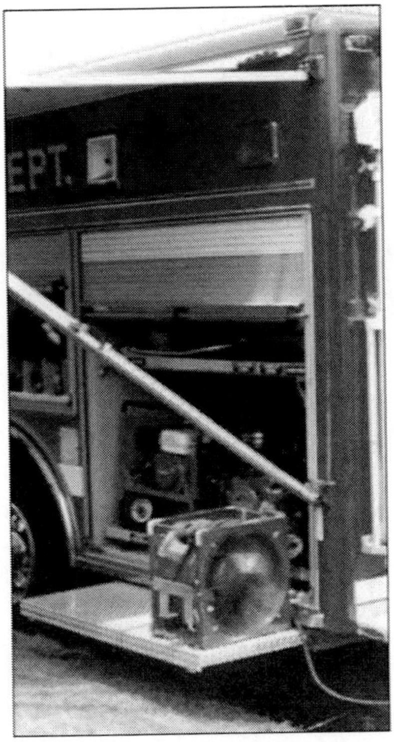

Figure 4.41.

Regardless of which type of fan you choose to use, a source of electrical power will be required for its operation. Most commonly, an electric generator on a piece of fire apparatus will provide power. However, if a ground supply source of power is available, it will create less noise for the rehab area than running a generator.

Lighting and Electric Generation Equipment

Virtually any rehab operation will require a source of electrical power in order to run the variety of powered equipment that will be used there. This includes items such as blowers, portable heaters, floodlights, food preparation appliances, and similar devices. The first choice for operating electrically powered devices should always be a ground supply source of electrical power. This eliminates the use of noisy, fume-producing portable generating devices. If a ground supply source is not readily available, some type of portable electrical generating device will be required.

Fire departments typically rely on three types of electrical power generating equipment for supplying power needs at incident scenes. These are inverters, portable generators, and vehicle-mounted generators. Inverters are step-up transformers mounted to the apparatus that convert the vehicle's 12- or 24-volt direct current into 110- or 220-volt alternat ing current. Since the inverter doesn't have a separate motor, they don't use any more fuel than is already used by the idling vehicle and they generate virtually no noise during operation. On the downside they typically have small power supply capacities (5 kW or less) and they may not beoperated remote from the vehicle.

Portable generators are powered by gasoline or diesel engines and generally have 110- and/or 220-volt capacities (**Figure 4.42**).They may be operated from their storage location on the vehicle or they can be carried or wheeled to their needed location. Most portable generators have a capacity of 7.5kW or less. When used for rehab operations it is most desirable to locate them somewhat away from resting firefighters to reduce noise and exposure to exhaust fumes.

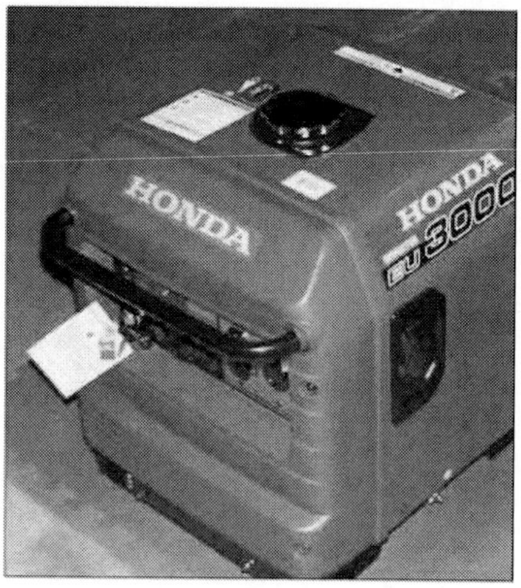

Figure 4.42.

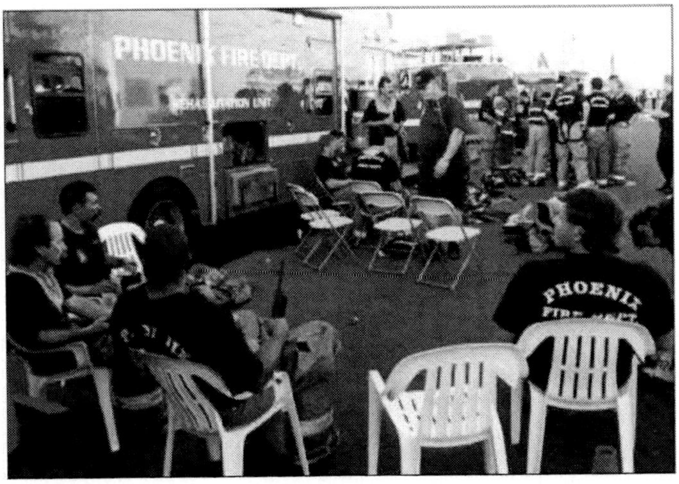

Figure 4.43. Courtesy of Phoenix, *AZ* Fire Department.

Vehicle-mounted generators have substantially larger power production capabilities than inverters or portable generators. Capacities of up to 75 kW commonly are found on rescue or utility service vehicles (**Figure 4.43**). Units ranging from 5 kW to 20 kW commonly are found on engine and truck companies. Vehicle-mounted generators can be powered by auxiliary engines or vehicle hydraulic or power takeoff systems. Fixed electrical equipment on the apparatus containing the generator often is wired permanently into the generator for quick deployment. Vehicle-mounted generators that are powered by auxiliary engines are noisy and should be parked as far away from resting firefighters as practically possible.

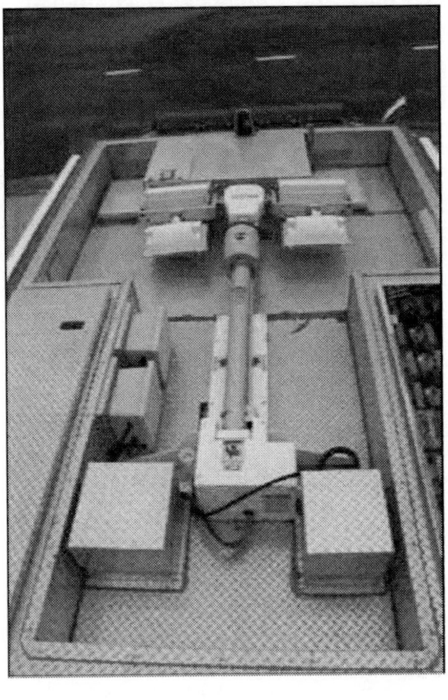

Figure 4.44.

Lighting equipment may also be needed to illuminate the rehab area during nighttime operations. Fixed lighting systems on apparatus provide the most effective means of lighting a large area (**Figure 4.44**). If the rehab area is too far away from apparatus for fixed floodlighting to be effective, portable floodlights may be used. When using portable floodlights firefighters must take care not to come into direct contact with the equipment as is gets very hot and can burn the person severely. When using either type of light, make sure that you are aware of the generating capacity of the power source for the lights. Trying to power too much equipment will overtax the generator and possibly damage both it and the lighting equipment.

In order to use electrical generating equipment and floodlighting equipment, as well as any other electrically-powered equipment that may be required, a variety of other electrical distribution equipment may be needed. Suitable extension cords, cord reels, junction boxes, and related devices will be needed to connect the electrically-powered equipment to the power source. Such equipment used for fire department service is typically much heavier than that used for residential or commercial use. Electrical cables must be adequately insulated and waterproofed and must have no exposed wires. It should be checked regularly to ensure it is in safe operating condition. If departments that regularly work together use different types of electrical connections for their equipment, each should carry adaptors that allow equipment to be interconnected when required.

Rehab Recording Equipment

Depending on the procedures used for tracking personnel in rehab by a particular fire department, a variety of recording and timekeeping equipment may be needed. It is most efficient to collocate all of this equipment on an apparatus that is likely to be involved in rehab operations. By having all the necessary items collocated together, the personnel assigned to establish the rehab area will be able to begin the process more quickly than if they first have to locate and assemble these items separately. Depending on the procedures used by a fire department, the following equipment may be used for information recording and timekeeping:

- handheld or laptop computers;
- bar code readers;
- logbooks;
- rehab forms or tags;
- EMS report forms;
- clipboards;
- writing implements; and
- clocks, stopwatches, or other time recording/stamping equipment.

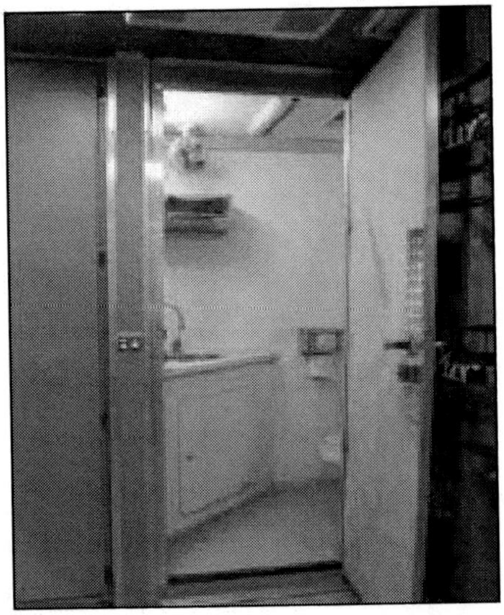

Figure 4.45. Courtesy of Phoenix, AZ Fire Department.

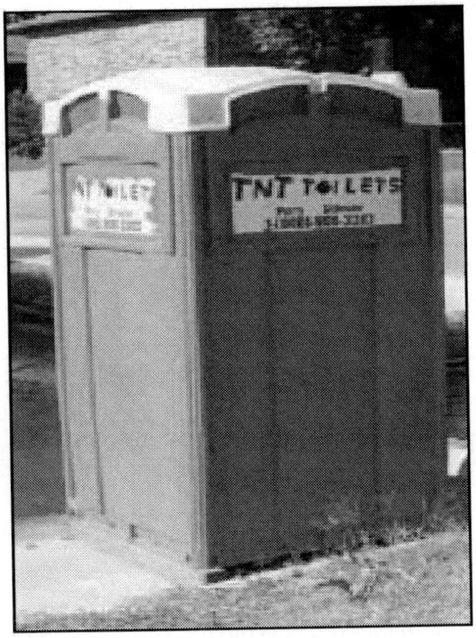

Figure 4.46.

Spare Clothing/Personal Protective Equipment

In the "old days," many fire departments, particularly volunteer fire departments, carried all of their turnout equipment on the fire apparatus. If a firefighter's gear got wet or damaged at an incident, it was often possible to return to the apparatus to switch our their gear for a dry set. This is no longer a common practice in any portion of the fire service.

Some fire departments do carry a limited supply of dry clothing and PPE on rehab vehicles or service apparatus that may be placed in rehab areas for responders to change into as the need arises. Some departments also have procedures in place to bring equipment to a scene from storage locations when needed. Departments that provide this service should have defined procedures for collecting the items after an incident. The spare equipment should be washed and inspected before it is placed back on the apparatus or in storage.

Portable Toilets

Portable toilets may be required if the rehab area is not located close to a facility with accessible restrooms. It is becoming common practice for fire departments to equip rehab, service, and Command vehicles with restrooms that are similar to those found in buses or recreational vehicles (**Figure 4.45**).

If neither of these options are available, or if the portable restroom is in a Command vehicle and constant use will be disruptive to Command functions, other portable restrooms may need to be brought to the scene. Fire departments should have preincident arrangements in place with a portable restroom provider so that these devices may be delivered any time they are needed (**Figure 4.46**). Some portable toilets are trailer-mounted and can be brought to the scene and set up quickly. Others must be unloaded off a truck and placed at the desired location. If the incident will last more than 24 hours, arrangements should be made for the provider to return periodically to empty and service the toilets.

Hand Washing Equipment

Every emergency response and scene will expose firefighters and other responders to a variety of dirt and germ hazards. The vast majority of responders who will show up at a rehab area will be dirty and sweaty. To counteract this fact, rehab areas must include the means for firefighters to wash their hands and faces (at least) before resting, eating, and/or drinking (**Figure 4.47**). All responders should be required to wash their hands and faces before beginning the rest and replenishment portion of the rehab process. If the rehab area is not accessible to facilities with restrooms, sinks, or other means of cleaning off firefighters, these supplies must be brought to the rehab area. Such supplies include these:

- potable water;
- soap or other cleansers—preferably antibacterial soap;
- catch basins or dispensing equipment;
- premoistened towelettes; and
- paper towels.

Chairs and Tables

Chairs and tables will be useful during rehab operations. Some personnel find it more appealing and comfortable to sit on a chair or bench when resting rather than sitting on the ground. Many departments who operate rehab vehicles or service vehicles carry a supply of chairs for use Figure during rehab operations. Because firefighters are often large people wearing heavy protective clothing, any chairs that are used for this purpose need to be extremely sturdy. Sturdy folding chairs or stackable, resin-type patio chairs tend to work best.

Some fire departments are using chairs that are specially designed for rehab operations. These chairs are typically of a "pop-up" design and they contain special fluid-holding wells in the arm rests of the chair. The design intent of these chairs is for the arm rest wells to be filled with ice water during rehab operations. When a firefighter sits in the chair he or she submerges his or her arms into the ice water baths. This process cools the blood that is flowing through the person's arms and assists in cooling the body core temperature. It has been shown to be an effective means of reducing body core temperatures. Departments that do not have these special chairs can have firefighters submerge their hands and lower arms into buckets of ice water that are placed on either side of them.

Drink Dispensing Equipment

One of the primary functions of a rehab area is to provide fluids for the rehydration of firefighters. Fire departments who are establishing a rehab capability must take this into consideration and ensure that they have the proper equipment to provide these fluids. There are two basic means for providing fluids in rehab operations: by using individual serving containers or by using bulk beverage coolers and cups.

Individual serving containers of water or sports drinks are very convenient and they have very long shelf lives under a wide range of atmospheric conditions (**Figure 4.48**).Their primary downside is that they tend to be a little more expensive than bulk beverages. Fire departments need to establish a procedure for ensuring that these drinks get to the rehab area when needed. Some of the following items must be considered in this procedure:

- Identify what vehicle will carry the drinks. Depending on the department this may be a rehab vehicle, air/ power/light unit, rescue apparatus, ambulance, or a chief officer or Safety Officer vehicle.
- Assign an inventory check of these drinks to someone as a regular duty.
- Have ice chests and ice available for cooling down these beverages when needed. Determine what vehicle will carry this equipment or who will be responsible for getting it when needed.

Departments that use bulk beverages for rehab operations typically dispense them from large, insulated containers where water or sports drinks and ice are kept (**Figure 4.49**). If this method is employed, disposable cups for personnel will be required also. It is recommended that cups used for serving beverages have a capacity of at least 16 ounces. Cups of this size allow firefighters to get reasonable-size drinks and then sit down and relax. The advantage of using these containers is cost; their use is usually less expensive than that of individual containers.

As with single serving containers, departments that use bulk beverage equipment need to have SOPs for ensuring that they are ready to go when needed. Career fire departments should determine which vehicle these containers will be carried on and the containers should be dumped, rinsed, and refilled at the beginning of every shift. Departments that use sports beverages in these containers typically do so by mixing powder into ice water. From an economic standpoint it makes more sense to fill the container with ice water on each shift and only mix in the powder when readying the equipment for use at an incident. Volunteer departments will have to determine a method for deploying this equipment that works best for their situation.

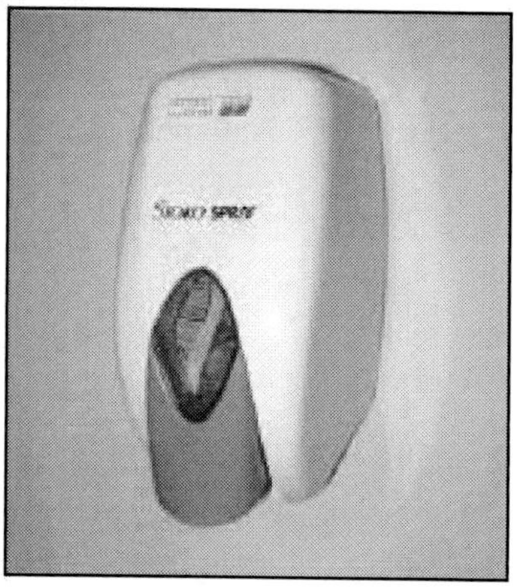

Figure 4.47.

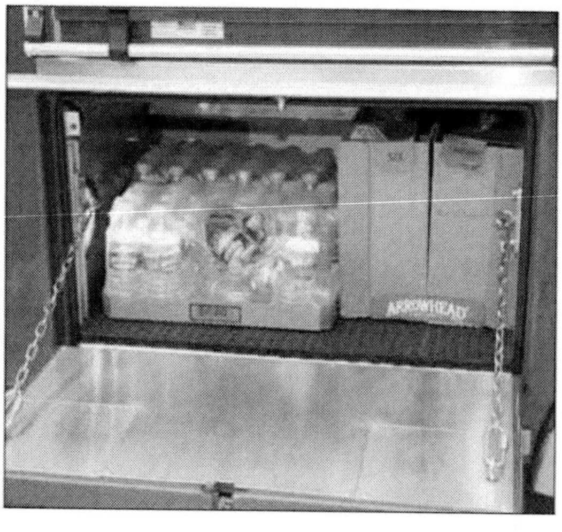

Figure 4.48.

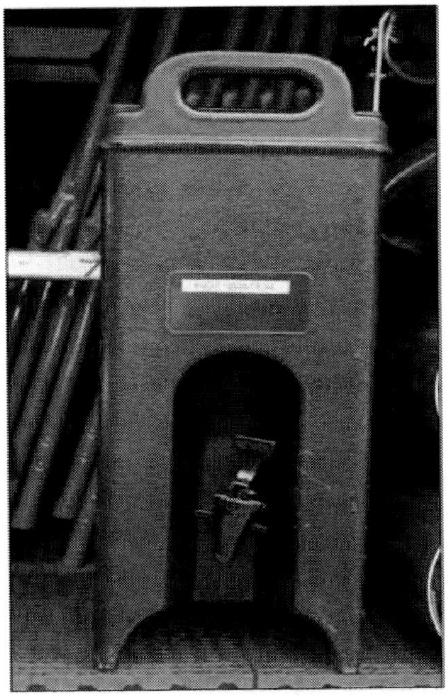

Figure 4.49.

Trash Collection Equipment

Rehab areas will quickly accumulate a relatively large amount of trash. This includes cups, drink containers, food serving supplies, ice bags, and a wide variety of other items. The fire department needs to provide a means for capturing and disposing waste items. Vehicles that carry rehab supplies should be equipped with trash containers and/or trash bags. Trash collection equipment should be deployed as soon as the rehab area is set up and the trash that is collected must be disposed of appropriately. Keep in mind that simply throwing the trash in the nearest dumpster may not be the best option, especially if the incident developed a large amount of waste. Some property owners are very sensitive about other people's trash being placed in their trash bins, as they may be paying a "per load" fee for trash removal. It is usually best to haul the trash back to a department waste collection location.

In: Rehab, Protection and Safety Measures or Firefighters … ISBN: 978-1-60741-566-4
Editor: Andreo Rios

Chapter 5

CARING FOR FIREFIGHTERS DURING REHAB OPERATIONS

There is much more to establishing an effective rehab area than selecting a good location and having the right vehicles and equipment. The whole purpose of establishing the rehab operation is to ensure optimum care of the firefighters and other responders who will be operating at the incident. In order to do this there must be effective means for operating the rehab area, established procedures for requiring firefighters to enter the rehab area, and a solid plan for providing the services that are required.

This chapter examines means for minimizing the amount of stress placed on firefighters during incident operations. This includes establishing safe work-to-rest ratios and monitoring personnel for signs of problems. Detailed information on performing both self-rehab and formal rehab functions is provided also. The latter half of the chapter details medical evaluation and treatment considerations for rehab operations, as well as principles of hydration and fluid and nutritional support.

ESTABLISHING REQUIREMENTS FOR REHABBING FIREFIGHTERS

Setting up the most elaborate and well-prepared rehab area in the world will have no impact on the safety of responders unless that area is used appropriately. In other words, we have to find ways to ensure that responders actually will go to the rehab area and use the services as appropriate during the course of the incident. This is not as easy as it may seem.

Firefighters are notoriously proud people and a hearty machismo attitude is pervasive within the fire service. Pride and macho can be a dangerous combination. This combination is often responsible for firefighters failing to recognize the dangers posed by overexertion at an emergency scene or training situation. The end result is often one of two unnecessary outcomes:

1. The firefighter continues to operate at the incident or training session until he/she either becomes injured or is completely unfit to go on.

2. The firefighter is in such poor shape by the time he/she gets to the rehab area that his/her medical wellness is at risk and he/she will not be able to be rehabbed to the point where he/she can continue operating at this incident or training session.

Simply stated, in many cases, if we simply leave it up to individual firefighters to decide when to take a break and enter the rehab operation, most will either avoid it completely or go there too late. Fire departments must establish and enforce mandatory policies for personnel to participate in rehab functions at all appropriate incidents and training sessions. Anything short of this enforced requirement likely will result in many firefighters' failure to seek appropriate rehab services when they should.

Prior to the development of the National Fire Protection Association (NFPA) 1584, *Recommended Practice on the Rehabilitation of Members Operating at Incident Scene Operations and Training Exercises*, (2003 ed.), the requirements for sending firefighters to rehab varied widely from fire department to fire department. Perhaps the most common rule of thumb for structural firefighting was the requirement that firefighters enter rehab following the expenditure of two 30-minute SCBA cylinders. Requirements for nonstructural firefighting incidents were either nonexistent or inconsistent.

NFPA 1584 provided the first standards-driven direction on recommended work-to-rest ratios and guidelines at structure fires or similar incidents.The NFPA 1584 requirement essentially has two parts:

1. The company or crew must perform self-rehab (rest with hydration) for at least 10 minutes following the depletion of one 30-minute self-contained breathing apparatus (SCBA) cylinder or 20 minutes of intense work without wearing an SCBA (**Figure 5.1**). Following the self-rehab period it is up to the Company Officer (CO) or crew leaders to determine the readiness of the other crewmembers to return to duty.
2. The company or crew must enter a formal rehab area, receive a medical evaluation, and rest with hydration for a minimum of 20 minutes following:

   - the depletion of two 30-minute SCBA cylinders;
   - the depletion of one 45- or 60-minute SCBA cylinder;
   - whenever encapsulating chemical protective clothing is worn; and
   - following 40 minutes of intense work without an SCBA.

The reason that the preceding guidelines are based on SCBA use is that this is the easiest thing for firefighters to remember. They almost always know how many SCBA cylinders they have expended. If they have used more cylinders than they can remember, they probably shouldn't be on the scene anymore. Monitoring rehab needs strictly by time is somewhat of a challenge. Time tends to compress for those who are involved in emergency operations and firefighters often lose track of time. It may be necessary to have someone who serves as a time recorder during the incident to ensure that crews are rotating out as necessary.

It should be noted that the above two requirements are progressive in nature. They are not optional choices. A common structure fire scenario can be used to highlight how this works.

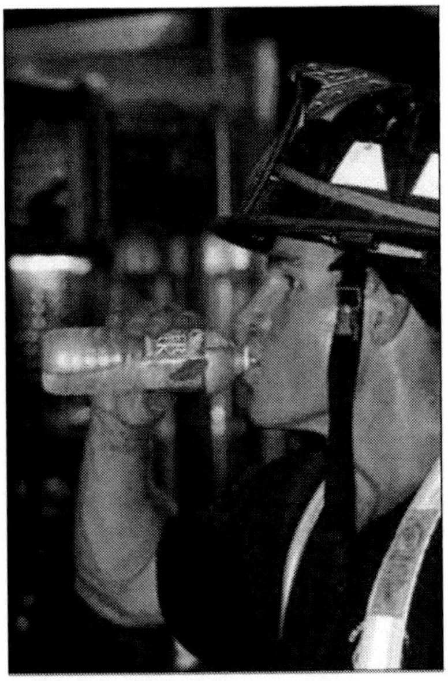

Figure 5.1. Courtesy of Dennis Wetherhold Jr., Allentown, PA.

Engine 65 is engaged in a fire attack at a garden apartment fire. Their firefighters are equipped with 30-minute SCBAs. After attacking the fire for some time the company is forced to retreat when one of the members'low air-pressure alarm begins to sound.The crew exits the structure and reports to a utility vehicle in order to change out SCBA cylinders. While at the utility vehicle the crew also drinks some water that is provided there and rests for about 10 minutes. Following this period Engine 65's captain deems the crew ready for reassignment and requests orders from the Incident Commander (IC).The IC assigns the Engine 65 crew to perform overhaul operations inside the structure.

Engine 65 s crew enters the structure and begins overhaul activities. After operating for a period of time the crew is again forced to exit the structure when one member's low air-pressure alarm sounds. Upon exiting the structure for the second time (after having expended two SCBA cylinders) the crew reports to the designated rehab area. Once at the rehab area they doff their protective clothing and SCBAs, receive a medical evaluation, drink the provided beverages and eat some snacks, and rest for a minimum of 20 minutes. If the firefighters remain engaged at the incident they will need to report to rehab after every subsequent SCBA cylinder use or following 20 more minutes of intense work.

It should also be noted that NFPA 1584 states that any firefighters entering the rehab area prior to going through two SCBA cylinders or performing 40 minutes of intense work should receive the same medical evaluation and rehab services as would firefighters who had met that criteria.

The guidelines from NFPA 1584 should be considered minimums and individual fire departments may choose to establish different parameters. One example of a modified protocol can be found in the International Association of Fire Fighters' (IAFF's) T*hermal Heat Stress Protocol for Firefighters and Hazmat Responders*. This document recommends a 30-minute work period followed by 30 minutes of rest in a rehab area. The firefighter's heart rate should be assessed as soon as he/she enters the rehab area. Some agencies allow the firefighter to assess his/her own rate. If his/her pulse exceeds 75 percent of his/her age-adjusted maximum heart rate (AAMHR), the responder worked too long and his or her next work cycle should be decreased by one third (from 30 minutes to 20 minutes). The AAMHR is calculated by subtracting the person's age from a constant of 220 (220 - age = AAMHR). If the AAMHR is impractical to use, a value of 110 beats-per-minute may be substituted. This value is low, but it should ensure that all responders who are at risk of dehydration are adequately identified. Under the AAMHR, a young responder would be "allowed" a much higher pulse, but will suffer no penalty in adhering to this 110 action level, other than being observed during his rest cycle.

Regardless of which one of the above procedures is implemented, it is absolutely crucial that all responders follow these guidelines. No one, including officers, should be allowed to skip the rehab process. Enforcement of this policy will have a measurable affect on the long-term well-being of all the firefighters.

The Rehab Process

Assuming that we have assembled the proper equipment and established requirements for firefighters to participate in the rehab process at an incident scene or training session, we must then ensure that all the mechanisms are in place to run the rehab operation in an organized and structured manner. Rehab operations should be viewed and managed as a process, rather than a single event. There are various parts to the rehab process and each has its own importance in the overall well-being of the firefighters who are participating in the process.

This section examines the various parts of the rehab process. They are covered in a logical manner, the same order in which firefighters should proceed through the process. The overall rehab process includes both self-rehab and formal rehab components. Each of these is detailed below.

Self-Rehab

In the previous section it was noted that NFPA 1584 suggests that firefighters enter a formal rehab operation only after depleting their second SCBA cylinder or exceeding 40 minutes of otherwise strenuous work. The vast majority of incidents to which firefighters respond will not require this level of activity and thus will not contain a formal rehab area operation. In these incidents or training activities it will be incumbent on the firefighters to take care of themselves, or perform self-rehab. Self-rehab refers to the process of firefighters getting some rest and replenishing their fluid levels outside the constraints of a formal rehab area. In many cases self-rehab may be the only rehab activities performed at those short-duration events.

In most cases the self-rehab process will contain two simple components: taking a break and drinking fluids to replenish personal hydration levels. During training activities self-rehab is often built into the rotation process for firefighters working their way through a series of training ground evolutions. After every so many evolutions or on a time-measured basis, the firefighters will report to a rest area for a prescribed period of time. While at the rest area the firefighters will doff appropriate protective clothing, sit down, and drink fluids that are provided at that location. These may either be water or sport beverage-type fluids. At a minimum, firefighters should drink 2 to 4 ounces of an appropriate beverage after every 20 minutes of training or emergency scene activities. Greater amounts may be required depending on the activity level, atmospheric conditions, and the needs of each individual firefighter.

At incident scenes, self-rehab generally will occur whenever firefighters go for their first SCBA cylinder change or following a period of work at the incident scene. In either case the firefighters are relieved momentarily of the duties they were performing and have some time to rest and drink some fluids. NFPA 1584 recommends that the self-rehab period should be at least 10 minutes. Local conditions and policies may require this period to be longer.

Fluids for self-rehab at incident scenes may be found in a number of locations, depending on local Standard Operating Procedures (SOPs). The following is a sample of the common methods that are employed for providing fluids for self-rehab:

- Bulk-storage containers often are located on utility (air/power/light) vehicles, as this is where firefight ers will report when they need to replace or refill SCBA cylinders **(Figure 5.2).** In departments that have cascade cylinders on different vehicles, such as rescue apparatus, drink containers may be located on those vehicles.
- Bulk-storage containers or individual serving containers of fluids may be carried on all apparatus. They may be carried in the cab of the apparatus or a compartment. Some departments locate individual serv ing containers at the same location on the apparatus as spare SCBA cylinders.This encourages firefighters to drink some fluid when they retrieve the spare cylinder.
- Bulk containers or individual serving containers may be carried in command vehicles, other apparatus, or may be brought to the scene as needed **(Figure 5.3).**

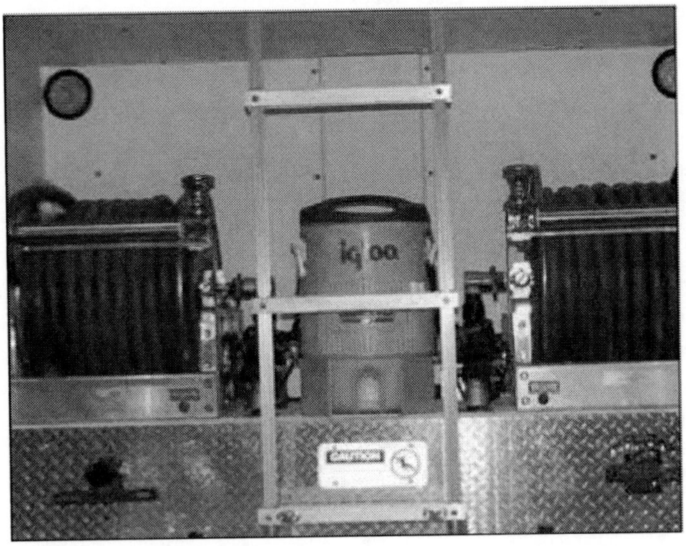

Figure 5.2.

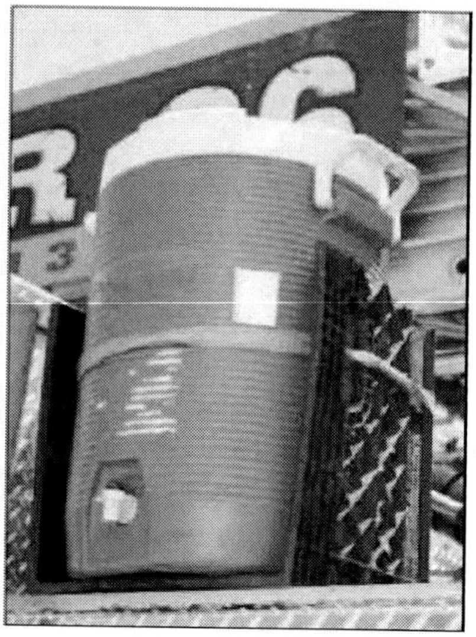

Figure 5.3.

Firefighters who self-rehab at an incident typically will do so in the area where they are servicing their SCBAs. It is most desirable to have other firefighters available to service the SCBA so that the rehabbing firefighters can rest and drink some fluids. After the firefighters have rested for at least 10 minutes and their equipment is ready for service, they may seek reassignment at the incident through the command system that is in place. COs or crew leaders should check all of their members to make sure they appear fit for further service. Should any of the crewmembers not appear fit, they should be referred to the formal rehab area or to medical personnel who are on the scene for further evaluation and rest. The remainder of the crew may be reassigned according to local SOPs.

Formal Rehab Operations

Formal rehab area operations will be established in situations where emergency incidents or training sessions will extend firefighters beyond the physical point where self-rehab activities are sufficient to ensure their well being. Once the decision to establish rehab operations has been made, it is important that the appropriate equipment and personnel are assembled to meet the need. The equipment needed to set up a rehab operation was covered in Chapter 4 of this publication. In this section we will discuss the personnel staffing needs for formal rehab operations and then highlight the progression of services that firefighters entering the rehab area will encounter once they are assigned there.

Rehab Area Staffing

Effective rehab operations cannot be established unless sufficient numbers of appropriately-qualified personnel are assigned to operate the rehab area. There are no set formulas for how many people will be required to run an effective rehab area. This will depend on a variety of factors, including

- the number of firefighters and other responders who will require rehab services;
- the duration of the incident;
- the environmental conditions at the time of the incident (more severe conditions will require more personnel); and
- the condition in which responders accessing the rehab are in when they arrive at the rehab area. The worse shape they are in, the more people that will be required to care for them.

The medical aspects of a rehab operation require that at least some of the personnel assigned to rehab operations be certified emergency medical personnel. In particular, the personnel assigned to perform both the initial assessment and medical evaluation/treatment functions should at least be certified EMT-Bs **(Figure 5.4).** When advanced life support (ALS) personnel are available, it is desirable that they be assigned to the rehab function as well. If the EMS personnel who are assigned to work in the rehab area are non-fire-service providers, it is important that they understand how to work in the incident management system that is being used at the incident and that they have radio communications with the fire department personnel with whom they are assigned.

The availability of ALS personnel is crucial at large-scale incidents, incidents that require firefighters to operate at the limits of their endurance, and those incidents in conditions where serious heat- and stress-related illnesses are likely. In these situations, ALS personnel should evaluate and treat the responders in rehab who appear to be in need of a higher level of care than EMT-Bs can provide. This care includes the establishment of intravenous (IV) lines for severely dehydrated personnel and advanced care of individuals with heat- or stress-related illnesses. In some cases, particularly at long-term, large-scale incidents, extended rehab operations may call for the use of medical doctors and/or registered nurses with the rehab operation. These people can provide a level of on scene care for responders with serious symptoms that exceeds that which standard EMS personnel may provide.

It must be re-emphasized that the EMS personnel who are assigned to operate in the rehab area must be different than those who would be assigned to transport patients who need to be seen at a hospital. It is not acceptable to strip the rehab operation of essential medical personnel in order to transport a patient to the hospital.

There are plenty of functions to be carried out within the rehab operation that do not require personnel to have emergency medical training, such as food and beverage service and servicing breathing apparatus. In many jurisdictions, members of the fire department's Ladies' Auxiliary, members of an Explorer Post, or departmental civilian staff members fill this function. In addition, agencies such as the American Red Cross and the Salvation Army, local civic organizations such as the Lion's Club and the Rotary Club, local food retailers, or fire buff organizations offer additional nutritional support **(Figure 5.5).** As mentioned above for third-service EMS organizations, if these other personnel are not members of the fire department it is important that they know how to operate in the command system that is in place at the incident and that all fire department policies for rehab operations be adhered to strictly. No one should attempt to provide services for which they are not explicitly qualified to perform.

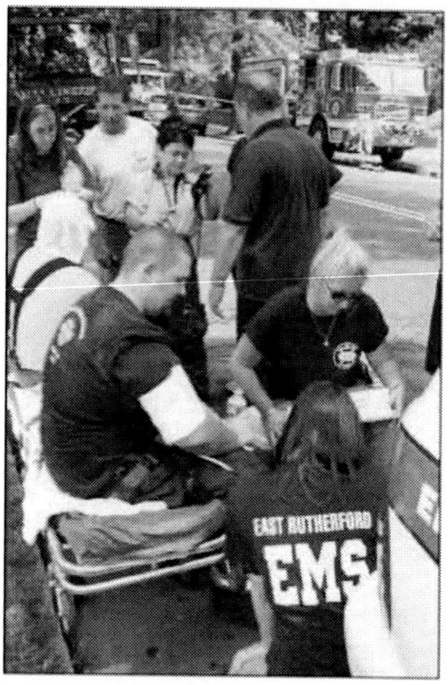

Figure 5.4. Courtesy of Ron Jeffers, Union City, NJ.

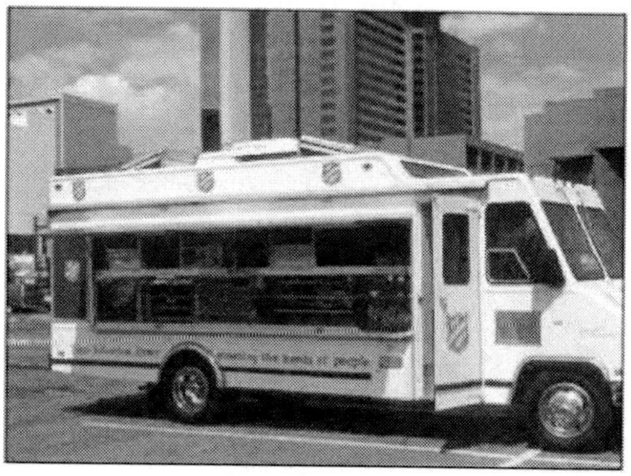

Figure 5.5.

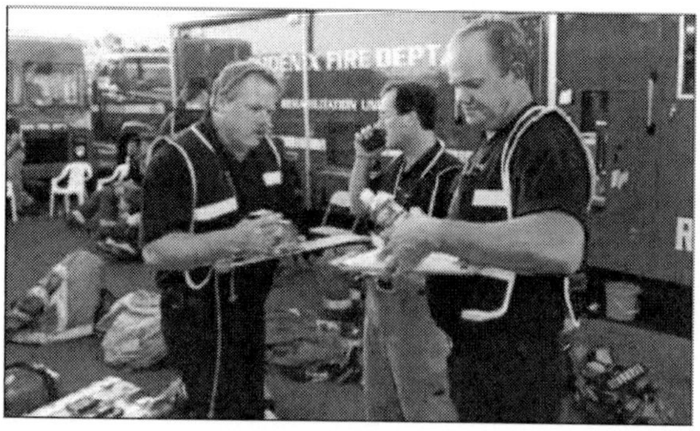

Figure 5.6. Courtesy of Phoenix, AZ Fire Department.

Entry Point/Initial Assessment

The first point of contact for all responders who are assigned to report to a rehab area must be with the designated Entry Point for the rehab operation. All rehab operations must have a single, designated Entry Point through which all responders will report when accessing the area. This ensures that all personnel will be logged in according to local procedures, their accountability markers will be collected, and they will receive an initial assessment of their medical condition and well-being **(Figure 5.6).** From an accountability standpoint, it is most desirable for crews or companies to report to rehab as a whole group. This eliminates the need to hunt for scattered groups should a rapid head count be required.

The individual collecting the accountability tags and logging personnel into the rehab area needs only to be familiar with the accountability system and login procedures used in that jurisdiction. It does provide an extra layer of observation if the login person has some emergency medical training, but it is not required, as long as other personnel in the entry area are capable of performing an initial medical assessment of the personnel once they arrive.

Once the firefighters have logged into the rehab area they should shed their SCBA, if they are wearing one, as well as any other special protective equipment. The exceptions to this statement are people who have been wearing chemical protective garments and potentially had been exposed to hazardous materials. Those personnel should go through decontamination and remove the chemical protective clothing before they proceed to the rehab area.

Ideally, the rehab area will be located in an area whose climate allows the firefighters to remove there regular turnout clothing as well.This is important in warm weather situations, as there is a need for the firefighter's body temperature to be cooled as much as possible. Turnout coats, protective hoods, gloves, and helmets should be removed completely. Protective trousers and boots should also be removed if possible. At the very least, protective pants should be rolled down over the boots, if the boots are to be left on **(Figure 5.7).** This allows the lower body to cool faster than if the pants remain on.

Once the firefighters have shed their gear they should be given an initial assessment to check for signs of injuries and/or heat- and stress-related illnesses. This initial assessment should be performed by at least an EMT-Basic; if higher trained medical personnel are available they should be used. The initial assessment must include obtaining entry vital signs, including blood pressure, pulse, and temperature. The results of this assessment will be used to determine whether the firefighter simply needs some rest and rehydration, or if he/she needs more detailed medical evaluation and treatment.

Each fire department needs to establish criteria in their SOPs on vital signs that require medical treatment or on the minimum rehab time needed on the basis of various levels of vital signs. NFPA 1584 does not provide any requirements on these levels. Various publications and research studies suggest slightly different criteria for triggering further medical evaluation and treatment. In general, the following criteria may be used, unless locally validated criteria are established

- pulse in excess of 120 bpm;
- body temperature in excess of 100.5 °F (38 °C);
- diastolic blood pressure above 90 mmHg; and
- systolic blood pressure above 130 mmHg.

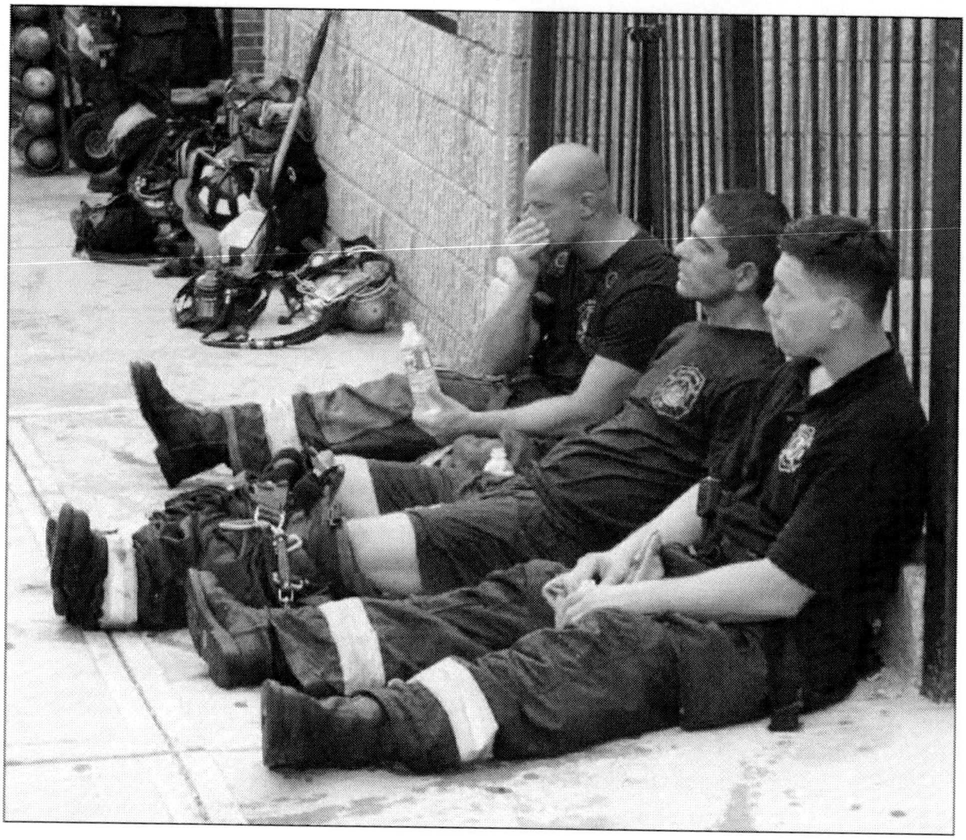

Figure 5.7. Courtesy of Ron Jeffers, Union City, NJ.

In addition to simply taking vital signs, the rehab personal should also look for other possible clues of injury or distress, including chest pains, shortness of breath, altered level of consciousness, extreme fatigue, poor skin color, and similar symptoms. It is a good idea to talk to the firefighters while they are being evaluated to determine how they respond. Any members who have unacceptable vital signs or who exhibit any other signs of an injury or illness should be sent to the Medical Evaluation/Treatment Unit for further evaluation and treatment. Responders who appear to be in relatively good condition should be directed to the Rest and Refreshment Unit.

Rest and Refreshment Unit

The Rest and Refreshment Unit is responsible for three functions that are extremely important in allowing tired, but otherwise medically fit, firefighters to be ready to return to duty: providing rest, fluid replacement, and nutritional support. It is important for resting firefighters to replace body fluids that were lost through sweating during their work period so that they will be able to maintain their general well-being and be able to report back for duty, if so required by the demands of the incident.

During warm weather operations, the Rest and Refreshment Unit may be in an air conditioned area, such as a building, rehab unit, or a bus. It is important for firefighters to first allow their bodies to cool down somewhat before entering the air conditioned area. This will prevent an extreme thermal shock load on the body that could result in the body's inability to help cool itself. Before entering the air conditioning, the firefighter can rest in a shaded area (if during daylight hours), which may be equipped with fans or misting equipment to help their bodies cool down for a few minutes at the ambient temperature before entering the chilled environment (**Figure 5.8**).

On the contrary, when operating in cold weather conditions there should be no delay in allowing firefighters to enter a heated environment, if one is available. The process of heating a cooled body does not provide the same level of thermal shock on the system as does rapid cooling of a heated person.

The amount of time that firefighters need to spend in the Rest and Refreshment Unit varies depending on a variety of conditions, including.

- the responder's level of physical conditioning;
- the atmospheric conditions;
- the nature of the activities the responder was performing before entering rehab; and
- the time needed for adequate rehydration and/or eating.

NFPA 1584 states that the minimum amount of time that must be spent in rehab following the initial assessment is 10 minutes. This amount of time is increased to 20 minutes if the responder has depleted two 30-minute SCBA cylinders or one 45- or 60-minute SCBA cylinder, was wearing encapsulating chemical protective clothing, or was otherwise performing hard labor for 40 minutes. Many doctors and experts actually recommend longer rest periods than the minimums provided by NFPA 1584. Each jurisdiction should develop and validate criteria for their personnel. More detailed information on work-to-rest ratios was discussed earlier in this chapter and may be followed when developing local policies.

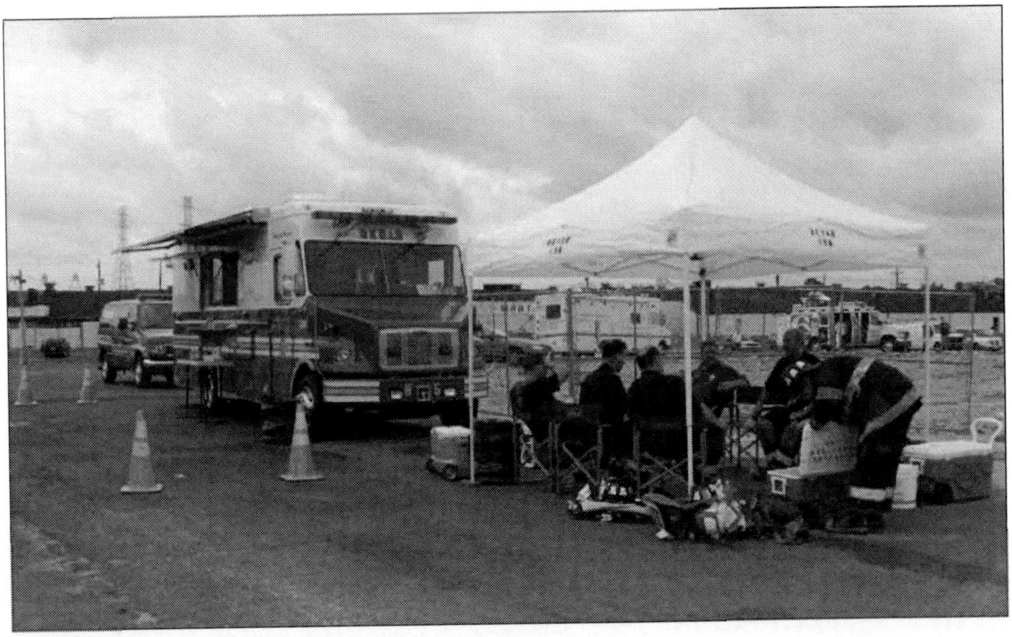

Figure 5.8. Courtesy of Cherry Hill, NJ Fire Department.

While there are a variety of opinions and sources of information on minimum rest times; little information exists on maximum rest times. Obviously, the longer we can allow personnel to rest, the better off they will be in the long run. However, the maximum amount of time that we can afford to have people in the rehab area will depend on a variety of factors, including the demands of the incident and the number of available personnel. It is a generally accepted principle that any responder who does not appear to be in a condition suitable for returning to action following 30 minutes of rest should be sent to the Medical Evaluation/Treatment Unit for further evaluation. Depending on the results of that evaluation the firefighter may be ordered to rest a little longer, seek medical treatment, or simply ordered to return to quarters or home.

The second important function carried out in the Rest and Refreshment Unit is the provision of fluids for rehydrating firefighters. The signs and dangers of dehydration were covered in detail earlier in this document. While rehab personnel can do little to ensure that personnel are prehydrated adequately before an incident or training exercise occurs, they certainly can ensure that firefighters maintain adequate hydration during the course of the incident. Maintaining sufficient levels of water and electrolytes in firefighters' bodies is a major step towards the prevention of heat- and/or stress-related illness and injury. Information on proper hydration and prehydration levels, as well the appropriate type of fluids for rehab operations, is discussed in detail later on in this chapter of the manual.

The manner in which drinks will be served in the rehab area depends on local resources, departmental preferences, and in some cases the scope if the incident. Regardless of what serving manner is used, the beverages should be readily accessible to the firefighters who are in this unit **(Figure 5.9).** In general, there are two ways to serve rehab beverages: individual serving containers (cans or bottles) or from large service dispensers using drinking cups. There are advantages and disadvantages of each of these methods.

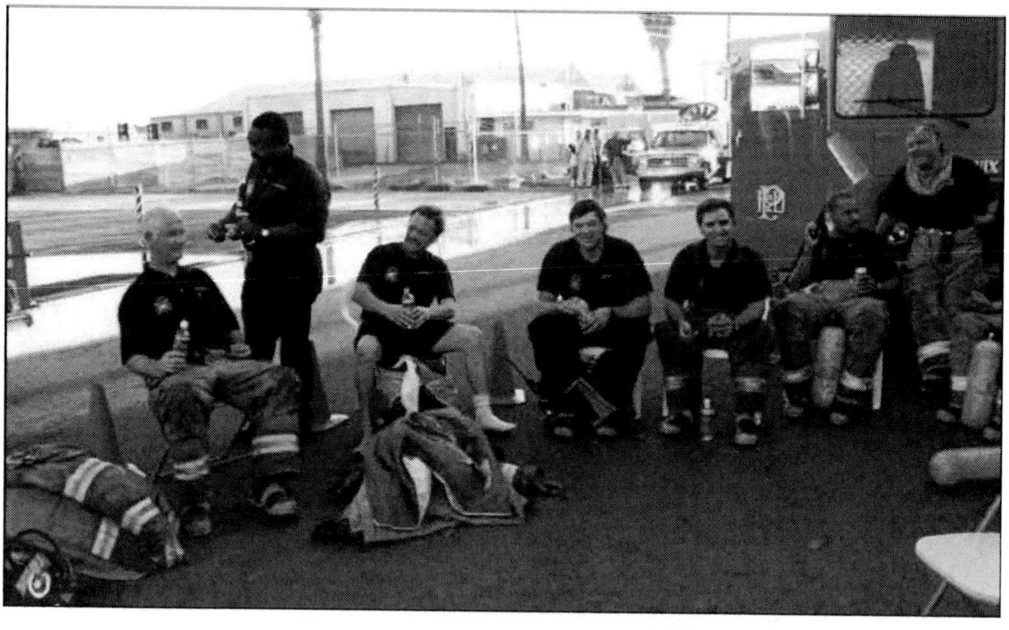

Figure 5.9. Courtesy of Phoenix, AZ Fire Department.

Individual serving containers are extremely convenient and sanitary. Firefighters drink straight from the container so additional cups are not needed. The drinks typically have long shelf-lives and can be stored on apparatus or in supply rooms for extended periods of times and still be acceptable for use. There are, however, several drawbacks to using individual serving containers. Many doctors recommend that sport beverages be mixed with even parts of plain water (a 50/50 concentration) before serving to firefighters. When using individual serving containers this is only possible if the firefighter first pours out half of the sport beverage and then refills it with water. This is inconvenient and wasteful. Individual containers also require a substantial amount of storage space and may not be practical on large scale incidents. They are best suited for short duration incidents with small numbers of rehabbing firefighters.

Serving fluids in large drinking dispensers is best suited for large-scale incidents with high numbers of rehabbing firefighters. Most approved sports beverages can be provided in a powdered form and mixed with water when needed at an incident. Make sure that the drinking containers are kept clean and that only suitable drinking water is used in the containers when put into service. Make sure that reasonably-sized drinking cups are made available with the dispensing containers. Regardless of whether individual containers or large dispensers are used, make sure waste collection equipment is nearby to collect the trash that accumulates when cups and containers are emptied.

The third function of the Rest and Refreshment Unit is the provision of nutritional support, or food, when needed at an incident. While every incident that requires rehab operations will require beverages to be served to firefighters, a lesser number of events will require food support. Most jurisdictions have established criteria for when food services will need to be provided within the rehab function.This often is based on the expected duration of the incident or the time of day at which the incident occurs. A common incident duration time that is used to trigger the response of food services is 3 or more hours. This may be adjusted down if the incident occurs early in the morning or over a meal time. In these situations it may have been an extended period of time since the firefighters had their last meal and they may require the energy boost.

Who serves the food at incidents and what type of food is served highly depends on local resources and SOPs. Some fire departments have their own canteen apparatus that respond to the scene and provide food services **(Figure 5.10).** In other jurisdictions there are service organizations such as the Red Cross, Salvation Army, or fire buff organizations that provide these services. Regardless of who provides the food and what type of food they provide, it is crucial that all food services follow proper sanitary and health guidelines for food service. State or local health department guidelines may apply to these operations. Failure to follow these guidelines could risk making responders ill. More details on the appropriate types of food that can be provided at incidents is covered later in this chapter.

Medical Evaluation/Treatment Unit

When personnel performing the initial assessment at the rehab entry point determine that a firefighter needs a more thorough examination or some type of medical treatment, the firefighter is assigned to the Medical Evaluation/Treatment Unit. For ease of discussion, this unit will herein be referred to simply as the Treatment Unit. Before getting any further into this section it is important to note that the Treatment Unit in the rehab operation should not be confused with the Treatment Unit (usually in the Operations Section) for victims at a mass casualty incident. They are two distinctly different operations: one caters only to incident victims and the other (rehab's) only to firefighters and other first responders requiring medical attention.

NFPA 1584 requires that the Treatment Unit be staffed by the highest level of emergency medical care providers on the scene. When available, ALS personnel such as paramedics, cardiac technicians, EMT-Intermediates, or physician's assistants should staff the Treatment Unit. On large-scale and long-term rehab operations it may be possible to have medical doctors assist in staffing this function.

Firefighters who are referred to the Treatment Unit should receive a thorough medical evaluation that is based on the symptoms they present and standard local emergency medical services (EMS) protocols. This should include the establishment of medical documentation for each person sent to the Treatment Unit. Standard EMS patient forms/reports can be used for this purpose. When illnesses or injuries are identified, aggressive procedures to stabilize or correct the problems also should be initiated according to the protocols. This may include functions such as heart monitoring, oxygen administration, active body cooling, establishing IVs, and standard splinting and bandaging.

In many cases the firefighter's condition and vital signs will improve once they have rested, cooled down, and received some fluid and nutritional support. If this is not the case, the firefighter typically should be transported to an appropriate medical facility, per local protocols, for further evaluation and treatment. Any firefighter that requires ALS treatment, such as the establishment of an IV, in the rehab area should be transported to a medical facility to be seen by a doctor **(Figure 5.11).**

In summary, there are three basic dispositions for firefighters who are sent to the Treatment Unit within a rehab operation:

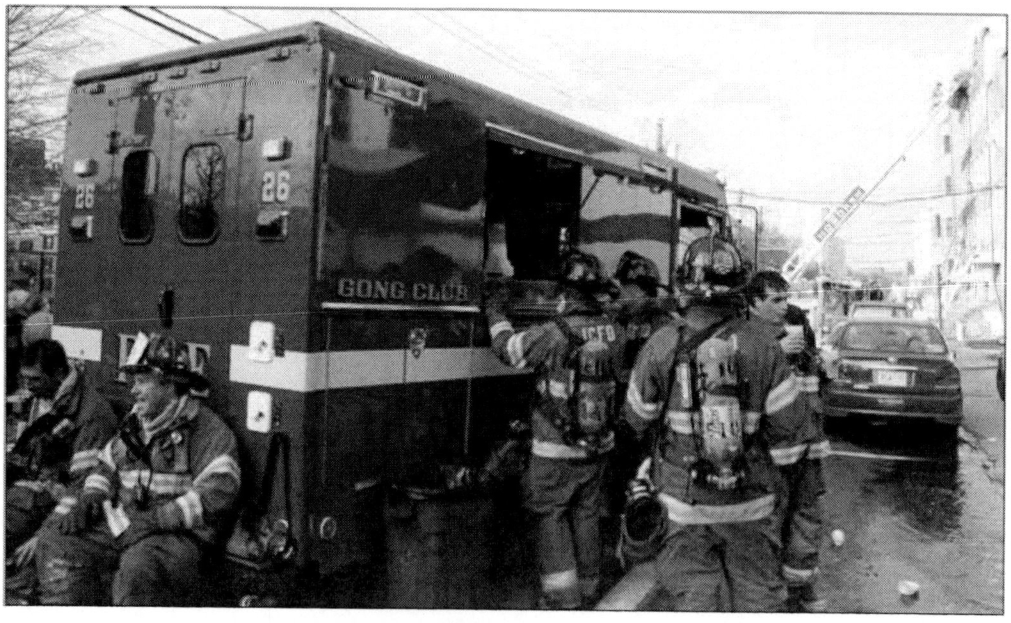

Figure 5.10. Courtesy of Ron Jeffers, Union City, NJ.

1. The responder responds appropriately to rest and rehydration and is able to return to action or return to quarters. The person often is moved from the Treatment Unit to the Rest and Refreshment Unit before leaving the rehab area.
2. Standard, basic EMS treatment procedures are initiated and the firefighter is monitored to see if the treat ment corrects the situation they are facing.
3. Advanced medical treatment, followed by transport to a medical facility, is required. Make sure that any paperwork that is started on the patient is transported to the hospital per local protocols.

Fire departments should develop a policy for filing medical paperwork that is developed on personnel who enter the Treatment Unit in the rehab operation. Copies of this information may be placed in the firefighter's personnel file, may be attached to the incident report, or may be otherwise filed according to local EMS protocols. More detailed information on common injuries and illnesses encountered in rehab operations and their basic treatments is covered later in this chapter.

Responders in the Treatment Unit should have access to fluids and food as their condition allows. In many cases, the symptoms that forced their assignment to the area are corrected easily with fluids and rest. In some instances, however, responders' conditions will not improve without more significant medical intervention. Responders whose signs and/or symptoms indicate potential problems should be treated and transported in accordance with local protocols established by the medical director. Any responders who require ALS procedures, such as IV rehy-dration, must be removed from the action for the duration of the incident.

Appropriate documentation for every responder assigned to the Treatment Unit is essential. The standard forms used on routine EMS calls can be used in the Treatment Unit. The responder's name and agency should be recorded, along with vital signs, pertinent medical complaints, and treatment information. If a responder eventually is transported to a hospital, this paperwork should be given to the transporting crew. If the responder is not transported, the forms should be made part of the incident report.

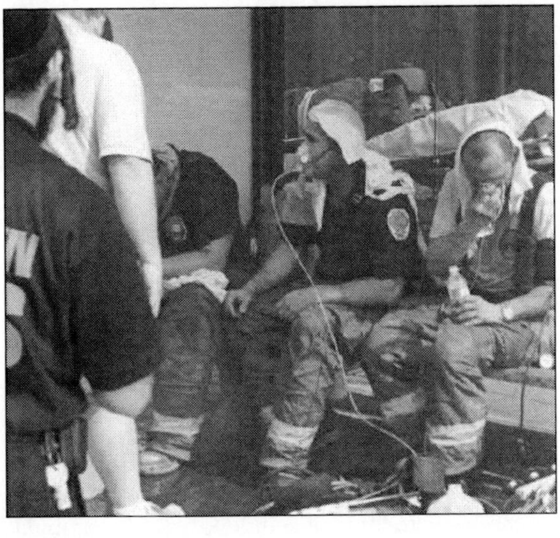

Figure 5.11. Courtesy of Ron Jeffers, Union City, NJ.

Personnel who respond favorably to treatment in the Treatment Unit may then be allowed to go to the Rest and Refreshment Unit or to report for reassignment. More detailed information on the medical evaluation and treatment of responders can be found in Chapter 4.

Transportation Unit

The Transportation Unit is responsible for transporting firefighters to an appropriate medical facility who need greater attention than can be provided by the Treatment Unit. As discussed above in the Treatment Unit section, the Transportation Unit within the rehab operation should not be confused or commingled with any Transportation Unit that is established in the Operations Section for incident victims. A Transportation Unit Leader should be assigned to coordinate this function.

It is also important to note that it typically is not good to commingle Treatment Unit and Transportation Unit resources within the rehab operation. In other words, whenever possible, personnel who are staffing Treatment Unit functions should not be responsible for transporting firefighters requiring further medical attention to the hospital. To do this will strip the Treatment Unit of the personnel they need to perform their duties. This compromises the efficient care of later arriving firefighters in the Treatment Unit.

The following is a summary of the major responsibilities of the Transportation Unit Leader, based on the Transportation Unit's role in the rehab operation:

- Determine and arrange all transportation needs for the rehab operation.
- Determine the availability of medical facilities with special capabilities, such as trauma centers, burn units, and/or hyperbaric centers.
- Allocate patients to medical facilities in consultation with the Treatment Unit Leader and personnel at the receiving facilities.
- Establish a site from which to manage patient transportation from the rehab area to appropriate medical facilities.

The amount of resources assigned to the Transportation Unit function within the rehab operation will depend on the overall size of the rehab operation, the number of firefighters cycling through rehab, and the level of risk or physical exertion posed to the firefighters working at the incident. At a minimum, at least one ambulance should always be on scene and available to transport any firefighter requiring medical treatment at a hospital. Multiple ambulances will be required for larger rehab operations. All resources, such as ambulances, that are needed for the Transportation Unit should be ordered through the Incident Command System (ICS) that is in place for the incident.

The Transportation Unit Leader should notify local medical facilities when major rehab operations are initiated. This allows the medical facilities to activate internal plans for the potential of accepting significant numbers of patients. It is also important to do this from a protocol standpoint, as ALS patients will be treated according to standing protocols with these facilities. Medical facilities should be updated on incident status as the incident progresses.

Local policies and preferences will dictate whether ambulances assigned to the rehab Transportation Unit are staged in direct proximity to the Rehab Area or at a remote Staging Area. On smaller incidents, where only a single or a few ambulances are required, the ambulance(s) may be positioned at the Rehab Area as space allows. In larger incidents it may be necessary to stage the ambulances at a remote Staging Area. This may be the standard Staging Area for all incident resources or it may be a separate area specifically for ambulances assigned to the Transportation Unit. If the Staging Area is remote from the Rehab Area, it is important that access and egress routes for the ambulances be kept open and clear at all time. The Transportation Unit Leader also may anticipate the need for air medical evacuation and should identify potential landing sites for helicopters in the event they become needed.

When the Treatment Unit determines that a firefighter in rehab will need to be taken to a medical facility for further evaluation and/or treatment, the Transportation Unit Leader must be notified of the need. The Treatment Unit should advise the Transportation Unit Leader of any special requirements (need for a burn unit, air medical evacuation, etc.) when making the request. The Transportation Unit Leader then assigns an ambulance to make the transfer to the hospital. Once the firefighter is ready to be transported, the transporting ambulance crew or other Transportation Unit members move the firefighter to the ambulance or helicopter. The Transportation Unit Leader also determines where the person will be transported and alerts that facility of the inbound patient. All parties must make sure that any medical reports/documentation that was started on the patient remain with him/her and are transported to the hospital along with the patient. As patients are transported from the scene, hospitals should be advised of estimated arrival times and of basic patient information.

When firefighters are transported by staged ambulances from the incident, the Transportation Unit Leader should request a replacement ambulance to assume the standby role. The number of ambulances on standby may be reduced as the number of personnel on the incident decreases during the normal course of operations. However, at least one should remain on site until all firefighters clear the scene.

Reassignment Unit

The Reassignment Unit is responsible for releasing personnel from the Rehab Unit. According to NFPA 1584, there are three basic dispositions for personnel who have been assigned to the Rehab Unit:

1. If they are in suitable condition they may be reassigned to another function on the emergency scene.
2. If they are in good condition, but their services at the emergency scene are no longer required, they can return to service and be sent back to the station or home, as the case may be.
3. If deemed necessary, they can be transported to a hospital for further evaluation and/or treatment.

In most cases the Reassignment Unit will be dealing with firefighters who fall into one of the first two disposition criteria discussed above. Firefighters who required significant medical treatment within the Rehab Unit or who had been transported to a medical facility must not be reassigned to the same incident.

On smaller incidents the Reassignment Unit actually may be a single person. In these cases an individual person assigned to the function should be able to verify that the crews are ready to return to duty, return their accountability markers, and log them out of the Rehab

Unit. On large-scale incidents it may be necessary to assign multiple people to manage these tasks to ensure that none of the steps are missed. If there are people with emergency medical training checking on the firefighters as they leave the Rest and Refreshment Area, it is not necessary that the personnel in the Reassignment Unit be emergency medical personnel. However, regardless of the level of their EMS training, Reassignment personnel should be alert for firefighters who say they are ready to return for duty, but appear otherwise.

Although as had been stated previously there is a desire to always keep whole crews intact through the rehab process, there may be occasions where one member of the crew is not ready to return to service when the remainder of the crew clearly is fit for duty and ready for reassignment. In these situations the following options are available to the Reassignment Unit Leader:

- The remaining crew members may be paired up with another group of firefighters and one crew leader can be designated for the new crew.
- The remaining crew members may be reassigned as a single crew to a function that can be handled with the remaining number of crew members. If the missing crew member was the leader of the crew, such as a CO, then a new crew leader must be established.
- If the member that did not return to service was injured severely or is suffering from a serious illness, the remaining crew members may need to be removed from service, particularly if the crew members were involved in treating the victim. In these situations it might be difficult for the remaining crew members to maintain a safe focus on emergency functions and they may be in need of starting the criti cal incident stress management (CISM) process.

Once a crew has been determined to be fit for duty, the Reassignment Unit Leader should notify the appropriate ICS entity of their availability. Depending on what portions of the ICS toolbox have been activated, this may be the IC, Operations Section Chief, or the Staging Officer. On large-scale incidents it most likely will be the Staging Officer and the crew will report to Staging until another assignment is given to it. On smaller incidents the crew may be ordered to a new tactical assignment location directly upon leaving the Rehab Area. Regardless of where the crew is directed to go, they should collect the accountability tags or markers from the Reassignment Unit Leader and pass them on to their new assignment according to departmental protocols.

Demobilizing Rehab Operations

Remember that the Rehab operation should remain proportional with the size of the incident as the incident progresses through its normal stages. As the incident grows, so should the ability to rehab greater numbers of firefighters. Conversely, as an incident begins to wind down, the rehab operation may be scaled back as well. However, some prudence in scaling back rehab operations is warranted. While it may be tempting to drastically scale back or shut down rehab operations once the major part of the emergency operations have been concluded, the ability to provide all the necessary rehab services must be maintained until the very end of the incident. If these services can be maintained with a smaller number of rehab crew members, it is fine to release some of them to return to service.

Although the number of firefighters may decrease as an incident is brought under control, clearly the work is not yet done. In many cases the work that remains when a fire is brought under control is actually the most demanding part required of firefighters at that incident. Activities such as salvage and overhaul operations are physically taxing on firefighters, especially when those firefighters have been operating at the incident for an extended period of time already. The Rehab Unit must be ready to service those firefighters who remain on the scene performing these activities.

Once rehab crews have been released from service at the incident, they should make sure that their apparatus is readied for service, all supplies are restocked, and they are available to initiate rehab operations at another incident when the next one occurs. Final remaining Rehab crew members should also police the area where rehab operations were held and make sure that all trash and other debris is picked up and properly disposed of. The area should look better following the rehab operation than it did before the incident. This is very important from a public relations standpoint. It is also important from a public health standpoint, should discarded medical supplies be left and picked up by children or other people who use the area following this incident. More information on demobilizing and terminating rehab operations is contained in Chapter 6 of this document.

Medical Evaluation and Treatment for Rehab Operations

Ensuring that firefighters who require medical attention get expedient and proper treatment when they arrive at the rehab area is certainly one of the most important functions of the overall rehab operation. All efforts must be made to ensure that the highest level of available EMS is positioned within the rehab operation Medical Evaluation and Treatment Unit so that firefighters who require aggressive medical care procedures receive them as soon as possible.

It is not the purpose of this chapter to be a detailed guide for the treatment of injuries and illnesses that may be encountered in a rehab area. Appropriate treatment of these injuries and illnesses is based on evolving current medical practices and standard protocols used within local EMS systems. This section of the report will, however, provide information on the most common types of injuries and illnesses encountered in rehab operations and highlight some suggestions for how they should be handled when they are encountered.

Medical personnel assigned to operate in the rehab operation may be faced with an almost endless variety of injuries and illnesses. However the most commonly encountered conditions that may require treatment can be broadly lumped into four categories:

- Traumatic injuries such as cuts, bruises, burns, sprains, fractures, and similar injuries.
- Thermal injuries such as heat-related illnesses, frostbite, and hypothermia.
- Stress-related illnesses such as heart attacks, strokes, or other cardiac-related problems.
- Respiratory illnesses related to exposure to heat, smoke, and toxic gases or chemicals.

Traumatic Injuries

Traumatic injuries such as cuts, sprains, strains, burns, and eye injuries are, by far, the most common medical conditions encountered in rehab operations. The vast majority of these injuries are minor in nature and can be treated using standard basic life support (BLS) procedures and protocols. Because of the dirty nature of firefighting operations and the other types of emergency scene environments in which firefighters operate, extra attention must be paid to ensuring that open wounds and eye injuries are cleaned extremely well before bandaging and other treatments.

Minor cuts typically can be cleaned and bandaged. More severe cuts also should be cleaned and covered. EMS personnel will need to determine whether the cut warrants further medical attention at a medical facility. Burns that cover less than 10 percent of the firefighter's total body surface should be covered with moist, sterile dressing. Burns exceeding that size should be covered with dry dressings. Again, local protocols on advanced life support procedures and further treatment for burns should be followed. Generally, all burn injuries, regardless of the size, should be evaluated by physicians at a medical facility.

Any suspected sprains, strains, or possible fractures should be splinted according to local EMS protocols **(Figure 5.12).** Anyone with this type of injury should be required to seek further medical attention at a hospital. X rays or other tests will need to be performed in order to determine the actual nature and severity of the injury.

Medical personnel working in rehab operations commonly will encounter eye injuries to firefighters. These injuries may be as a result of the eye being struck by a foreign object or from small pieces of foreign debris becoming stuck in the eye opening area. Without proper treatment, relatively minor eye ailments quickly can become serious. With proper treatment, even serious eye injuries may be mitigated before a permanent loss of sight occurs. Local protocols for handling eye injuries will vary depending on the level of emergency medical care that is provided. However, there are some basic steps that can be followed to ensure proper care in most cases.

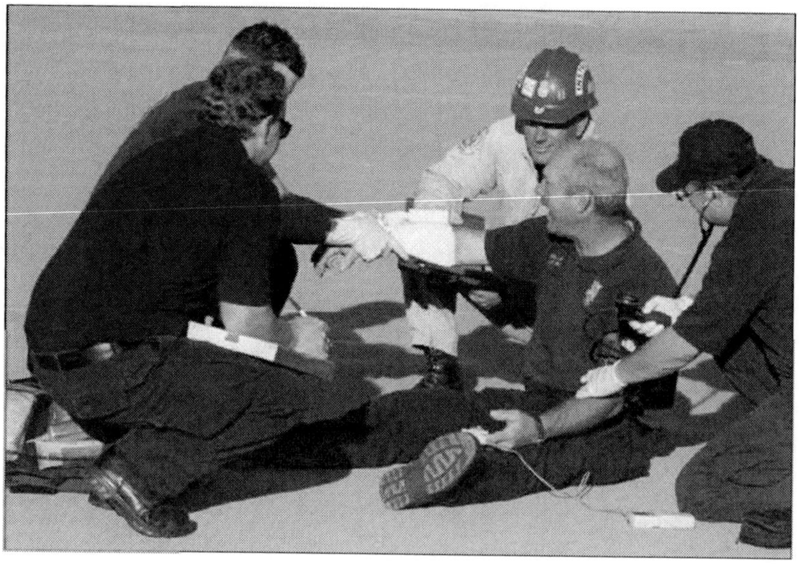

Figure 5.12. Courtesy of IFSTA/Fire Protection Publications.

Any small foreign debris that has become lodged around the eye should be irrigated with copious amounts of saline solution or sterile water. If minor scratches or abrasions are suspected, at least the affected eye should be covered with a clean dressing or eye patch. Some local protocols require both eyes to be covered. If there is a more serious laceration, imbedded object, or possible rupture of the eye ball, a rigid eye shield should be used to cover the eye during transport to a medical facility. If the eye has been exposed to a chemical agent, it should be irrigated continually with saline or sterile water on the scene and during transport to a medical facility.

Firefighters are a dedicated, hearty group of people who do not like to be pulled from an incident until the job is done. Medical personnel who are treating rehabbing firefighters with apparently minor traumatic injuries will need to determine whether the injured firefighter can be allowed to return to the incident, needs immediate treatment at a medical facility, or should be released from service and required to seek further medical evaluation before being able to return to duty. In many cases local EMS protocols will dictate the disposition of the firefighter based on the severity of their injury. In cases where this is not so clear and the firefighter wishes to return to duty, two criteria may be used to determine whether or not it is prudent for the firefighter to do so. First, if there is any chance that the injury may be worsened or subject to infection by participating in further emergency operation, the firefighter should not be allowed to continue. Secondly, if the injury is such that it impairs the firefighter from completely and safely performing their duties, they also should be removed from service.

Thermal Injuries

Other than minor traumatic injuries, the next most common medical problem that will be encountered by firefighters in rehab operations are typically those involving heat- or cold-related problems. In emergency response or training situations that are conducted in moderately to severely hot/humid or cold conditions it is likely that the vast majority of firefighters accessing the rehab area may be suffering from at least minor symptoms of exposure to these conditions.

Severe cold conditions that might endanger firefighters who are exposed to them typically are limited to specific portions of the U.S. and certain times of the year (winter). Moderate to high heat conditions and high humidity atmospheres can affect almost any portion of the U.S. and may do so over a greater portion of the calendar year. In reviewing firefighter injury and death statistics, heat-related problems historically are responsible for a much larger number of firefighter health and safety problems than are cold weather conditions (**Figure 5.13**).

EMS personnel assigned to all portions of the rehab operation, and particularly at the initial entry point and Medical Evaluation and Treatment Unit, must be alert for signs of possible heat- or cold-related medical problems. Heat-related problems, in particular, require immediate, aggressive treatment in order to minimize the long-term affects on the victim. For detailed information on the dangers, symptoms, and treatment of heat-related illnesses, see Chapter 2 of this document. Similar information for cold-related emergencies can be found in Chapter 3.

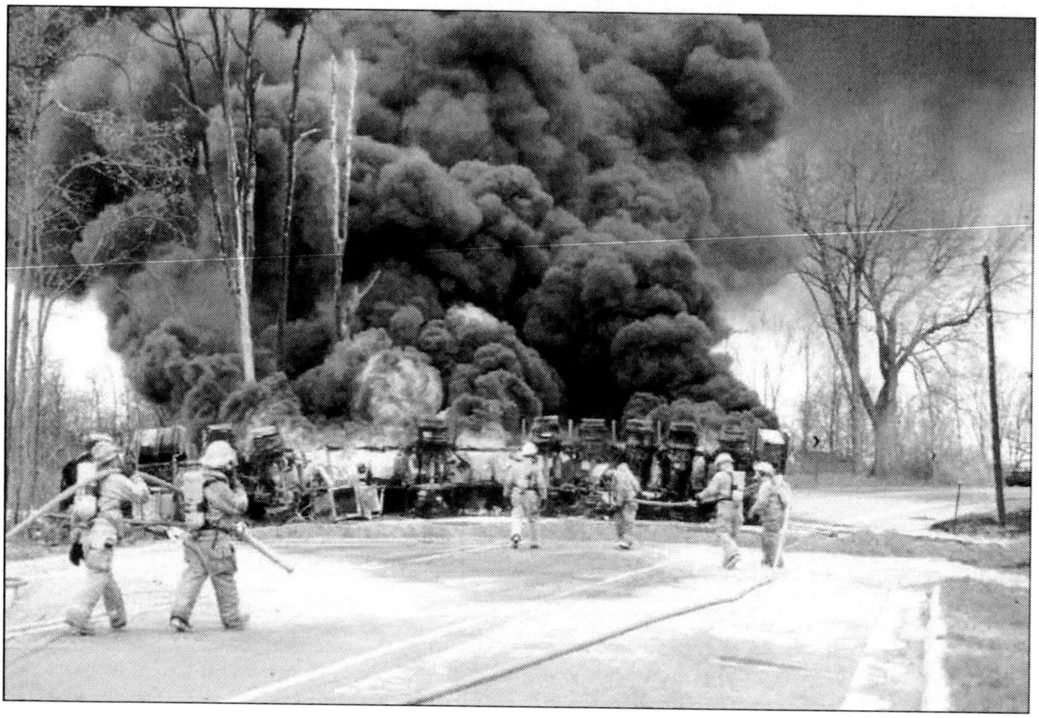

Figure 5.13. Courtesy of Rich Mahaney.

Stress-Related Illnesses

By its nature, firefighting imposes a significant amount of both psychological and physiological stress on firefighters. Increasingly, medical studies are showing that the negative impacts of both types of stress are related.

Statistically, the overall percentage of firefighters who suffer stress-related illnesses, such as heart attacks and strokes, at the emergency scene is actually very low. Annual firefighter injury statistics that are kept by both the NFPA and the U.S. Fire Administration (USFA) report that less than 2 percent of all firefighter injuries are stress-related. On the contrary, those same recordkeeping organizations report that 40 to 50 percent of all firefighter fatalities each year are as a result of stress-related illnesses. What this tells us is that while stress-related illnesses at emergency scenes are fairly uncommon, when they do occur they tend to be very severe. In fact, on average, about 1 out of every 1,500 firefighters who receive traumatic injuries will die as a result of those injuries. On the other hand, about 1 out of every 25 who suffer a stress-related illness will die as a result of that event.

Because of the life-threatening severity of stress-related illnesses when they do occur, it is incumbent on all fire service medical personnel operating at emergency scenes and training exercises to be alert for early signs of these problems in both themselves and the other personnel at the scene. Early intervention in these types of events greatly increases the survivability of the episode. The following section briefly discusses the various types of stresses and stress-related illnesses that may be encountered during rehab operations.

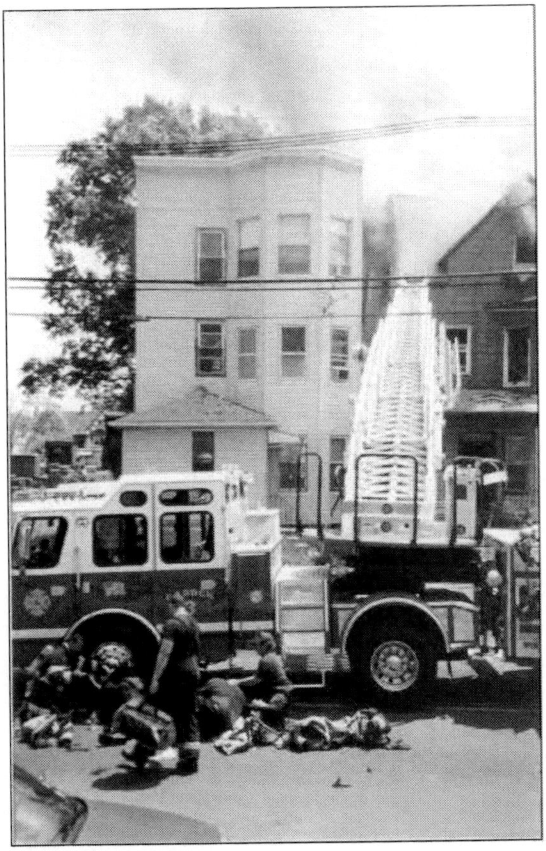

Figure 5.14. Courtesy of Ron Jeffers, Union City, NJ.

Psychological Stress

Historically, the identification of firefighters who may be suffering from the effects of excessive psychological stress was viewed solely as a function of the CISM process. In the same vein, the primary purpose tied to identifying and treating this stress was strictly for the long-term psychological well-being of the firefighter. Now that we recognize the link between psychological and physiological stress, it is important to identify victims of psychological stress before it manifests itself in physiological symptoms.

Of course, our most immediate concern for reducing the effects of psychological stress at emergency operations is to minimize the chance of a stress-induced cardiac event from occurring. But there are other concerns as well. Overly-stressed personnel often do not make the best decisions when faced with choices and might choose a course of action at an incident that creates undue danger to them or the other personnel whom with they are working. There also are potential long-term effects on the physiological well-being of overly stressed firefighters that may manifest in a variety of ways, including

- a decreased ability to mobilize the fight-or-flight response of the sympathetic nervous system of the firefighter;
- increases or decreases in the firefighter's appetite, either of which can result in long-term negative heal consequences;

- suppression of the firefighter's autoimmune system, resulting in a reduced capacity to fight off common infections; and
- an alteration in the perception of the severity of pain.

There is little that can be done to reduce the potential psychological stresses that will face firefighters at emergency scenes. Much of what firefighters do involves dealing with difficult, emotional situations (**Figure 5.14**). The best way to counteract these stresses is to ensure that the firefighter is emotionally stable and healthy prior the occurrence of a significant incident. This includes regular evaluation and participation in ongoing stress reduction programs. Firefighters who appear to be suffering the effects of psychological stress during everyday life need to be evaluated and treated accordingly before being allowed to participate in emergency operations.

The second way that psychological stresses can be minimized is to properly manage incidents that may expose firefighters to troubling conditions. When faced with an incident that may be difficult or troubling to firefighters, limit the number of firefighters dealing directly with the worst parts of the incident to the minimum number safely possible. Then rotate out personnel frequently to reduce the amount of time they are in the stressful situation. Proper rehabbing and CISM defusing during the rest periods will help reduce the stress level. More information on CISM programs is covered in Chapter 6 of this book.

Proper management of psychological stressors at emergency scenes also includes ensuring that the rehab area, where CISM debriefing may be taking place, is located in a place that does not add to the stress of the situation. This is one reason why most professionals advocate locating the rehab area well apart from the emergency operations. Clearly, it should not be in view of disturbing sights and it should provide a calm haven for personnel who have been working in stressful environments. This includes making sure that rehab is not located in close view to gruesome incident scene sights, victim treatment areas, field morgues, and similar locations.

Personnel working in rehab operation should be watchful for rehabbing firefighters who are showing signs of suffering from acute psychological stress.This stress can be manifested in a variety of ways, but some of the following are the more common ones:

- inappropriate levels of angry or aggressive behavior, in general or directed towards other people;
- obvious emotional symptoms such as crying, yelling, or a sense of panic, often in an uncontrolled manner; and
- signs of being withdrawn, in a state of shock, or being depressed.

Any firefighters who are noted to have any of these or other signs of significant psychological stress should be referred to the CISM personnel at the scene or required to seek counseling assistance per agency protocols. These personnel should not be allowed to resume emergency operations until they have been evaluated by appropriately-trained personnel and have been determined fit to resume duties.

Physiological Stress

This section will focus on the two most severe potential physiological stress illnesses that may be encountered during rehab operations: heart attacks and strokes. As mentioned above, though relatively rare on the emergency scene, the severe, often fatal, consequences associated with suffering one of these two illness warrants their discussion at this point in this chapter.

Because of the heavy equipment firefighters wear to perform their duties and the extremely physically demanding nature of the activities they are often required to perform, tremendous levels of stress are placed on the firefighter's body (**Figure 5.15**). The effects of this stress will include increased heart rates, elevated blood pressures, and raised body core temperatures, among other things. The impacts of these changes typically are more significant in firefighters who were not in good physical condition before the incident occurred, but in extreme situations they will eventually negatively affect even the most physically fit firefighter. Regardless of the level of fitness in a firefighter, it also must be recognized that many firefighters have pre-existing medical conditions, known or unknown to the individual, that may be exacerbated by the activities on the emergency scene and lead to a physiological emergency.

Clearly, the best way to lessen the chance of suffering a physiological illness during emergency operations, or at any other time for that matter, is to live a healthy lifestyle that includes exercise, proper nutrition, and plenty of rest (**Figure 5.16**). This gives firefighters higher levels of energy and fitness and increases their capacity for work. The goal is to avoid overextending the firefighter during periods of heavy work. In addition to possible cardiac-related illnesses, overexertion eventually will lead to exhaustion and dehydration. These conditions impair gross- and fine-motor skills, as well as impair cognitive abilities, such as rationalization and decisionmaking. Many minor injuries, such as trips and falls, are caused by reduced motor skills or lowered cognition.

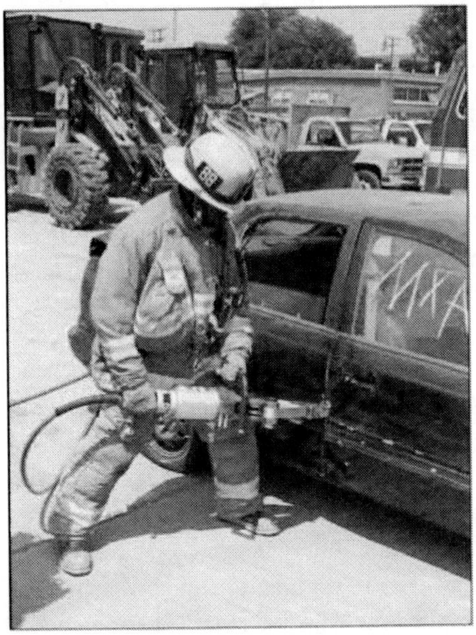

Figure 5.15.

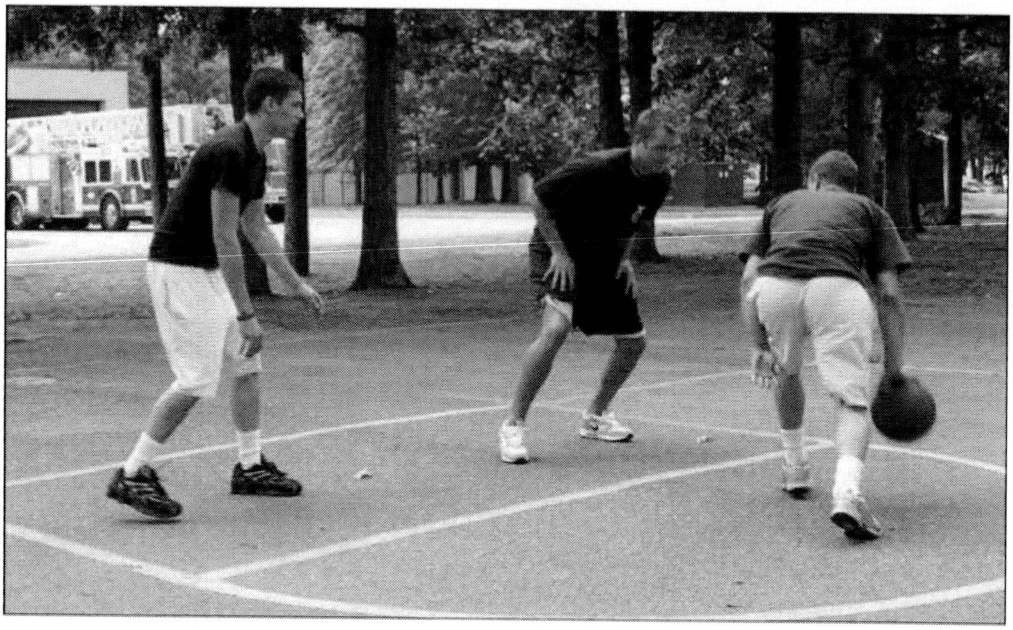

Figure 5.16. Courtesy of IFSTA/Fire Protection Publications.

Heart attacks—The human cardiopulmonary system consists of the heart, the lungs, circulatory vessels, and other related organs. In order for the cardiopulmonary system to operate properly, two basic functions must occur:

1. The lungs must function properly in order to ensure that adequate oxygen is delivered to the circulatory system and the rest of the body, and also to scrub carbon dioxide that accumulates in the bloodstream from the body.
2. The heart must operate correctly and pump a sufficient amount of blood through the circulatory system to ensure proper perfusion of all of the body's organs.

The combination of these two functions allows a person's body to function properly both under normal conditions and during periods of heavy exercise or other high physiological stresses placed on the body. A person's health, and life, will be endangered if either of these functions is compromised due to a chronic condition or an acute illness or injury.

The most common chronic (preexisting) condition that negatively impacts the circulatory system is coronary artery disease. This occurs when arteries that supply blood (perfusion) to the heart muscle become progressively narrowed over time by deposits of harmful materials such as cholesterol. The result is reduced blood flow to the heart muscle that can trigger a serious cardiac emergency, such as angina pectoris, an acute myocardial infarction (AMI), and dysrhythmias. Firefighters with this preexisting condition become particularly at risk during emergency or training operations because of the high amounts of physiologic stress that are placed on the body by this heavy exercise. This requires the heart to pump faster in order to supply increased amounts of blood needed to support the body. When the heart works faster, it requires greater amounts of oxygen to function properly. Narrowed arteries prevent sufficient blood flow to meet the increased demand. If the demand for blood flow exceeds the vessels' capacity to supply it, a condition called ischemia may occur. The symptoms of ischemia include shortness of breath and chest pain (angina pectoris). Ischemia also may lead to a disruption of the heart's electrical system, which may result in dysrhythmias such as ventricular fibrillation (VF). VF can result in sudden death, if not corrected.

If blood flow through one or more coronary arteries becomes completely blocked, not only will ischemia occur, but possibly also infarction, which is death of cardiac tissue. This may result in an AMI, or heart attack, that causes a lethal dysrhythmia.

Because of the serious nature of these illnesses, medical personnel staffing the rehab operation must be acutely aware of personnel who are exhibiting signs of potential cardiac emergencies. While the range of symptoms for people suffering a cardiac emergency are fairly broad, some of the most common ones include

- shortness of breath, beyond that of someone who simply has been working hard and is tired;
- tightness in the chest or chest pain, often radiating to the back, abdomen, or down one or both arms; and
- unusually rapid, slow, or otherwise irregular pulse and/or the sensation of heart palpitations.

Any firefighter who shows any signs of suffering a cardiac emergency should receive immediate treatment according to local protocols, by the highest-trained medical personnel on the scene. This treatment should include, at a minimum, the administration of high-flow oxygen and connection to an automated external defibrillator (AED), if available. If ALS personnel are available, the firefighter should be hooked to an electrocardiogram (EKG) monitor, should have a normal saline IV started, and may be administered cardiac drugs, according to local protocols. Once these actions have been taken, the firefighter should be transported to a medical facility as soon as possible. Strict adherence to these recommendations may make the difference between life and death for the firefighter.

Strokes—Cerebrovascular accidents (CVAs), also called strokes, typically result from the blockage of a cerebral artery in the brain.This blockage, typically a small blood clot, travels through the bloodstream and lodges in a vessel supplying blood to a particular part of the brain. This reduction or cessation of blood flow quickly affects that part of the brain. How it affects the brain, which in turn determines what symptoms will be present, varies greatly depending on the normal function of the affected portion of the brain. Some of the more common signs and symptoms include

- severe headache;
- difficult, slurred, or lost speech ability;
- facial droop; and
- weakness or paralysis on one side of the body, typically on the opposite side of the body from any pres ent facial droop.

As with heart attacks, the symptoms of a possible stroke have potentially fatal consequences and any firefighter who presents these symptoms should receive aggressive medical treatment by the highest-trained personnel on the scene, as soon as possible. Local protocols for this treatment will vary depending on the level of emergency medical care that is provided. At a minimum, efforts to ensure an open airway and the provision of supplemental oxygen must be initiated. Immediate transportation to a medical facility is crucial. Recent advances in medical technology, including the use of thrombolytic (clot-busting) medications, can greatly improve the outcome for stroke patients if they are administered within 3 hours of the onset of symptoms. This can only be accomplished following tests that must be performed in a medical facility.

Respiratory Illnesses /Emergencies

There are two primary respiratory illnesses or emergencies associated with fire emergency or training scenes: thermal injuries and smoke inhalation. In reality, in this day and age there is little or no reason for firefighters to suffer the effects of any respiratory illness or injury. Most fire departments are equipped with adequate numbers of SCBA. When used appropriately, this equipment will protect the firefighter from virtually any type of respiratory illness or injury. Firefighters who do suffer respiratory illnesses or injuries at an incident or training scene typically do so because of one of three reasons:

1. They fail to follow fire department SOPs requiring the use of available SCBA whenever operating in a potentially toxic atmosphere **(Figure 5.17).**
2. They do not to follow safe fireground tactical principles or otherwise become entrapped in a hazardous atmosphere and fail to exit the atmosphere prior to the depletion of the air in their SCBA.
3. They do not have functional SCBA and engage in tactical operations that should not be attempted unless properly equipped.

In jurisdictions where safe fireground operating procedures are frequently ignored, the potential for seeing personnel exhibiting signs of respiratory injury in the rehab area is fairly commonplace. In jurisdictions where good safety procedures are observed, these problems are not as common, and in some cases actually are quite rare. In either case it is important that medical personnel in the rehab operation be familiar with the signs and treatment for respiratory illness or injuries that may be encountered.

Thermal Injuries

Thermal injuries to the respiratory system typically occur when a firefighter who is not wearing a functional SCBA is exposed to, and breathes in, high levels of heat being generated from a fire. The majority of fireground thermal respiratory injuries occur to the upper airway, causing mucosal damage with erythema, ulceration, and edema. Visible signs of these injuries can include blistering or edema of the oropharynx and soot deposits in the nose or mouth. Stridor, dyspnea, and respiratory distress typically do not occur immediately, but often develop several hours after the thermal injury. Upper airway edema usually becomes apparent within 24 hours of injury and resolves itself within 3 to 5 days. Chest x rays of a victim suffering thermal respiratory injuries may appear to be normal. However, the combination of a moderate to severe thermal injury coupled with the presence of pulmonary infiltrates is associated with a poor prognosis for the patient.

Smoke Inhalation

The term smoke inhalation is associated with injury or illness as a result of breathing in the gases or par-ticulates that are discharged from a fire and contained in the smoke. Some of these byproducts of the combustion process are merely irritants, while others are highly toxic. Those that are toxic generally fall into one of two categories: lung toxins and systemic toxins.

Lung toxins encompass a variety of different toxins present in smoke that are highly irritant or directly toxic to the bronchial mucosa causing airway inflammation. Symptoms of exposure to lung toxins may include a cough, breathlessness, wheezing, and excessive bronchial secretions. These symptoms may start relatively soon after exposure to the smoke and may continue to develop for up to 36 hours after exposure. Adult respiratory distress syndrome or delayed pulmonary edema may occur in severe cases of exposure to lung toxins.

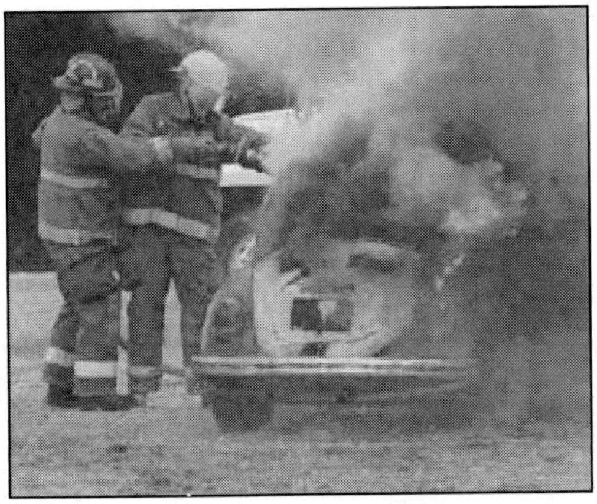

Figure 5.17.

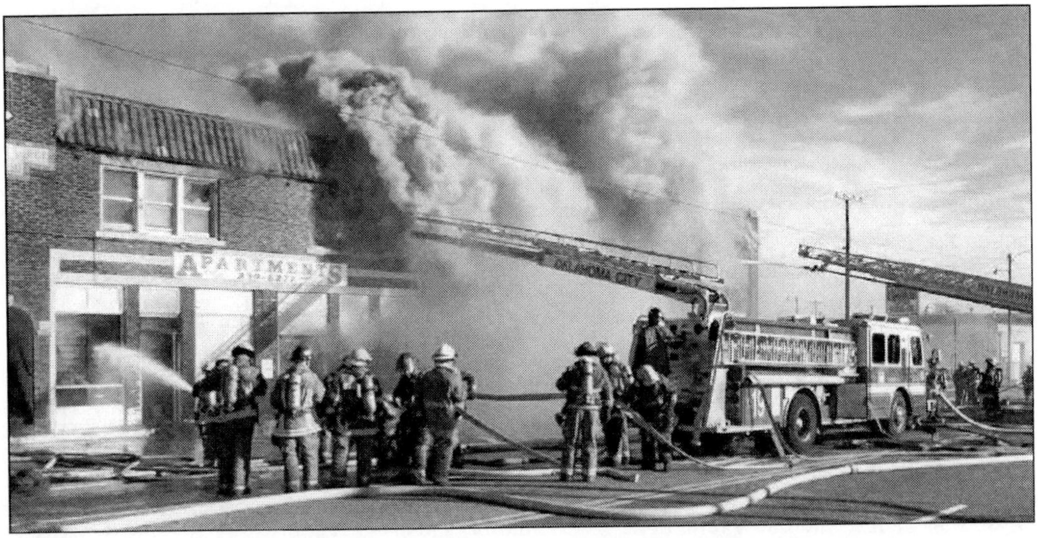

Figure 5.18. Courtesy of Danny Atchley, Oklahoma City Fire Department.

Firefighters who breathe in smoke may also be exposed to a variety of systemic toxins. As opposed to the direct contact effect that lungs toxins have, these substances are absorbed into the firefighter's entire body system and can have serious and fatal effects on the person. The two most common systemic toxins associated with exposure to smoke during firefighting operations are carbon monoxide and hydrogen cyanide.

Carbon monoxide (CO) is contained in relatively high amounts in smoke from almost every burning material. Higher levels of carbon monoxide are associated with fires that contain incomplete combustion (**Figure 5.18**). This includes smoldering phase fires and postextinguishment smoldering that is occurring during overhaul operations. This is why it is extremely important that SCBA continue to be worn during overhaul operations.

Carbon monoxide is an asphyxiant in humans. When inhaled into the system, carbon monoxide readily binds to hemoglobin, reducing the blood's oxygen carrying capacity, and increasing the concentration of carboxyhemoglobin in blood. The reduction in oxygen-carrying capacity of the blood is proportional to the amount of carboxyhemoglobin formed. All factors that speed respiration and circulation accelerate the rate of carboxyhemoglobin formation; thus, the type of exertion that occurs during firefighting operations will enhance carbon monoxide absorption into the system if proper respiratory protection is not worn. Several other preexisting medical conditions also will increase a firefighter's susceptibility to carbon monoxide poisoning, including hyperthyroidism, obesity, bronchitis, asthma, heart disease, and alcoholism.

Personnel performing medical duties in the rehab operation should be alert for firefighters exhibiting symptoms of possible carbon monoxide poisoning. Symptoms of a potentially mild exposure include headache, nausea, vomiting, drowsiness, red/flushed skin appearance, and poor coordination. Most people who develop mild carbon monoxide poisoning recover quickly when moved into fresh air. Moderate or severe carbon monoxide poisoning causes confusion, unconsciousness, chest pain, shortness of breath, and coma. Because of the severity of these symptoms, it is unlikely these people would present themselves to a rehab operation, but more likely they would have to be assisted there by other personnel. Severe poisoning is often fatal. Rarely, weeks after apparent recovery from severe carbon monoxide poisoning, symptoms such as memory loss, poor coordination, and uncontrollable loss of urine (which are referred to as delayed neuropsychiat-ric symptoms) develop. Information on treating these victims is discussed a little later in this section.

Hydrogen cyanide (HCN) is released during combustion of materials such as polyurethane, nylon, and acrylonitrile. Cyanide is an inhibitor of cellular respiration and energy production. Hydrogen cyanide is lighter than air. Hydrogen cyanide is readily absorbed from the lungs; symptoms of poisoning begin within seconds to minutes. The bitter almond odor of hydrogen cyanide is detectable at 2 to 10 parts per million (ppm) (OSHA PEL =10 ppm), but does not provide adequate warning of hazardous concentrations. Perception of the odor is a genetic trait and 20 percent to 40 percent of the general population cannot detect the odor of hydrogen cyanide.

Hydrogen cyanide acts as a cellular asphyxiant. By binding to mitochondrial cytochrome oxidase, it prevents the use of oxygen in cellular metabolism. The central nervous system (CNS) is particularly sensitive to the toxic effects of cyanide. CNS signs and symptoms usually develop rapidly. Initial symptoms are nonspecific and may be confused with CO poisoning. These include excitement, eye irritation, headache, confusion, dizziness, nausea, vomiting, and weakness. As HCN poisoning progresses, drowsiness, tetanic spasm, lockjaw, convulsions, hallucinations, loss of consciousness, and coma may occur.

After systemic HCN poisoning begins, victims may complain of shortness of breath and chest tightness. Pulmonary findings may include rapid breathing and increased depth of respirations. As poisoning progresses, respirations become slow and gasping; a bluish skin color may or may not be present. Accumulation of fluid in the lungs may develop.

As mentioned above, because of the similarities with symptoms associated with CO poisoning, hydrogen cyanide poisoning is often difficult to diagnose in the field. Definitive diagnosis will have to occur in a hospital setting. Measurement of carboxyhemoglobin concentration and blood cyanide concentrations will help to differentiate between HCN and CO poisoning. Plasma lactate measured at the time of admission to the hospital has been shown to correlate with HCN toxicity. A high plasma lactate (> 10.0 mmol/L) in the absence of severe burns or hypotension may suggest cyanide toxicity which can be confirmed subsequently by measuring blood cyanide concentrations.

Regardless of toxins firefighters may have been exposed to, the following procedures are recommended for emergency medical care at the scene. Of course local EMS protocols should prevail in all cases.

- Give high flow humidified oxygen **(Figure 5.19).** If hypercapnia is secondary to coma or respiratory insufficiency, intubation and ventilation may be required.
- Early intubation should be considered if there is stridor or respiratory distress. Consider immediate or early intubation if there are facial or neck burns, erythema, blistering or edema of the oropharynx. It often is better to intubate electively at this stage than try and perform an emergency intubation several hours later when the upper airway may be extremely swollen.
- If ALS personnel are available, start IV therapy according to local protocols.
- Transport the victim to an appropriate medical facility as soon a possible. Preference should be given to trauma centers and those facilities that specialize in the treatment of burn victims and respiratory ailments. Treatment within a hyperbaric chamber may be required in extreme cases.

Once at the hospital, medical personnel may be required to perform any or all of the following functions in order to adequately treat a possible smoke inhalation victim:

- If there are any signs of thermal injury to the face/ oropharynx, patients must be monitored closely for 24 hours in a facility where emergency airway care can be provided if required.
- Perform arterial blood gases and check carboxyhemoglobin concentration and lactate concentrations. Consider measuring blood cyanide concentrations.
- Perform a chest x-ray.
- Nebulized bronchodilators may be of benefit if bronchospasm present.
- Corticosteroids are not of proven benefit.
- If lactate concentration exceeds 10 mmol/L in absence of significant burns and after correction of hypotension, consider the possibility that cyanide poisoning is present and treat accordingly.

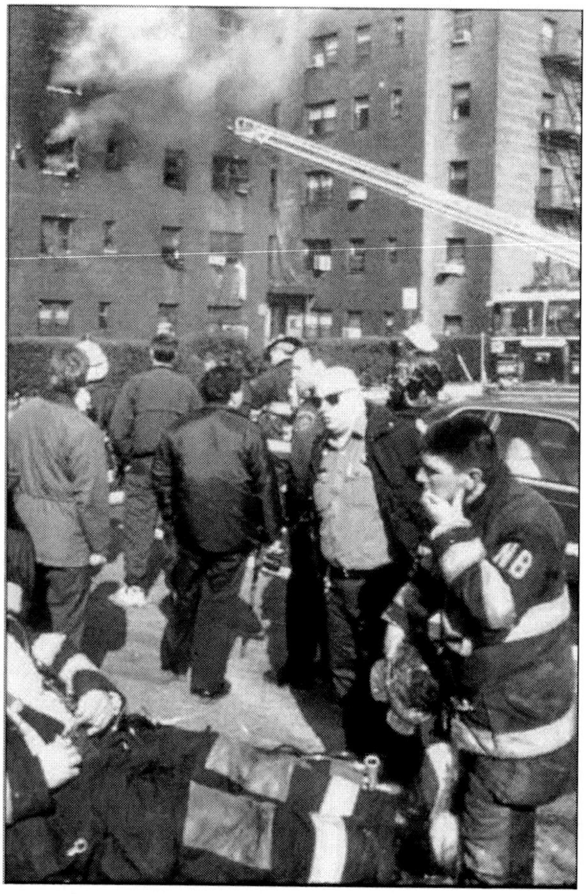

Figure 5.19. Courtesy of Ron Jeffers, Union City, NJ.

Hydration and Dehydration Concerns in Rehab Operations

Other than treating personnel who show signs of a physical illness or injury, perhaps the most important function carried out in the rehab operation is ensuring that firefighters receive adequate hydration to support their body's need to replenish fluid lost during emergency operations or training evolutions. In this section we will examine the body's need for proper hydration and the consequences of failing to meet those needs.

The Body's Need for Hydration

Every cell within the human body is comprised, in part, with varying amounts of water. The amount of water contained in individual cells varies depending on the type cell. Muscle cells typically contain a greater percentage of water than do fat cells. In total, the typically human body is composed of about 60 percent water. Because so much of the body of comprised of water and proper functioning of most bodily functions is dependent on water, the need to keep the body properly hydrated at all times becomes one of the most essential functions in ensuring the well-being of the firefighter.

A basic definition for the term "hydration" is simply the amount of water contained by the human body. Under normal circumstances a body is kept hydrated properly by ensuring that the water lost from the body through normal functions is adequately replaced through oral intake of fluids and by water that is contained in foods that are eaten. The whole goal of a proper hydration strategy is to ensure this intake versus discharge balance is always maintained.

The human body loses water through four basic means: in urine, in stool, during exhalation, and through sweating. In normal, nonstrenuous conditions the majority of water is discharged from the body through urination. Though not totally precise, one basic way in which a person can monitor their own hydration level is by observing the characteristics of their urine during discharge. A properly hydrated body will discharge urine that is relatively clear in color, with little or no odor, and in a reasonable volume. Urine that is dark (typically yellow) in color, has a strong odor, and is low in volume is indicative of body whose hydration level is low and in need of fluid replacement. Likewise, overly frequent large volumes of clear urine can indicate a body that is over hydrated.

During periods of extreme work or when exposed to high atmospheric temperatures, the majority of water lost from the body is as a result of sweating. Sweating occurs as a result of the body's attempt to maintain a constant temperature by cooling itself through the evaporation of perspiration. The amount a person sweats will vary depending on a number of factors, including the:

- individual's metabolism and level of physical fitness;
- level of exertion the individual is performing;
- atmospheric temperature the person is operating in; and
- amount of clothing and protective equipment being worn.

During periods of extreme exertion, some people may lose as much as 1 liter (about 1 quart or 2.2 pounds) of sweat per hour (**Figure 5.20**). People who are relatively fit and have a lower percentage of body fat are actually more susceptible to early dehydration because muscle cells contain more water than do fat cells and therefore require more frequent replenishment.

Regardless of the level of fitness of the individual, failure to adequately replace fluid that is lost during strenuous activity will cause the body's water balance to go into a negative situation and ultimately result in dehydration. The person's performance may begin to be affected adversely before serious dehydration. Serious consequences can result if as little as 4 percent of the body's total weight is lost in water from sweating. This includes increasing the body's core temperature, which is particularly harmful to firefighters who are wearing heavy protective clothing and operating in high temperature atmospheres. This drastically increases their chance of suffering a heat-related illness.

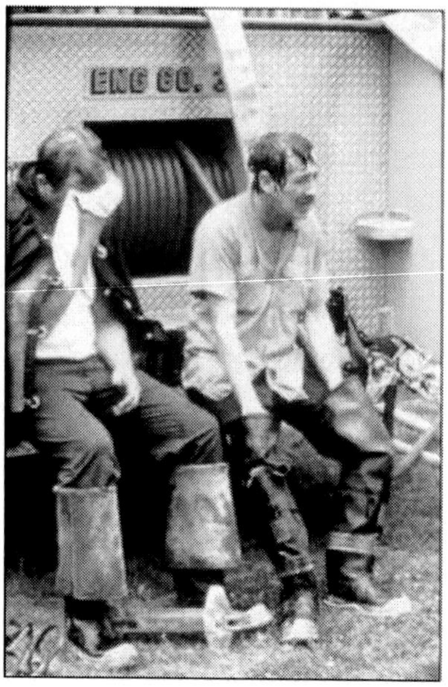

Figure 5.20. City, NJ. Courtesy of Ron Jeffers, Union.

Firefighters must be trained to monitor themselves for signs of negative water balance or dehydration. Many people assume that thirst is the first indicator of a need to rehydrate, but this is not always the case and thirst in and of itself is not necessary an accurate indicator of hydration levels. A more reliable method is to monitor urine output for the characteristics described earlier in this section. There are two exceptions to the urine characteristics previously described. A properly hydrated person may still have very yellow or odorous urine if they have recently taken high doses of Vitamin B supplements or if they have recently eaten asparagus. Onset of a headache is also often an early sign of dehydration.

The Body's Need for Electrolytes and Carbohydrates

To this point in this section we have focused solely on the importance of proper water balance to the functioning of the human body. While water balance is indeed crucial, so too are the levels of electrolytes and carbohydrates present in the body. Electrolytes are chemically-charged elements essential to proper cellular function in most parts of the human body. Among the more important electrolytes needed by the human body are sodium, potassium, calcium, and magnesium.

Water and electrolyte imbalance often are discussed together because they are closely linked and both are lost from the body in relatively the same manner. Most electrolytes are lost during urination or sweating. As with water, during strenuous activities electrolytes are lost primarily through heavy sweating. That is why sweat has a salty taste to it; the salt taste is a result of sodium being lost from the body.

To fully explain the importance of electrolyte balance in the human body is beyond the scope of this document. However, suffice to say that electrolytes have a major impact on a wide variety of cell activities, including allowing the movement of skeletal muscles and maintaining a properly beating/functioning heart. Failure to maintain adequate levels of electrolytes will negatively impact these functions and potentially endanger the firefighter. Using the two examples above, large losses of sodium will negatively impact skeletal muscle function, typically manifesting itself in cramps. Failure to maintain adequate levels of potassium in the blood may result in the heart's electrical system losing its ability to properly generate and conduct electrical impulses. This disruption of electrical activity in the heart can cause potentially lethal cardiac arrhythmias, including ventricular tachycardia and ventricular fibrillation. Death by cardiac arrest is a possibility in these circumstances.

As with water loss, all firefighters, regardless of their physical condition can be subject to significant electrolyte losses during periods of strenuous activities or exposure to high temperature conditions. Firefighters who are taking diuretic medications, such as Lasix®, will be especially susceptible to excessive amounts of electrolyte loss. These firefighters should be monitored closely during high activity or heat situations.

The most common way for firefighters to replace electrolytes lost during emergency scene or training exercises is to drink sports beverages that contain replacement electrolytes. These will be discussed in more detail later in this chapter.

Carbohydrates exist in two basic forms: simple and complex. Simple carbohydrates are sugars such as glucose, sucrose, dextrose, lactose, and fructose that are found in variety of natural foods such as fruits, milk, processed sugar, and honey. Complex carbohydrates are molecules made up of three or more sugars. Complex carbohydrates are typically found in starchy foods, such as bread, pasta, and potatoes.

The human body uses primarily simple sugars as sources of energy for vital organs and muscles. Complex carbohydrates are broken down into simple sugars by the body in order to be used as fuel for the body. Of the various types of simple sugars, glucose is perhaps the most important from a metabolic standpoint. Insufficient amounts of glucose in the human system will cause cellular dysfunction. In severe glucose deficiency situations, particularly in insulin-dependent diabetics, hypoglycemia or insulin shock may occur. Hypoglycemic symptoms include confusion, altered level of consciousness, and unconsciousness.

The human body has a very limited ability to store carbohydrates. During strenuous activities the body will accelerate the amount of carbohydrates it burns to fuel muscles and organs. Because of this limited storage ability and increased demand during heavy physical activity, firefighters who are rehabbing at extended incidents will likely need to replace lost carbohydrates as much as they will water and electrolytes. For short to medium duration incidents it is better to provide foods and sports drinks that contain simple carbohydrates, because of the extended time it takes the body to break down complex carbohydrates. Starchy foods containing complex carbohydrates are more suited for extended duration incidents.

Prehydration Strategies

In many cases it is preparation prior to an emergency incident that makes the difference between a successful outcome and a not-so-successful outcome. Preincident planning of target hazards allows incidents to be conducted with fewer surprises. Good physical conditioning of firefighters reduces their chance of suffering an injury or illness at the emergency scene or training exercise. So too is the case with hydration. It is better if firefighters enter into operation with an even or slightly positive water balance. This prevents them from quickly lapsing into a negative water balance or dehydrated state during the early stages of an incident.

The concept of ensuring that firefighters are hydrated properly prior to the onset of emergency or training operations is referred to as prehydration. Firefighters must be encouraged to regularly drink appropriate beverages during the course of the day so that their bodies are prepared for strenuous activity should it occur (**Figure 5.21**). At a minimum, firefighters should drink 6 to 8 ounces of fluids every 6 hours, in addition to fluids taken with meals. In reality most firefighters will require even more fluids than that to stay properly hydrated.

The following is a list of other suggestions for an effective prehydration strategy that may be used by firefighters:

- Use the guidelines for monitoring urine output discussed earlier in this section to determine level of prehydration. Dark or odorous urine is an indication that fluid intake should be increased.
- Avoid excessive amounts of caffeinated beverages while on duty or prior to training activities. Caffeinated beverages cause increased urination and make it more difficult to maintain adequate hydration.
- Excessive amounts of alcohol used within the previous 24 hours often causes dehydration. In fact, dehy dration is one of the factors in creating a hangover.
- If performing strenuous activities while on duty, such as physical training or practical training exercises, make sure to drink adequate fluids following these activities to restore hydration levels in the event an emergency response occurs.

Appropriate beverages to be used for prehydration will be discussed later in this section.

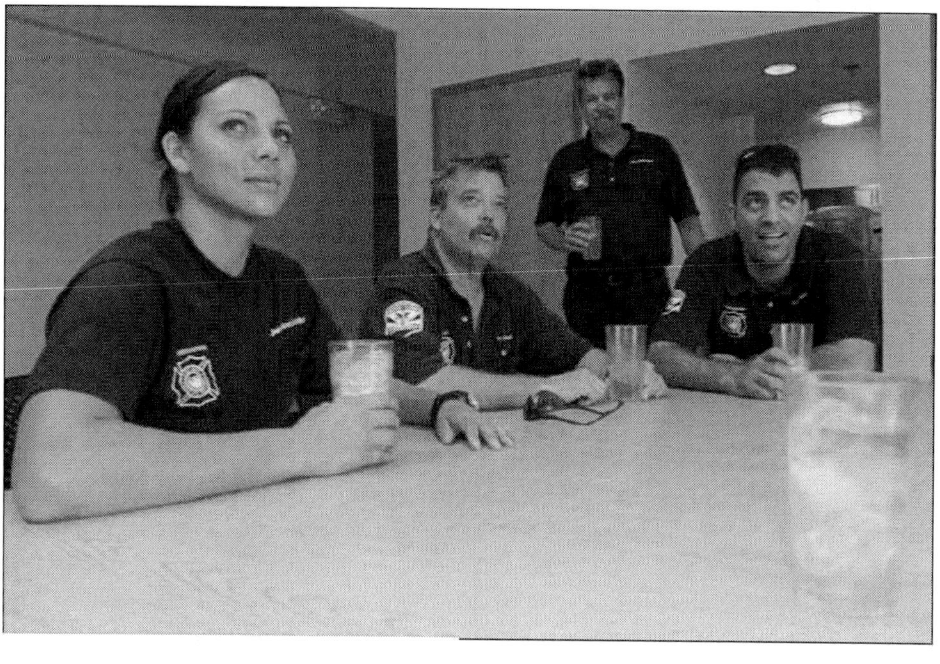

Figure 5.21. Courtesy of Phoenix, AZ Fire Department.

Rehydration Strategies

Regardless of how well firefighters have prehydrated prior to an emergency incident or training exercise, it will be necessary for them to take on additional fluids during and after the incident to maintain their level of hydration and be able to operate at optimum levels. Fluids for rehydrating firefighters should be a part of both self-rehab and formal rehab processes.

The principles of self-rehab were discussed earlier in this chapter. Self-rehab is performed on short duration incidents, or after depletion of the first SCBA cylinder or 20 minutes of strenuous work at larger incidents. Self-rehab is performed outside and independent of a formal rehab operation. The most common locations for self-rehab to occur include at the companies own apparatus or at a utility vehicle where SCBA cylinders are replaced and/or refilled. COs or crew leaders must ensure that all members of the team assigned to them drink an appropriate amount of fluid during self-rehab periods.

The amount of fluid a firefighter drinks during self-rehab will typically be less than that which would be taken in during a formal rehab period. NFPA 1584 recommends 2 to 4 ounces of liquid during self-rehab. This is roughly the amount contained in a bathroom Dixie cup. Some departments recommend slightly larger amounts in the 6 to 8 ounce range.

Fluids for consumption during periods of self-rehab may be provided in a number of ways. Some departments chose to carry individual serving size bottles of water or sports beverages on each apparatus. They may be carried in the cab or a compartment. Some departments carry these bottles at the same location as spare SCBA cylinders as a reminder to use them when changing out cylinders **(Figure 5.22).** Other departments have bulk beverage containers and cups on the apparatus. Beverages also may be carried in command vehicles or on utility vehicles. Utility vehicles are a natural choice, as that is where firefighters will go to replace or refill their SCBA cylinders. In some cases bulk serving containers and cups are stored on the utility vehicle. If bulk containers are used, they should be refilled and cleaned on a regular basis.

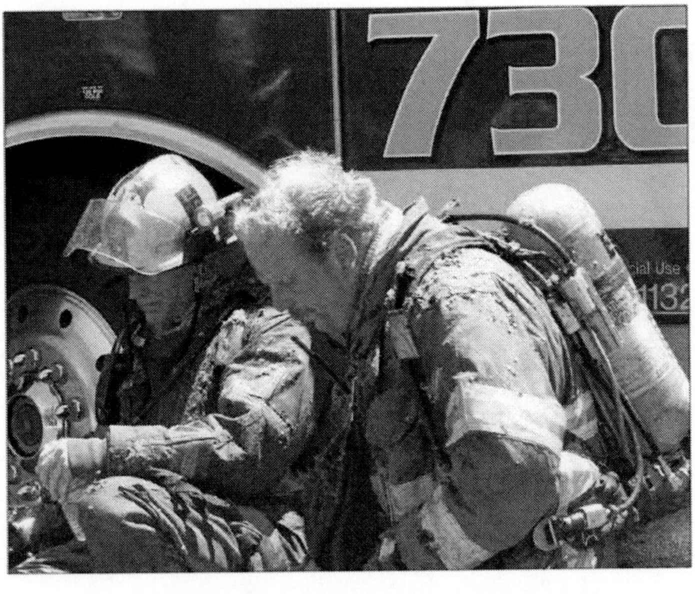

Figure 5.22. Courtesy of Phoenix,AZ Fire Department.

Other than attending to recognized medical needs, the administration of fluids for rehydration is perhaps the most important function carried out in a formal rehab operation. Firefighters who enter the rehab area should be required to begin drinking fluids as soon as they have been logged in, given their medical evaluation, and removed their protective clothing. Fluids should be readily accessible within the Rest and Refreshment Unit of the rehab area. Again, fluids may be served in individual serving containers or from bulk dispensing units, depending on local preferences.

The amount of fluids that firefighters in rehab will require depends on a number of variables, including their individual metabolic needs, the level of exertion they were operating at, ambient conditions, and their level of thirst. On average, firefighters who have been fairly active prior to entering rehab will require anywhere from 12 to 32 ounces of fluids during their rehab period. These amounts may be increased during operations in extreme hot or cold temperatures.

On the other hand, firefighters should not drink so much fluid that they become uncomfortable and bloated. This could result in them becoming ill and at the very least will impair their future performance for a substantial period of time. Most adults are capable of emptying no more than 1.0 to 1.5 liters of fluid from their gastric system per hour. This rate will be reduced during strenuous activity, exposure to high temperature conditions, and even by the early stages of dehydration itself. Although it might seem to defy common sense, very hot, tired firefighters actually are capable of handling lesser amounts of liquids in their systems than are firefighters who were not exposed to such extremes.

Firefighters who show up at the rehab area with an altered level of consciousness or feelings of nausea should not be given liquids orally. ALS personnel should start an IV on these firefighters according to local protocols. These firefighters should receive a more detailed medical evaluation and should not be allowed to participate in further operations during the course of this incident.

It should be noted also that the hydration process does not end in the rehab area or when firefighters are returned to quarters. In many cases even properly rehabbed firefighters will leave the scene in a state of minor dehydration. It is important for firefighters to continue drinking appropriate beverages for up to two hours after the event has been concluded. Self-monitoring of urinary output will be one way to ensure that a proper fluid balance has been restored.

Fluids for Rehab Operations

When determining what beverages to serve in a rehab operation, there are two primary factors that must be taken into consideration: how the beverages will be served and what type of beverages will be served. Both of these have been discussed, in part, previously in this publication. In this section we will examine these issues in more detail.

Methods for Dispensing Rehab Fluids

There are two primary methods for dispensing fluids in rehab: individual serving containers and bulk storage containers. Each of these methods has their own advantages and disadvantages.

Water and most sports type beverages used for rehab purposes are available in individual serving size containers. These containers commonly range in size from 6 to 32 ounces. Table 5.1 lists some of the advantages and disadvantages of using individual serving containers for rehab operations.

In general, most jurisdictions find that using individual serving containers is best suited for self-rehab activities and small-scale rehab operations. In these situations the needs of the rehab operation typically can be handled with the bottled beverages that normally are carried on the apparatus or in Command vehicles.

Bulk-serving containers are the dispensing method of choice for many jurisdictions. Most jurisdictions that use this method employ large, insulated beverage containers equipped with shutoff spouts for dispensing either water or sports beverages. These containers typically range in size from 2 to 15 gallons. Drinking cups must be supplied to allow firefighters to drink the fluid in the containers. Table 5.2 lists some of the advantages and disadvantages of using bulk-serving containers for rehab operations.

Bulk-serving containers are well suited for all types of rehab operations if the containers are kept full at all times. Most departments that keep bulk containers prefilled with liquids do so with ice water. If the need for sports beverages becomes evident at an incident, they then mix in an appropriate amount of powder or concentrate into the ice water. By doing this they do not waste sports beverage mix when containers are regularly emptied and sanitized. When using bulk serving containers it will be necessary to provide drinking cups for the firefighters to use. These cups should be relatively sturdy and disposable. They should be of sufficient size that eliminates the need from frequent returns to the beverage dispenser, as this works against our desire for the firefighters to sit and rest.

Table 5.1. Advantages and Disadvantages of Using Individual Serving Beverage Containers in Rehab Operations

Advantages	Disadvantages
This is a very sanitary method of dispensing drinks, unless containers are shared.	Typically, serving from individual serving containers will be more costly than serving from bulk containers.
Individual containers may be stored in small places on the apparatus, including with spare SCBA cylinders.	Storing large quantities of individual serving containers takes considerable space.
Beverages are ready-to-go and require no preparation.	Moving large quantities of individual serving containers to incident scenes can be a cumbersome process.
Bottled beverages of this type have a fairly long shelf life.	Individual serving containers generate larger quantities of trash at the rehab site than do the cups used with bulk containers.
Portion control can be built into the size of the containers that are selected.	

Table 5.2. Advantages and Disadvantages of Using Bulk-Serving Containers in Rehab Operations

Advantages	Disadvantages
Large quantities of fluids can be dispensed for extended periods of time at major incidents.	Containers must be filled before use and sports beverages may need to be prepared using concentrates or powders.
This method is more cost-effective than individual serving containers.	Containers must be emptied and cleaned on a regular basis.
The cups used with this method generate less trash than individual serving containers	In some cases there may be difficulty finding a placeto quickly fill empty containers at the rehab site.
Less storage space is required to provide liquids for large-scale incidents.	

Regardless of which dispensing method is used, appropriate trash containers should be placed in the rehab area to collect the empty cups or bottles when firefighters are through with them. Personnel assigned to rehab should police the area once operations are complete to ensure all waste is picked up. The trash containers then should be emptied in an appropriate bulk trash bin.

Types of Beverages for Rehab Operations

The type of beverages used in rehab operations has been a source of debate for as long as rehab and incident scene canteen operations have been conducted. Well-intentioned providers commonly brought drinks to the scene that they thought firefighters would enjoy: coffee, tea, soda, hot chocolate, etc.; however, in some cases these drinks were not the best choices from a health standpoint. In this section we will review the various factors that go into selecting an appropriate beverage for rehab operations.

There are three primary considerations when choosing appropriate drinks for rehab operations: taste, tol-erability, and nutritional value. Appropriate rehab beverages must be acceptable, to some extent, in all three of these areas.

Some may question the role of taste in whether or not a fluid is acceptable for use in rehab. In reality, taste's role is pretty simple. If firefighters do not like the taste of a beverage that is provided, they are less likely to drink enough of the beverage in order to adequate rehydrate their bodies. If they enjoy the taste, they will drink more and are more likely to effectively replace fluids and nutrients that were lost from their bodies. Certainly, taste is a matter of individual preference and not every firefighter will like a given drink that is provided. That is why it is better to provide as least two different kinds whenever possible.

Tolerability is also an important consideration. In this sense we are referring to the body's ability to tolerate and absorb the fluid into its system. There are a number of factors related to how well a particular fluid may be tolerated. First, of course, is the temperature at which the beverage is served. Most rehab operations serve cool beverages regardless of the weather conditions. During particularly hot conditions it is important the drinks not be served ice cold, as this can cause painful spasms of the esophagus or even slow the heart rate. Drinks should be cool (50-60 °F), but not ice cold. In cold weather some jurisdictions serve warm drinks. Again, they should be warm, not piping hot. If the liquids are too hot they will burn the person's mouth. Another issue with serving warm drinks is that often firefighters will sip them to make themselves feel warm inside, but may not drink enough to properly rehydrate themselves. Firefighters should follow warm drinks with appropriate rehydrating drinks.

The second important factor in the tolerability of a fluid is its thickness, which is commonly referred to as its osmolarity. The osmolarity of a fluid is a measure of the number of particles in a solution. The higher the osmolarity, the longer the time it will take to absorb the fluid and the harder the fluid will be to digest. In a drink, these particles are comprised of carbohydrates, electrolytes, sweeteners, and preservatives. In blood plasma the particles are comprised of sodium, proteins and glucose. Blood has an osmolarity of 280 to 330 mOsm/kg. Drinks with an osmolarity of 270 to 330 mOsm/kg are said to be in balance with the body's fluid and are called isotonic. In general, it is recommended that rehydration solutions served in rehab do not exceed an osmolarity of 350 mOsm/kg. In some cases commercially available sports beverages have osmolarities in excess of 350 mOsm/kg. In these cases those fluids should be diluted with water before serving.

Drinks that are too thick, such as a milk shake, will not be tolerated easily by the body and will take an extensive amount of time to absorb into the system. During periods of heavy exercise this will cause feelings of bloating or nausea and may even lead to vomiting. All of this works against the goal of rehydrating the person. Consuming fluids with a low osmolarity, such as water, results in a fall in the blood plasma osmolarity and may reduce the drive to drink well before sufficient fluid has been consumed to replace losses.

The third factor to be considered when selecting a fluid for rehab operations is the nutritional value of the fluid. As noted previously in this document, when firefighters are engaged in heavy manual labor for extended periods of time, their bodies lose water, electrolytes, and carbohydrates. Ideally the jurisdiction will select a fluid for rehab operations that replaces all of these elements. This will be discussed in more detail in the sections regarding specific types of beverages below.

Water

Water is perhaps the most commonly used fluid for rehab operations. This is probably due to the fact that it is readily available almost anywhere and it is inexpensive (free actually, if you are filling containers with tap water). While water is an excellent choice for use in rehab situations, it actually is not perfect and it does have some drawbacks.

Water is the principle fluid being lost from the body during hard work and exercise. However, in addition to losing water the body is also losing electrolytes and burning carbohydrates, which it does not store efficiently to begin with. Using plain water for rehab operations will meet the body's need to replenish hydration levels, but it will do nothing to replace lost carbohydrates and electrolytes, as plain water contains neither of these.

Some people prefer the taste of water over other drinks, but most people find it relatively bland. In many cases this will cause them to stop drinking water before becoming fully hydrated. Drinking a lot of plain water causes bloating, which will suppress thirst and again cause the person to stop drinking before they may be fully hydrated.

Most research and sources suggest that water is perfectly fine for low intensity work situations that last one hour or less. There is not enough carbohydrate or electrolyte loss in the first hour to require other types of fluid, though they certainly may be used if available. If the incident involves heavy labor and extends more than one hour, plain water will not be the most suitable choice.

If commercial sports beverages are not available, personnel can make water more effective by adding a little sugar (carbohydrates) and salt to the water before serving. The U.S. Army field guidelines for high heat situations recommend adding about 1-1/2 teaspoons of salt per gallon of water when field mixing the preparation. This will not affect the taste of the water, but will improve its performance in the body when ingested. It is best to mix the salt up in a small container of water to get it dissolved before adding and mixing in the larger container. This water can further be enhanced by adding 1-1/4 cups of sugar per gallon. This will provide an effective carbohydrate level (6 percent) as well.

Sports Drinks

The term sports drink is applied to a variety of commercial beverages that are specially formulated to help athletes rehydrate during and after engaging in strenuous athletic training and competition **(Figure 5.23).** Sports drinks have been available to the public since the introduction of Gatorade® in 1966. Because of the similarity in the physical demands of firefighting when compared to athletic endeavors, sports drinks have become an important part of firefighter rehab operations.

As mentioned above, replacing water that is lost through sweating and other bodily functions is important, but water is not the only thing being lost by the body during work and exercise. As well, if too much plain water is consumed during periods of work or exercise, a condition called water intoxication may result. Overconsumption of plain water reduces levels of electrolytes, such as sodium and potassium in the body by dilution, interfering with the proper functioning of nervous system. Serious illness or death may result in extreme cases.

Sports drinks are formulated carefully to ensure that they provide the user with Figure 5.23—Courtesy of Cherry Hill, NJ Fire Department, needed water, electrolytes, sugar (carbohydrates), and other nutrients. This mixture ensures that all the body's replacement needs are met and that electrolyte and carbohydrate levels are kept in balance with water intake and retention. Most sports drinks have an osmolarity that is very similar to blood and therefore they are easily absorbed into the body system. Because of the variety of flavors that are available, it is more likely that firefighters will find choices that they find more appealing than drinking plain water.The typical sweet-tart taste combination doesn't quench thirst, which combined with the more appealing taste, means that in many cases firefighters will continue drinking the sports drink long after water has lost its appeal.

Commercial sports drinks are available in individual drinking containers, bulk-serving bottles, and in powdered mixes that can be stirred into water in large-serving containers. The nutritional content of a sports drink will vary depending on the manufacturer of the drink. Table 5.3 shows the nutritional content of a number of sports drinks available commercially. Most research shows that drinks with a carbohydrate concentration between 5 percent and 7 percent are preferred, although minor variances above and below that are acceptable.

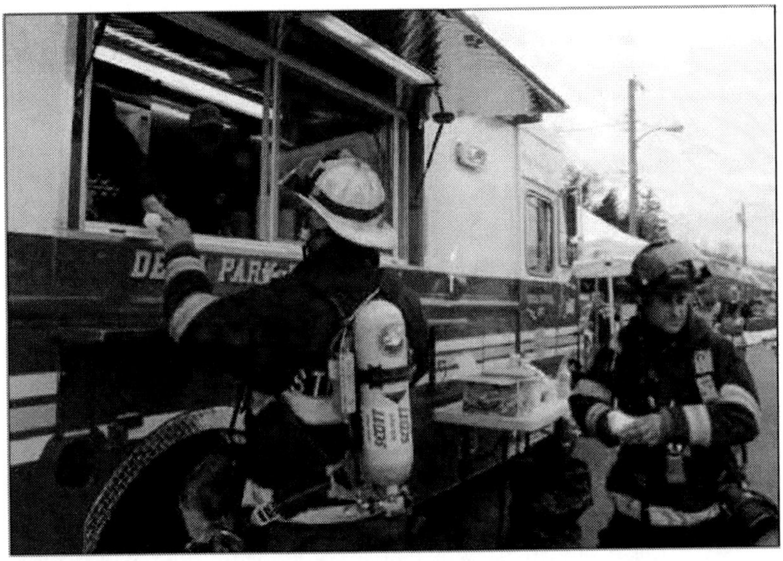

Figure 5.23. Courtesy of Cherry Hill, NJ Fire Department.

Before closing this section it is important to make one clarification. Sports drinks should not be confused with the wide variety of energy drinks that are available on the market today. These include drinks such as Red Bull®, Mountain Dew Amp®, and Monster Energy®. These energy drinks simply contain excessive amounts of sugar and caffeine and are not nutritionally balanced to meet the needs of firefighters (or athletes) who have expended a large amount of energy. They should not be used in rehab operations.

Firefighters also must be cognizant of the fact that because of the high levels of carbohydrates in these drinks, they will experience weight gain if these drinks are used on a regular basis without increasing exercise activity.

Table 5.3. Nutritional Content of Commercially Available Sports Drinks

Product (8 oz)	Calories	Carbohydrates (g)	Carbohydrate Concentration (percent)	Sodium (mg)
Accelerade®	105	19.5	8	142.5
Cytomax®	50	10	4	50
Gatorade®	50	12	5	110
GPUSH	25	6	2.5	170
GU2O	50	13	6	120
PowerBar® Performance Bar	60	16	7	110
Shaklee Performance®	100	25	10	115
SoBe® Sports System	70	19	8	70
Ultima Replenisher®	20	5	2	25
XLR8 Performance Drink®	50	12	5	40

Other Beverages

Well-intentioned volunteers, canteen providers, and other service organizations have long provided the fire service with a variety of other beverages on the emergency scene. Clearly water and sports drinks are the two best choices, yet others continue to be used in some jurisdictions. This section examines the issues associated with using other types of commonly provided beverages in a rehab setting.

Various types of juices or fruit drinks have been used historically in rehab operations. Juices are typically very nutritious, though most fruit drinks have less nutritional value. Neither of them are a great choice for rehydration use. The fructose, or fruit sugar, contained in these beverages reduces the rate of water absorption, so cells don't get hydrated very quickly. Juice is a food in its own right and it's uncommon for a person to drink sufficient quantities to keep hydrated. Juice has carbohydrates, vitamins, minerals, and electrolytes, but it isn't a great thirst quencher.

Carbonated soft drinks, or soda, are provided in rehab or canteen operations by some jurisdictions. These beverages have very little nutritional value and the acids used to carbonate and flavor these beverages will damage your teeth and may even weaken your bones. However, many people find the taste of these drinks most appealing and you are more likely to drink greater amounts of drinks that you enjoy the taste of. The large amounts of carbohydrates in these drinks will slow down the absorption of water into you body, but they will also provide an energy boost. Although many nutritionists probably would not agree, as long as the soda doesn't have excessive amounts of sugar or caffeine, they aren't really a bad choice for rehab operations.

Many jurisdictions serve hot coffee or tea during cold weather and iced tea during warm weather. Coffee and tea both work against effective measures to rehydrate the body. Both of these drinks are diuretics. Diuretics cause the kidneys to pull more water out of the bloodstream, even as the digestive system is trying to pull more water into the body. Milk or sugar added to these drinks further slow the rate of water absorption into the body. While they are better than nothing, neither of these is a solid choice for rehab operations.

While we are on the topic of alternative drinks for rehydration, it is probably appropriate to address the issue of alcoholic beverages, and more specifically beer. Certainly, no professionals or organizations advocate the provision of alcoholic beverages to firefighters before, during, or immediately after performing their duties. The negative consequences of alcohol impairment on judgment and performance have been widely documented. Endless cases where fire service personnel failed to heed these warnings and their tragic consequences can be cited.

Yet there remains an element in the fire service who still fails to recognize the adverse effect of mixing alcohol and fire department operations. Much misinformation has been spread through the years indicating that beer actually has some positive nutritional and rehydration value and when taken in moderation after heavy exercise or work is actually better for the body than a lot of other drinks. This often is used as the justification for some fire departments, particularly in the volunteer sector, to maintain supplies of beer on fire department premises.

The truth of the matter is that beer is not a good beverage for fluid replacement following heavy work or exercise. Any minor nutritional benefit that might be provided by some of its ingredients is more than counteracted by its alcoholic content. In addition to impairing judgment and performance, alcohol also dehydrates the body. It is this dehydration that is responsible for most hangovers. In effect, beer (or any alcohol) works against proper rehydration of the body. One expert notes that beer might be better than seawater for rehydration, but that is about it.

Food for Rehab Operations

The provision of food to firefighters and other emergency workers who are operating at extended duration incidents is a tradition that dates back almost as far as organized fire protection in the United States. In the early days this food was provided at the emergency scene in an impromptu manner by well-meaning citizens and frequently the spouses of the firefighters. The early part of the 20th century saw the formation of formal service organizations to carry out this function.

As we continue to do research and understand the importance of proper nutrition for optimum performance of people engaged in heavy work and exercise, we now know that the provision of nutritionally sound food to responders who have been operating for extended periods of time will allow them to restore energy levels, avoid illness or injury, and perhaps continue on with their work if necessary. This section briefly examines when food is needed in the rehab operation, who should provide that food, and what types of foods are best for these operations.

When to Provide Food in Rehab Operations?

Clearly, all rehab operations should include the provision of appropriate fluids for firefighters to drink while they are resting. Water and key electrolytes are quickly lost from the body when engaged in hard work and they need to be restored to maintain well-being. On the other hand, food may not necessarily be required at every incident in which rehab operations are established.

Different jurisdictions have different thoughts and policies on when to establish food provision at incident scenes. Most of these are based on the anticipated duration of incident operations. There are no set rules for when food operations should be established, but most jurisdictions typically plan for them if the incident will be more than 2 to 3 hours in duration. This may be adjusted based on a number of factors, including weather conditions and the time of day of the incident. Food services may need to be provided earlier in an incident if the firefighters were likely to have missed a meal just prior to responding to the emergency. For example, an incident that occurs early in the morning, before firefighters were likely to have eaten breakfast, may require earlier nutritional support. It may have been 10 to 12 hours since some firefighters had eaten their last meals.

Each agency must establish a policy on when food service operations should be initiated within the rehab operation. This policy also may outline what types of foods will be provided based on the duration of the incident. Short- to medium-duration incidents typically only require minor nutritional support in the form of prepackaged foods and other easy to serve and eat items. Long-duration incident may require more substantial, meal-like support operations.

Who Provides Food for Rehab Operations?

In addition to having established policies for when food is going to be provided for rehab operations, each jurisdiction also should have established plans for who will be providing this service as well. Preincident planning of who will be responsible for food service operations will ensure a number of things, including making sure that food actually does get to the scene and that the food that is brought is appropriate for the need.

The available options for providing food services at an incident will vary depending on the resources of the community, local customs or tradition, and the needs of the incident. The following is a summary of the more commonly used options for providing food services at emergency scenes.

- **Fire department canteen units**—Some fire departments operate their own apparatus that are designed to provide food services at incident scenes. These vehicles are referred to commonly as canteen units. The capabilities of a canteen unit will vary depending on local preferences. Some are simply equipped to provide beverages and prepackaged foods that require no preparation (**Figure 5.24**). Other canteen units have full kitchens and cooking equipment and are capable of providing hot foods prepared at the scene.

- **Independent service canteen units**—Fire departments may look to outside agencies to provide canteen units for food delivery at emergency scenes. These units may be operated by allied fire service organizations (fire buff associations, benevolent associations, etc.), local or national service organizations (Red Cross, Salvation Army, Rotary Club, etc.), or commercial catering operations (work site lunch wagons).

- **Nonvehicle-based operations**—Many jurisdictions do not have the availability of custom-designed canteen units to respond to their emergency scenes. In these jurisdictions, other arrangements will have to be made to have food provided to rehab operations when needed. In these situations some individual or group of people are designated to bring food to the scene. This includes members of the fire department, ladies auxiliaries, Explorer Post members, local service clubs or church groups, or restaurant employees. The food delivered in this manner may be prepackaged foods that require no preparation, may be prepared in a fire department or other kitchen facility, or may be prepared by a restaurant and then delivered to the rehab area.

- **Commercial caterers**—Organizations, that are involved in major long-term operations that frequently involve large numbers of firefighters and other responders, often use the services of special commercial caterers who move mobile kitchens and food service equipment to the scene. These caterers specialize in supporting long-term, but temporary incident operations.

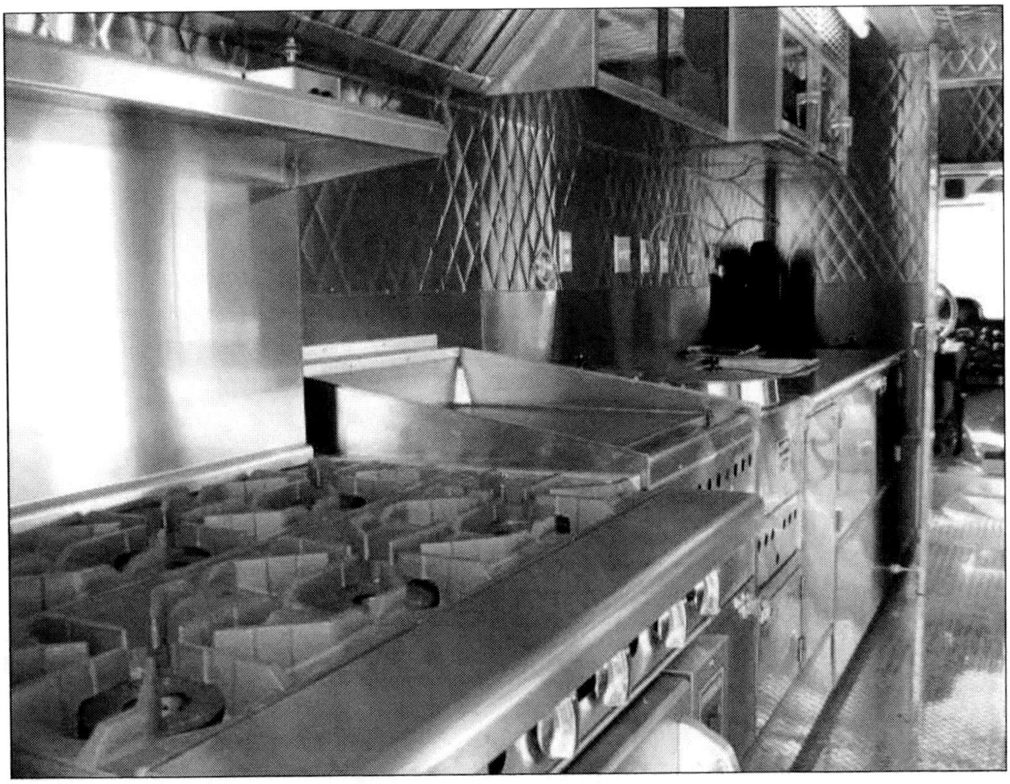

Figure 5.24.

When performing preincident planning of food services to support incident and rehab operations, fire departments must identify the resources that are available to them. These resources may be different depending on whether short-, medium-, or long-term operations need to be supported.They also may vary depending on the number of people that will need to be fed.

Selecting Foods for Rehab Operations

There is almost an endless variety of choices when it comes to selecting food to support incident rehab operations. The exact types of food to be served at the incident will depend on a variety of factors, including the service capabilities of the provider, the duration of the incident, and the preferences of the members of the fire department.

Throughout this document much has been said about the importance of a healthy lifestyle, including proper long-term nutritional habits. Certainly, these principles should be extended to the food selections that are chosen for incident rehab operations. Every effort should be made to ensure that food used at the incident is healthy, nutritional, and appropriate. However, in some jurisdictions it may not be that easy to get "ideal" foods to the rehab area. In some communities it is easier to get a bag of hamburgers from a fast food restaurant or a couple of pizzas from the local pizzeria. These foods are certainly better than nothing. While a long-term diet that consisted of these types of foods would not be ideal, there is nothing bad about eating them during an incident operation. The short-term benefits of providing food and energy to hungry firefighters clearly outweigh any alleged long-term negative health impacts of a one time serving of these types of foods.

Agencies that do have the benefit of tailoring their food selections to meet incident nutritional needs should put a lot of thought and planning into their food selections. They should work with the agencies or organizations that will be providing the food services at the incident to ensure that those people provide the types of foods that best meet the firefighter's needs. When making these selections it is important to consider the three basic types of nutrients that make up a normal diet: carbohydrates, fats, and proteins.

As discussed earlier in this chapter, carbohydrates have a vital metabolic role in producing energy for the body. The body also has a very limited ability to store carbohydrates. Thus, food containing large quantities of carbohydrates should be served to firefighters at medium and long-duration incidents. This includes breads, potatoes, pasta, rice, and other high starch foods.

While too much fat in the diet and on a person's body certainly is not good, some fat in the diet and on the body is necessary for a healthy lifestyle. The body stores fat much more easily than carbohydrates. Burning fat will provide a certain amount of energy to the body and it will continue to be a source of energy even after all available carbohydrates are used up. While they are not as beneficial as high carbohydrate foods in rehab operations, foods with low to moderate fat contents are acceptable for these uses.

Proteins are not a major source of energy to the body. However proteins do support a variety of other metabolic functions, including developing muscles, repairing tissues, and helping transport other nutrients throughout the body. High protein foods include meats, fish, cheeses, and other dairy products. Protein-containing foods should be a part of the rehab area diet.

Unless the jurisdiction has the availability of a canteen provider with onscene cooking capabilities, most departments will support short- and medium-term incidents using simple foods that do not require preparation. These include things such as fruits, doughnuts, candy bars, and energy bars. Some of these items, such as the candy and energy bars, have long storage lives and may be carried on the apparatus or stored at the fire station until needed. Other types of food may need to be acquired from a local grocery store or restaurant.

Agencies that have fully equipped canteen units tend to provide food that is easy to prepare at the scene. These include things such as hot dogs, hamburgers, egg sandwiches, cold cut sandwiches, soups, stews, and similar easy-to-prepare and eat foods. Full-service, long-term caterers typically provide three full meal services per day.

Regardless of who is providing the food or what food is being served, the following principles must always be followed for incident scene food serving operations:

- Firefighters should wash their hands before eating any foods at the incident scene. If running water and soap are not available, use antibacterial premoistened towelettes, waterless hand cleaners, or handsanitizers.
- All food serving equipment must be sanitary and fully compliant with local health department regulations.
- All foods should be fresh and stored and served at appropriate temperatures. This reduces the risk of infecting responders with food-borne bacteria that may lead to a serious illness.

- Fire departments should have preestablished agreements with local grocery or food providers on how food will be provided when needed and how it will be billed and paid for. These agreements should take into account how food will be obtained if it is needed after normal business hours, assuming the business is not open 24 hours.
- These operations can generate a significant amount of trash. Provisions must be made for collecting and disposing of this trash. The area in which food is served should be at least as clean, if not cleaner, after the incident than it was prior to the incident.
- For medium- and long-term operations it may be necessary to rotate out personnel and volunteers who are serving food. This should be planned out ahead of time.

Well-fed personnel tend to have better morale and will have higher energy levels than hungry personnel. Every effort should be made to ensure that sound, appealing food service is provided in the rehab area when the situation calls for it.

In: Rehab, Protection and Safety Measures or Firefighters … ISBN: 978-1-60741-566-4
Editor: Andreo Rios

Chapter 6

POST-INCIDENT REHAB CONSIDERATIONS

The fire department's responsibility for safeguarding the well-being of their members does not end when the last firefighter leaves the rehab area at an incident. Policies and procedures must be in place to ensure that firefighters continue to receive restorative care after the incident. The fire department also must ensure that the resources used to provide rehab services are replenished and ready for the next incident where they may be needed.

This chapter briefly examines the de-escalation of rehab operations at an incident scene. It also provides information on care that firefighters should receive once they leave this incident scene. This includes medical evaluation, self-monitoring for hydration needs, and critical incident stress services, should they be required.

TERMINATING INCIDENT REHAB OPERATIONS

Most fire department incidents and operations run a fairly predictable life-span. There is an initial response to the incident, in some cases there are additional resources called to assist with the incident, and as the incident is brought under control there is a gradual scaling back of the number of resources and personnel on the scene. The establishment of rehab operations at an incident scene also should parallel these phases of the incident lifespan. Units on the initial response are often capable of self-rehab. If an incident expands in scope, additional resources are called to establish and operate a formal rehab area. As the incident winds down, rehab operations are scaled back and finally terminated altogether.

During the course of an incident, the individual assigned as the Rehab Group Supervisor, or Rehab Unit Leader as the case may be, monitors the growth and progress of the incident and builds the rehab operation accordingly. Similarly, as the incident winds down, the Rehab Group Supervisor must also monitor the de-escalation of activities and tailor the rehab operation to meet the remaining needs of the incident with a reasonable level of resources. While a large rehab operation using dozens of personnel and a significant inventory of equipment may have been prudent at the height of an incident that involved a large number of respond-ers, that same level of resources to staff the rehab unit should not be maintained when only a fraction of the total responders remains on the scene (**Figure 6.1**).

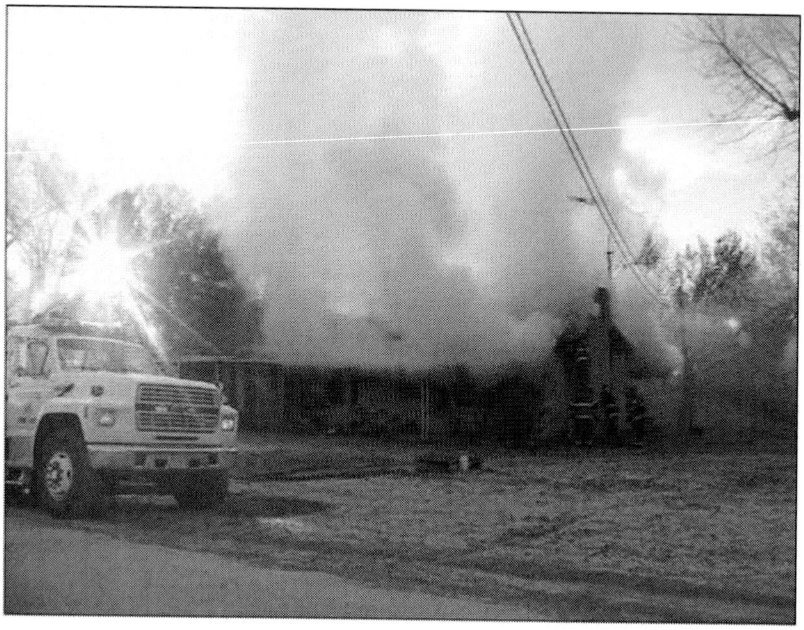

Figure 6.1.

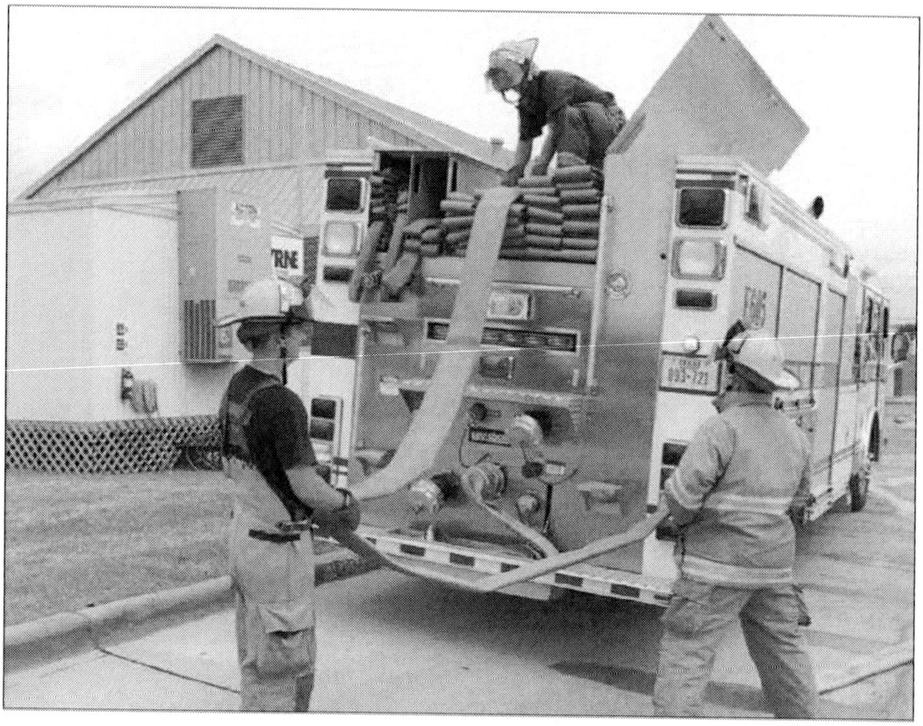

Figure 6.2.

Before getting too deep into any discussion on the scaling back and terminating of rehab services at an incident, it is important to recognize that we are talking about scaling back the number of resources assigned to the rehab operation; not the services that the rehab operation is capable of providing. All of the basic functions of the rehab operation that were discussed previously in this chapter must be provided to the end of the incident. They may not require as many people to perform each one of them as the number of personnel working at the incident scene decreases.

Many rehab concerns actually increase for those personnel remaining on the scene until the conclusion of an incident. Experienced fire service leaders recognize that some of the hardest work of the incident occurs after the fire is out or after a rescue has been completed. Salvage and overhaul operations, as well as retrieval of equipment are grueling tasks for personnel who may be very worn and tired already from the demands of the operational period of the incident (**Figure 6.2**). All rehab services must be available to these personnel to ensure their well-being.

Personnel charged with overseeing rehab operations should maintain frequent contact with the Incident Commander (IC) or Operations Section Chief to keep track of the level of personnel resources being held at the scene and the tasks those resources will be performing. On large-scale incidents it also may be necessary to coordinate with the Demobilization Unit Leader within the Planning Section (**Figure 6.3**).

The Rehab Group Supervisor can use this information gained from these sources to provide an appropriate level of rehab services as the incident winds down.

Maintaining an appropriate level of rehab resources will require some level of experienced judgment based on the number of personnel remaining on the scene and the tasks they will be performing. Decisions based on the number of personnel requiring services are fairly straightforward. However, the activities being performed by those people remaining on the scene require some level of examination in determining rehab needs. For example, a lesser number of personnel who will be performing heavy work such as salvage and overhaul operations actually may require a higher level of resources in rehab than a larger number of personnel who are performing simple fire watch duties.

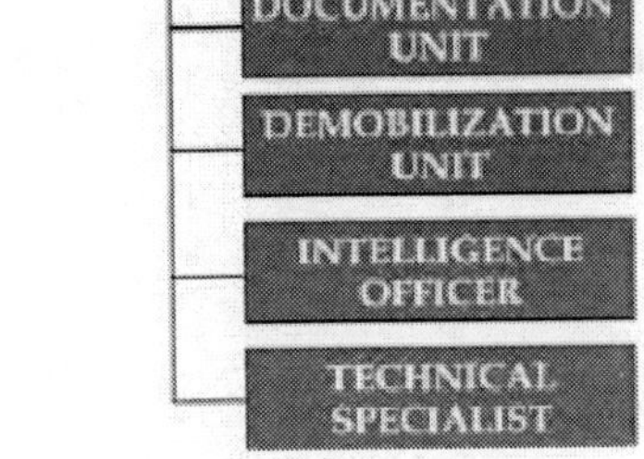

Figure 6.3.

There are several factors to evaluate when determining which resources should be left within the rehab operation and which may be returned to service:

- It is imperative that the people who remain within the rehab operation are qualified for the tasks that they will be expected to perform. This includes ensuring that appropriately trained and certified emer gency medical personnel remain assigned to staff those functions that require responder medical evaluation and treatment.
- Personnel who typically perform specialized functions within the department, such as rescue or hazmat companies, but who were assigned to rehab functions in this instance should be relieved and/or replaced as soon as possible so they are available to handle any responses that require their special capabilities.
- When all other things are equal, those personnel who have been operating in the rehab operation the longest should be the first ones to be released from service.This helps avoid the chance of overextending the rehab personnel.

Personnel who are being released from performing rehab functions should be treated the same as any other personnel who were operating at the scene. Other rehab personnel should evaluate the relieved personnel to determine their level of medical and emotional fitness before being released. Oftentimes personnel working in rehab have been performing those duties for an extended period of time and may be in need of rehab care themselves. Make sure that the rehab personnel are in good condition before they leave the scene.

Companies and personnel that are released from rehab duties should follow departmental procedures for restoring their apparatus and equipment to a state of readiness for the next call. All medical supplies should be inventoried and restocked. Any reusable equipment should be cleaned and sterilized according to standard operating procedures. Food handling and serving equipment must be cleaned and sterilized thoroughly according to local health department requirements (**Figure 6.4**). Any food that was prepared, but not served, should be disposed of in an appropriate manner.

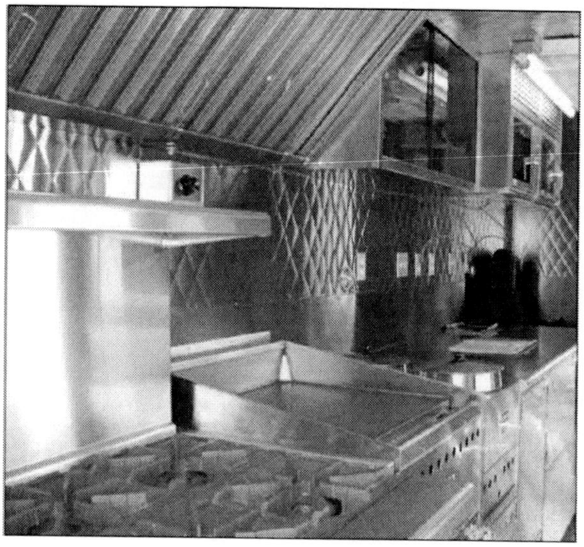

Figure 6.4.

Once it has been determined that the rehab operation can be shut down completely, all remaining units should follow the procedures described in the previous two paragraphs before clearing the scene. The last personnel on the scene should police the area to ensure that all trash, medical supplies, and other debris created by the rehab operation are picked up and disposed of properly. The IC should be advised when the rehab area is deactivated. All incident documentation, including medical evaluation and treatment reports, invoices for expendable supplies, and rehab accountability information should be routed and filed according to local Standard Operating Procedures (SOPs).

Critical Incident Stress Management

The basic foundation of this document is the care and well-being of firefighters and other emergency responders. The information to this point in the document has focused largely on the physiological aspects of this obligation. However, it must be recognized that the duties and activities that firefighters routinely perform also come with a heavy burden on the psychological well-being of these individuals. Fire and rescue operations can be extremely emotional events involving serious injury and death to civilians and firefighters alike (**Figure 6.5**). Regular exposure to dangerous situations and potential for harm also takes a toll on individuals and the combination of these factors can increase stress in daily family life. Fire departments and labor organizations must ensure that programs are in place to address and mitigate the psychological hazards of the job.

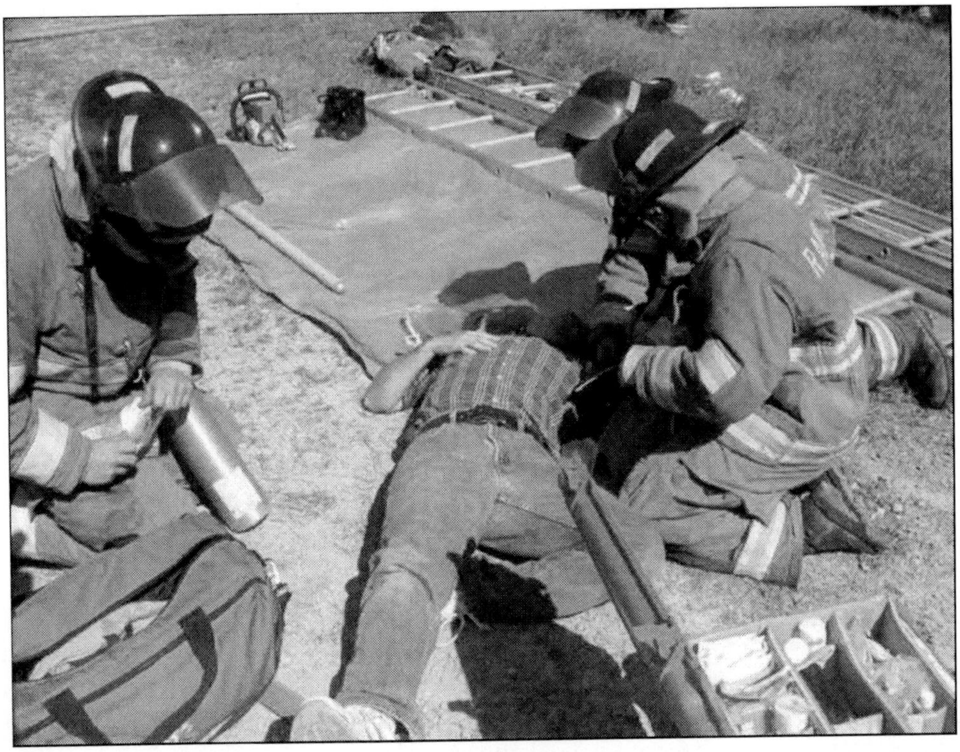

Figure 6.5. Courtesy of IFSTA/Fire Protection Publications.

This was not always the case. Previous generations of firefighters learned their trade at the heels of a smoke-seasoned 20-year captain who showed them both the nature of the work and the workings of the culture. It was in that context that traditions and values, as well as tactics and techniques, were learned, practiced, and reinforced. Those rookies often found themselves at some critical moment going for a walk with the captain who told them that this was difficult work in a difficult world, but that's what made it matter. They'd be told, most likely, that it hurts sometimes, but one had to "suck it in and stick it out" to survive in this service. That's how most would learn to cope with stress. Sometimes this method of coping would work and other times the peer pressure not to admit frailty would result in the use of alcohol, drugs, or other destructive behaviors as a way of handling the stress.

The nature of firefighters' work has changed dramatically in the last generation, adding new challenges to our profession. Contacts between contemporary fire service personnel and the people they serve—through emergency medical care, technical rescue, and other human services—have become increasingly personal and intimate. The challenges of these additional services have greatly expanded the rewards a fire service career can bestow. But while the rewards of mastering these challenges are more personally affirming, the consequences of perceived failure, limitation, or inadequacy can be painfully personal as well.

Attitudes and approaches that were once strong features in the firefighting culture can still be of help in dealing with these very personal human encounters. However, one cannot simply roll up hose, wash down the rig, and walk away from the most profound events of human life without being changed somehow by the experience. It has become progressively more important for fire service organizations and firefighting personnel to develop effective methods through which to successfully integrate these experiences into the fabric of their lives.

In response to this growing need, fire departments have developed critical incident stress management (behavioral health) programs to assist in the psychological well-being of their members. From their early days as relatively simple peer counseling programs, even the field of behavioral health continues to evolve as new understanding of how they need to work emerges. Behavioral health has progressed from informal discussions of individual events to our current understanding of the need for comprehensive programs of prevention, effective intervention, and followup care to prevent long-term effects.

The goals of a comprehensive critical incident stress management (CISM) program are to

- minimize the emotional impact of critical incidents on emergency responders;
- increase firefighters' resistance and resilience to this type of stress;
- prevent harmful effects following critical incidents by working with response personnel at or near the time of such incidents; and
- prevent any chronic effects, such as posttraumatic stress disorder, through the use of followup care and employee assistance programs.

Effective management of critical incidents involves a comprehensive approach to managing both incidents and the resulting stressors. The fire service must structure work and support mechanisms to enable fire service personnel to minimize the toll of career stress on themselves and their families while maximizing the personal rewards of the profession. Fire service personnel directly benefit from reduced stress and improved coping skills. In addition, reducing critical incident stress and its effects benefits the fire department and the municipality, as well as the family members of fire and emergency medical services (EMS) personnel. Benefits to the department may include

- decreased absenteeism;
- decreased physical ailments;
- increased morale;
- improved decisionmaking ability from reduced stress;
- reduction of poor coping strategies (e.g., substance abuse);
- longer retention of qualified personnel; and
- reduction of psychological problems.

Benefits of a comprehensive behavioral health program to the municipality may include

- a healthier fire/rescue service;
- reduced costs associated with absence, illness, and disability; and
- a more cohesive fire/rescue service.

In addition, a comprehensive approach to managing critical incident stress can benefit the families of fire service personnel by lessening the adverse effects on the firefighter and by providing direct support to the family as needed. This also has the effect of reducing families' feelings of helplessness.

Behavioral Health Integration into Rehab Operations

A well-designed comprehensive behavioral health program is multifaceted and involves a myriad of inter-ventional approaches. Each of these approaches increases in formality and have been designed to prevent the full impact of harm once exposure to a disturbing incident has occurred. Assistance should always be offered in as informal a manner as possible, depending on the needs of the company or individual being assisted. Interventions near the time of the incident include the following:

- informal discussion and support at the company level;
- defusing with a behavioral health professional or other behavioral health team member; and
- formal debriefing with a behavioral health professional and other behavioral health team members.

Members requiring long-term care will do so under the care of licensed mental health professionals.

Covering all the aspects and components of a well-designed, comprehensive behavioral health program is beyond the scope of this document. This document's purpose is to highlight those parts of the system that might be activated within a formally-established rehab area at an incident. Realistically, only the earliest portions of the behavioral health program might be carried out in a rehab setting. These include informal discussion among members and defusing sessions with behavioral health professionals or trained behavioral health team members. The remainder of the comprehensive behavioral health program functions would extend well beyond the scope of rehab operations.

Not every rehab operation will require a behavioral health component to be established within it. Standard firefighting incidents that are grueling to firefighters, but that do not have any accompanying psychological stressors such as injuries or deaths; most likely do not fall into the category of critical stress incidents. Experienced ICs and fire department leaders will be able to judge when the resources of a behavioral health operation will be required.

Most situations, even those involving serious losses, will resolve themselves informally over time, with or without intervention. Informal resources for support and discussion can be every bit as successful as structured sessions for many situations. There is also research that indicates that the use of informal avenues of support from peers can be very effective and assist in coping with the event. These informal discussions may occur in rehab or back at the station. If participants in these informal discussions have a general understanding of the nature and role of interpersonal support, the discussions can be particularly helpful. If the department regularly promotes this informal support, it becomes more likely that these discussions will take place in a helpful fashion as daily incidents occur. This atmosphere also provides a good foundation for any more formal interventions that may be needed. These informal discussions do not involve any outside professionals. There are times, however, when emergency responders may need more assistance in coping with job stress.

Defusing is an informal process to reduce immediately the pressure and anxiety surrounding a critical incident. It is not intended to encourage responders to ventilate feelings, but rather to provide some guidance about what to expect, describe resources, and establish a presence that may make future interventions easier. A defusing is informal and is sometimes conducted in a brief one-on-one discussion, at the scene, in the rehab area, or when the companies return to the station. Defusings also can be conducted in a more private location if requested by the emergency responder or if deemed appropriate by the critical incident stress management team member.

At this level of intervention, the organization's physician, behavioral health professional, clergy, behavioral health team members, or the Labor/Employee Assistance Program (L/EAP) provider may be involved. A defusing process must be guided by the needs of the emergency response personnel. A rigid approach to intervening that dictates only one way to discuss events will undoubtedly fail to meet the needs of individuals and the department as a whole. Often, reliable information about the outcome of an unknown event, such as the condition of an injured firefighter, is sufficient to reduce anxiety in personnel still operating at the scene. It is essential, however, to tailor the approach used to the culture of the department and the needs of individual emergency response personnel involved in the incident.

For more detailed information on conducting defusing sessions and overall behavioral health programs, consult the International Association of Fire Fighters' (IAFF's) *Guide to Developing Fire Service Labor/Employee Assistance & Critical Incident Stress Management Programs* or the IAFF/IAFC Fire Service Joint Labor Management Wellness/ Fitness Initiative.

Monitoring Postincident Hydration and Well-Being

Once the rehab operation has been terminated and all the resources returned to service, the job of those who were assigned to provide rehab services is complete. However, the firefighters and other first responders who received the services of the rehab operation must continue to monitor their own well-being. Make sure they complete the necessary rehydration, rest, and nourishment required to bring them back to a total state of well-being.

A properly run and used rehab area at the incident will go a long way towards making sure that personnel are medically evaluated, treated, rehydrated, and that they receive food when necessary. However, the job cannot be totally completed in a rehab setting. Additional rest, fluid intake, and in some cases, food intake will be needed after the incident to ensure that proper metabolic levels are restored.

In particular, in almost all cases require additional fluid intake after the incident. It is generally recommended that firefighters drink an additional 12 to 32 ounces of electrolyte- and carbohydrate-containing fluids within the 2 hours following the operation **(Figure 6.6).** One simple way to monitor if proper hydra-tion has been restored is to self-monitor one's urine output. A properly hydrated person should have a reasonable volume of urine output and that urine should be relatively clear and odor-free. Following an incident or strenuous training exercise, if the firefighter notices that his or her urine continues to be dark in color or strong in odor, then additional rehydration will be necessary to restore a proper water balance. Continue drinking fluids until the urine output appears to be normal.

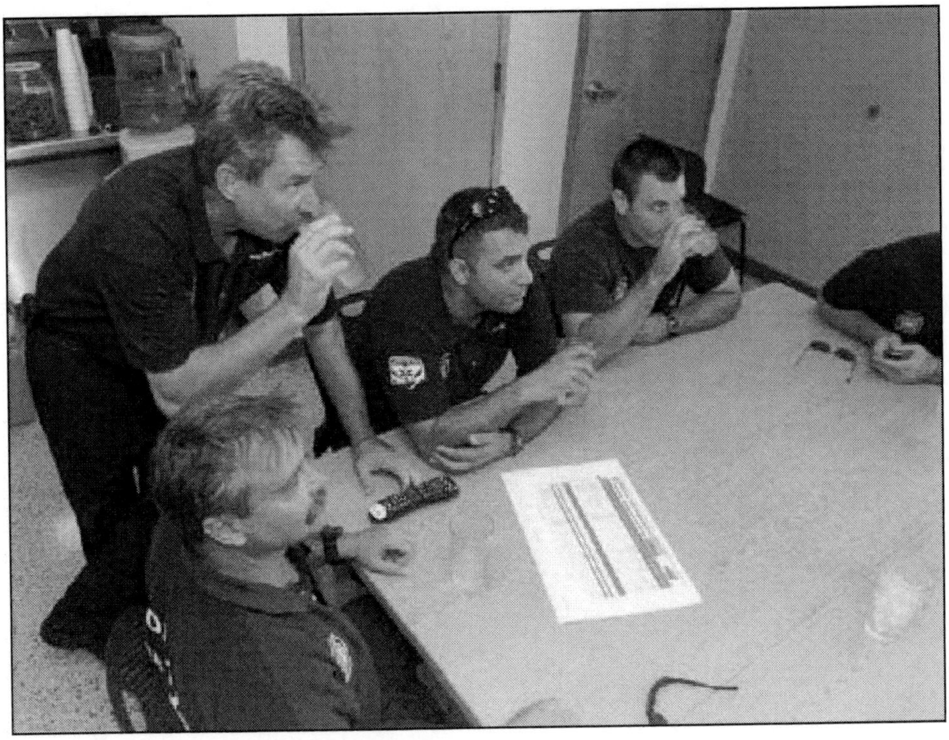

Figure 6.6. Courtesy of Phoenix, AZ Fire Department.

Firefighters also should monitor themselves and their fellow firefighters for signs of delayed medical problems following an incident or training exercise. Serious medical conditions, such as heart attacks, strokes, and other potentially fatal conditions can occur up to 24 hours following the activity. That is why most firefighter insurance and line-of-duty death programs recognize these injuries and deaths as line-of-duty related when they occur within 24 hours of the performed duty. Any members showing signs of an illness or injury should receive immediate medical attention following department SOPs and local EMS protocols.

Appendix A. Additional References and Resources

The purpose of this Appendix is to provide the reader with a wide array of additional sources of information on emergency incident rehabilitation and related topics. Some of these documents were used as information sources for this chapter.

ACSM Position Stand. (1996). Exercise and fluid replacement. Journal of Medicine and *Science, Sports, and Exercise*, *28* (1), January.

Alexander, D. A., & Wells, A. (1991). Reactions of police officers to body handling after a major disaster: A before and after comparison. *British Journal of Psychiatry*, *159*, 547-555.

Armstrong, L. E, et al. (1991). Prediction of the exercise-heat tolerance of soldiers wearing protective overgarments. *Aviation & Space Environmental Medicine*, July, 62, 673-777.

Augustine, J. (1990). In search of fatigue predictors. *Fire Command*, August, 12-13.

Avery, A., King, S., Bretherton, R. & Orner, R. (1999). Deconstructing psychological debriefing and the emergence of calls for evidence based practice. *Traumatic Stress Points*, 12(4), 7-10.

Beaton, R. D. & Murphy, S. A. (1993). Sources of occupational stress among firefighter/EMTs and firefighter/paramedics and correlations with job-related outcomes. *Prehospital and Disaster Medicine*, *8*, 140-150.

Becker, D. (2000) Rehabilitation operations. *Journal of Emergency Management Services*, *25* (11), 37-47.

Bisson, J. I. & Deahl, M. P. (1994). Psychological debriefing and prevention of post traumatic stress: More research is needed. *British Journal of Psychiatry*, *165*, 717-720.

Bisson, I. J., Jenkins, P. L., Alexander, J. & Bannister, C. (1997). A randomized controlled trial of psychological debriefing for victims of acute harm. *British Journal of Psychiatry*, *171*.

Borg, G. (1998) Borg's perceived exertion and pain scales. *Human Kinetics*. Champaign: IL.

Carlier, I.V. E., Lamberts, R. G., van Uchelen, A. J., & Gersons, B. P. R. (1998). Disaster related post-traumatic stress in police officers: A field study of debriefing on psychological distress. *American Journal of Psychiatry*, *154*, 415-417.

Casa, D. J., Clarkson, P. M. & Roberts, W.O. (2005). American college of sports medicine roundtable on hydration and physical activity: consensus statements. *Current Sports Medicine Reports*, *4*, 115-127.

Charlton, P. F. C. & Thompson, J. A. (1996). Ways of coping with psychological distress after trauma. *British Journal of Clinical Psychology*, *35*, 51 7-530.

Cheuvront, S. N., Carter, R., Haymes, E. M., & Sawka, M. N. (2006). No effect on moderate hypohydration or hyperthermia on anaerobic exercise performance. *Medicine & Science in Sports and Exercise*, *38*, 1093-1097.

Conner, D. R. & Hoopes, L. L. (1997). Elements of human diligence: Supporting the nimble organization. *Consulting Psychology: Practice and Research*, *49*, 1 7-24.

Cook, J. D. & Bickman, L. (1990). Social support and psychological symptomatology following a natural disaster. *Journal of Traumatic Stress*, *3*, 541-556.

Deahl, M. P. & Bisson, J. I. (1995). Dealing with disasters: Does psychological debriefing work? Journal of Accident and Emergency Medicine, 12, 255-258.

Deahl, M. P., Gillham, A. B., Thomas, J., Dearle, M. M. & Strinivasan, M. (1994). Psychological sequelae following the gulf war: Factors associated with subsequent morbidity and the effectiveness of psychological debriefing. British Journal of Psychiatry, 165, 60-65.

Dickinson, E.T. & Wieder, M. A. (2000). Emergency incident rehabilitation. Brady-Prentice-Hall Health, Upper Saddle River, NJ.

Dickinson, E.T. (2000). Protecting our own: refuel, recharge, rehab. *Journal of Emergency Management Services*, *25* (11), 25-35.

Echterling, L. & Wylie, M. L. (1981). Crisis centers: A social movement perspective. *Journal of Community Psychology*, *9*, 342-346.

Fahy, R. (2004). Sudden cardiac death. *NFPA Journal*, July/August, 44-47.

Fire Department Safety Officers Association (FDSOA). (1995). Don't let them crawl away to die: establishing rehabilitation sectors. *Safety-Gram*, *8* (10), October.

Foa, E. B. & Meadows, E. A. (1997). Psychosocial treatments for posttraumatic stress disorder: A critical review. *Annual Review of Psychology*, *48*, 935-938.

Fullerton, C. S., Wright, K. M., Ursano, R. J. & McCarroll, J. E. (1993). Social support for disaster workers after a mass-casualty disaster: Effects on the support provider. *Nordic Journal of Psychiatry*, *47*, 3 15-324.

Gist, R. & Lubin, B. (Eds.). (1999). *Response to disaster:Psychosocial, community, and ecological approaches*. Brunner/ Mazel: Philadelphia.

Gist, R., Lubin, B. & Redburn, B. G. (1998). Psychosocial, ecological, and community perspectives on disaster response. *Journal of Personal & Interpersonal Loss*, *3*, 25-5 1.

Gist, R. & Woodall, S. J. (1995). *Occupational stress in contemporary fire service. Occupational Medicine: State of the Art Reviews*, *10*, 763-787.

Gist, R. & Woodall, S. J. (1998). Social science versus social movements:The origins and natural history of debriefing. *Australasian Journal of Disaster and Trauma Studies*, 1998-1. Online serial at www.massey.ac.nz/~trauma.

Griffiths, J. & Watts, R. (1992). The Kempsey and Grafton bus crashes: The aftermath. *Instructional Design Solutions*. East Linsmore: Australia.

Grollmes, E. E. (1992). Postdisaster: Preserving and/or recovering the self. *Disaster Management*, *4*(2), 150-156.

Gump, B. B. & Kulik, J. A. (1997). Stress, affiliation, and emotional contagion. *Journal of Personality and Social Psychology*, *72*, 305-319.

Haigh, C. & Smith, D. (2006). Implementing effective on-scene rehabilitation. Fire Engineering, April.

Heightman, A. J. & O'Keefe, M. (2000). 20 tools to customize your rehab toolbox. J*ournal of Emergency Management Services*, *25* (11), 49-58.

Hobbs, M., Mayou, R., Harrison, B. &Worlock, P. (1996). A randomised controlled trial of psychological debriefing for victims of road traffic accidents. *British Medical Journal*, *313*, 1438-1439.

House, J. R., Holmes, C. & Allsopp, A. J., (1997). *Prevention of Heat Strain by Immersing the Hands and Forearms in Water*. Royal Naval Medical Service.

Hytten, K. & Hasle, A. (1989). Firefighters: A study of stress and coping. *Acta Psychiatrica Scandinavia, 355* (supp.), 50-55.

International Association of Fire Fighters, *Thermal heat stress protocol for firefighters and hazmat responders*. Washington, DC.

International Association of Fire Fighters. *Thermal stress and the firefighter*. Washington, DC.

International Fire Service Training Association (IFSTA). (2001) *Fire Department Safety Officer*, 1st Edition, Fire Protection Publications, Stillwater, OK.

Jankovic, J., Jones, W., Burkhart, J., Noonan, G. (1991). Environmental study of firefighters. *Annals of Occupational Hygiene, 35*, 581-602.

Kenardy, J. A. & Carr, V. (1996). Imbalance in the debriefing debate: What we don't know far outweighs what we do. *Bulletin of the Australian Psychological Society, 18*(2), 4-6.

Kenardy, J. A., Webster, R. A., Lewin, T. J., Carr,V. J., Hazell, P. L. & Carter, G. L. (1996). Stress debriefing and patterns of recovery following a natural disaster. *Journal of Traumatic Stress, 9*, 37-49.

Kenney, W. L. (1997). Fluid intake during cold weather. *Penn State University Sports Medicine Newsletter*.

Lee, C., Slade, P. & Lygo, V. (1996). The influence of psychological debriefing on emotional adaptation in women following early miscarriage: A preliminary study. *British Journal of Medical Psychology, 69*, 47-58.

McCrae, R. R. (1984). Situational determinants of coping responses: Loss, threat, and challenge, *Journal of Personality and Social Psychology, 46*, 919-928.

McEvoy, M. (2005). Biomedically speaking: measuring exhaled CO. *Fire EngineeringsFireEMS Magazine*, May, 6-7.

McEvoy, M. (2005). Averting oxygen hazards with oximetry. *Fire Engineering s FireEMS Magazine*, June, 8-11.

McEvoy, M. (2006). Biomedically speaking: Interpreting carboxyhemoglobin SpCO findings. *Fire Engineering's FireEMS Magazine*, April, 10-14.

McFarlane, A. C. (1988).The longitudinal course of posttraumatic morbidity: The range of outcomes and their predictors. *Journal of Nervous and Mental Disease, 176*, 30-39.

McFarlane, A. C. (1989). The aetiology of post-traumatic morbidity: Predisposing, precipitating, and perpetuating factors. *British Journal of Psychiatry, 154*, 221-228.

McLellan, T. M. & Selkirk, G. A., (2005). *The Management of Heat Stress for the Firefighter*. Defence Research and Development: Canada.

Meichenbaum, D. (1994). *A Clinical Handbook/Practical Therapist Manual for Assessing and Treating Adults with Posttraumatic Stress Disorder*. Waterloo, Ontario (Canada): Institute Press.

Mitchell, J. T. & Everly, G. S. (2nd Edition). *Critical incident stress management: A new era & standard of care in crisis intervention*. Ellicott City, MD: Chevron Publishing.

Mitchell, J.T. & Bray, G. P. (1990). *Emergency services stress: Guidelines for preserving the health and careers of emergency services personnel*. Englewood Cliffs, NJ: Prentice-Hall.

Mitchell, J.T. & Everly, G. S. & (1995). *Critical incident stress debriefing: An operations manual for the prevention of traumatic stress among emergency services and disaster workers*. Ellicott City, MD: Chevron Publishing.

Moran, C. C. (1998). Individual differences and debriefing effectiveness. *Australasian Journal of Disaster and Trauma Studies*, 1998-1. Online serial located at www.massey.ac.nz/~trauma

Motowidlo, S. J., Packard, J. S. & Manning, M. R. (1986). Occupational stress: Its causes and consequences for job performance. *Journal of Applied Psychology*, *71*, 618-629.

National Institute for Occupational Safety and Health (CDC). (1992) *Working in hot environments*. Washington, DC.

Ostrow, L. S. (1996). Critical incident stress management: Is it worth it? *Journal of Emergency Medical Services*, *21*(8), 28-36.

Pearson, D. (1999). Avoiding dehydration: What to drink. *Strength and Conditioning Journal*, June.

Raphael, B., Meldrum, L. & McFarlane, A. C. (1995). Does debriefing after psychological trauma work? Time for randomized controlled trials. *British Journal of Psychiatry*, *310*, 1479-1480.

Rubonis, A. V. & Bickman, L. (1991). Psychological impairment in the wake of disaster: The disaster-psychopathology relationship. *Psychological Bulletin*, *109*, 384-399.

Sachs, G. M. (2000). *The Fire and EMS Department Safety Officer*. Brady/Prentice-Hall Health: Upper Saddle River, NJ.

Sawka, M. N. & Pandolf, K. B. (1990). Effects of body water loss on physiological function and exercise performance. *Perspectives in Exercise Science and Sports Medicine*, Vol. *3*, Fluid Homeostasis During Exercise. Carmel, IN.

Sawka, M.N. (1992). Physiological consequences of hypohydration: Exercise performance and thermoregulation. *Medicine & Science in Sports and Exercise*, *24*(6), 657-669.

Skinner, J. S. (1985). Fighting the fire within. *Firehouse*, August, 46-48,66.

Shireffs, S. M. & Maugham, R. J. (2000). Rehydration and recovery of fluid balance after exercise. *Exercise and Sports Reviews (ACSM)*, *28*(1), January.

Smith, D. L. (2002). Acute effects of firefighting activity on coagulation. *Medicine and Science in Sports Exercise*. *34* (5), 194.

Smith, D. L. & Petruzzello, S. J. (1998). Selected physiological and psychological responses to live-fire drills in different configurations of firefighting gear. *Ergonomics*, *41*(8), 1141-1154.

Smith, D. L., Petruzzello, S. J., Chludzinski, M. A., Reed, J. J. & Woods, J. A., (2001). Effects of strenuous live-fire firefighting drills on hematological, blood chemistry, and psychological measures. *Journal of Thermal Biology*, *26*(4-5), 375-380.

Smith, D. L., Petruzzello, S. J. & Manning, T. S. (2001). The effect of strenuous live-fire drills on cardiovascular and psychological responses of recruit firefighters. *Ergonomics*, *44*(3), 244-254.

Stephens, C. (1997). Debriefing, social support, and PTSD in the New Zealand police: Testing a multidimensional model of organizational traumatic stress. *Australasian Journal of Disaster and Trauma Studies*, *1*. Electronic journal accessible at http://trauma.massey.ac.nz/issues/1997-1/cvs1.htm

Taylor, S. E. (1983). Adjusting to threatening events: A theory of cognitive adaptation. *American Psychologist*, *38*, 1161-1173.

Taylor, S. E. (1991). Asymmetrical effects of positive and negative events:The mobilization-minimization hypothesis. *Psychological Bulletin*, *110*, 67-85.

Taylor, S. E., and Brown, J. D. (1998). Illusion and well-being: A social psychological perspective on mental health. Psychological Bulletin, 103, 193-211.

Taylor, S. E. & Lobel, M. (1989). Social comparison activity under threat: Downward evaluation and upward contacts. *Psychological Review, 96,* 569-575.

Thompson, J. & Solomon, M. (1991). Body recovery teams at disasters: Trauma or challenge. *Anxiety Research, 4,* 235-244.

U.S. Department of the Army. (2003). *Heat stress control and heat casualty management* (TB Med 5 07). Washington, DC.

U.S. Department of the Army. (2005). *Prevention and management of cold weather injuries* (TB Med 5 08). Washington, DC.

U.S. Fire Administration. (1992). FA-114, *Emergency Incident Rehabilitation. Emmitsburg,* MD.

U.S. Fire Administration. (2002). FA-220, *Firefighter Fatality Retrospective Study.* Emmitsburg, MD.

Wenger, B. C. (2001). *Textbook of military medicine: Medical aspects of harsh environments.*

Wessely S., Rose, S. & Bisson, J. I. (1999). Brief psychological interventions ("debriefing") for treating immediate trauma-related symptoms and preventing post-traumatic stress disorder. *Cochrane Review.* The Cochrane Library, 1. Oxford, UK: Update Software.

Wieder, M. A. (1999). Operating a rehab area, part I. *Firehouse,* May.

Wieder, M. A. (2000). The evolution of rehab operations and rehab training materials. *Speaking of Fire,* January.

Wieder, M. A. (2000). Operating a rehab area, part II. *Firehouse.* February.

Wieder, M. A. (2000). Operating a rehab area, part III," *Firehouse.* June.

Wilcox, I. M., Cronin, J. B. & Hing, W. A. (2006). Physiologic response to water immersion—a method for sports recovery? *Sports Medicine, 36,* 747-765.

Woodall, S. J. (1994). *Personal, organizational, and agency development:The psychological dimension. A closer examination of critical incident stress management.* National Fire Academy Executive Fire Officer program, available through Learning Resource Center, National Emergency Training Center, Emmitsburg, MD [(800) 638-1821].

Woodall, S. J. (1997). Hearts on fire: An exploration of the emotional world of firefighters. *Clinical Sociology Review, 15,* 153-162.

Wright, R. M. (1993, May). Any fool can face a crisis: A look at the daily issues that make an incident critical. In R. Gist (Moderator), New information, new approaches, new ideas. Center for Continuing Professional Education, Johnson County Community College, Overland Park, KS.

APPLICABLE NFPA STANDARDS

NFPA 472, *Standard for Professional Competence of Responders to Hazardous Materials Incidents*

NFPA 1001, *Standard for Fire Fighter Professional Qualifications*

NFPA 1500, *Standard on Fire Department Occupational Safety and Health Program*

NFPA 1521, *Standard for Fire Department Safety Officer*

NFPA 1561, *Standard on Emergency Services Incident Management System*

NFPA 1581, *Standard on Fire Department Infection Control Program*

NFPA 1582, *Standard on Comprehensive Occupational Medical Program for Fire Departments*

NFPA 1583, *Standard on Health-Related Fitness Programs for Fire Fighters*

NFPA 1584, *Recommended Practice on the Rehabilitation of Members Operating at Incident Scene Operations and Training Exercises*

WEB SITE

www.firerehab.com—information on all aspects of emergency incident rehabilitation operations.

Appendix B. Fire Department Standard Operating Procedure Emergency Incident Rehabilitation

Purpose

The purpose of this procedure is to provide a framework for the establishment and operation of a Rehab Group/Sector to support the physiological needs of firefighters and other responders engaged in emergency operations, extended duration incidents, and training exercises.

Scope

This procedure identifies situations where the establishment of a Rehab Group/Sector is appropriate. It provides information on the operation of a Rehab Group/Sector, the tasks and procedures that are to be followed by those managing and those using a Rehab Group/Sector, and the equipment and staffing needs of these operations.

The Rehab Group/Sector provides firefighters and other emergency responders with fluids and food, shelter from the elements, and a medical evaluation to assure that the responder is ready to return to work in a safe and managed manner.

General Information

Firefighting and tasks associated with firefighting are among the most physiologically taxing activities that can be performed by humans. During the course of their work, firefighters are exposed to physiological stresses in the form of strenuous physical work. This work is most often performed within the confines of heavy structural firefighting personal protective clothing which further stresses the firefighter. The work is time-sensitive and often is performed under the psychological stressors of danger to the firefighter and others, the desire to do a good job, and the desire on the part of the firefighter to make an individual contribution to the work effort.

Proper implementation of this policy will ensure that members who may be suffering the effects of metabolic heat buildup, dehydration, physical exertion, and/or extreme weather (hot or cold) receive evaluation and rehabilitation during emergency and nonemergency operations.

Most heat and cold emergencies and injuries are entirely preventable. Rehab assists the Incident Commander (IC) with monitoring the health of firefighters and controlling the work/rest cycle to prevent environmental injuries.

The Rehab Group/Sector may be staffed by fire company personnel, emergency management services (EMS) responders, or responders specifically tasked with this function.

Policy

This procedure shall be implemented at all working fires, greater alarm emergencies or during extended operations. The Rehab Group/Sector is usually implemented during hot or cold environmental temperature extremes but may be used at any time at the direction of the IC.The situations that generally produce the need for the Rehab Group/Sector include, but are not limited to,

- greater alarm structural fire operations;
- wildland operations;
- hazardous materials incidents;
- trench rescue;
- confined space rescue;
- training exercises or special events; and
- any other situation deemed necessary by the IC.

The responsibility for the establishment of a Rehab Group/Sector rests with the IC. Other Command system positions, such as the Safety Officer, may assist the IC with recognition of the need for Rehab.

On smaller incidents, Rehab may be accomplished within an ambulance or protected area. Larger incidents require the commitment of resources to accomplish the necessary Rehab tasks.

It is the policy of the fire department that no member will be permitted to continue emergency operations beyond safe levels of physiological, medical, or mental endurance. The intent of the Rehab Group/Sector is to lessen the risk of injury that may result from extended field operations under adverse conditions.

Rehab Functions

The Rehab Group/Sector, radio designation REHAB, will be used to evaluate and assist personnel who could be suffering from the effects of sustained physiological or mental exertion during emergency operations. The Rehab Group/Sector will provide a specific area where personnel will assemble to receive:

- a physical assessment;
- revitalization—rest, hydration, and refreshments;
- medical evaluation and treatment of minor injuries;
- continual monitoring of physical condition;
- transportation for those requiring treatment at medical facilities;
- initial stress support assessment; and
- reassignment.

A Rehab team concept will be used wherever possible to establish and manage the Rehab Group/Sector. This team will be led by a Rehab Group/Sector Supervisor who has been appointed by the IC. The Rehab Group/Sector Supervisor should be wearing an appropriate Command vest that identifies him or her as this person. This full team will consist of:

- Designated Group/Sector Supervisor with crew;
- Rehab vehicle;
- utility (air/power/light) vehicle;
- canteen vehicle;
- one or more EMS transport vehicles;
- advanced life support (ALS) company/personnel; and
- critical incident management team member(s), as needed.

Rehab resources will be dispatched on all second alarm or greater incidents or when special-called by the IC. It will continue to be the responsibility of Incident Command to make an early determination of situations requiring the implementation of a Rehab Group/Sector. Given the time needed to assemble and deploy the needed resources, the IC should call for Rehab resources early.

At times, due to the incident size, weather conditions, or geographic barriers, it may be necessary to establish more than one Rehab Group/Sector. When this is initiated, each Group/Sector will assume a geographic designation consistent with the location at the incident site, i.e., Rehab South, Rehab North.

At incidents involving large life loss, or extended rescue operations (i.e., plane or train crash), the critical incident stress management (CISM) team should be contacted and be assigned to Rehab Group/Sector.

A city bus may be called to the incident scene to provide cooling or heat and shelter. Other considerations for selecting the exact location of the rehab site include

- ability to accommodate the number of personnel (fire, law enforcement, other) expected (including EMS personnel for medical monitoring) and accommodate a separate area to remove personal protective equipment (PPE).
- accessibility for an ambulance and EMS personnel should medical treatment or transportation be required.
- ability to be removed from hazardous atmospheres including apparatus exhaust, smoke, and other toxins.
- ability to provide shade in summer and protection from inclement weather at other times.
- accessibility to a water supply (bottled or running) to provide for hydration and active cooling.
- location away from spectators and media whenever possible.

The Rehab Group/Sector and vehicles should be located close to the Command Post (CP) whenever possible. The Rehab Group/Sector area boundaries will be defined with blue tape or blue traffic cones and will have only one entry point. It will be divided into the four Sections described later in this procedure.

Criteria for Reporting To Rehab

Personnel should perform self-rehab procedures as follows:

- following the use of one 30-minute SCBA cylinder;
- after 20 minutes of intense physical labor; and
- other times as necessary.

Personnel must report to the Rehab Group/Sector as follows:

- following the use of two 30-minute SCBA cylinders or one 45- or 60-minute cylinder
- after 40 minutes of intense physical labor
- after performing duties in hazardous materials encapsulating suits;
- when directed by an officer to do so; and
- when feeling the need to do so.

Section A: Entry Point

This is the initial entry point and decontamination area. Assigned personnel will collect accountability tags from crews and take a pulse rate on all crew members. Any member who has a pulse rate greater than 120 will report directly to Section C, Medical Treatment and Transport, where they will be treated appropriately. Members that do not require medical attention will then report to Section B, Hydration and Replenishment.

Section B: Hydration and Replenishment

This Section is staffed by the canteen driver and other personnel, as required. During warm weather conditions, all personnel in this area must remove coats, helmets, gloves, and protective hoods. Turnout pants also should be removed or at least rolled down over the boots. All personnel will be provided supplemental cooling devices, fluid and electrolyte replacement, and the proper amount of nourishment. For extreme heat, a misted area shall be provided for initial cool-down, with fans creating air movement. Hand-forearm immersion procedures to lower core body temperatures should also be used. Forearms should be submerged at least 10 and preferably 20 minutes. Air-conditioned areas for extended rehabilitation to which members can be moved after their body temperatures have stabilized should be provided. Initial CISM support will be provided in this Section, if needed.

The following other requirements pertain to personnel assigned to Section B:

- All personnel should spend a minimum of 20 minutes resting in this area.
- Personnel should consume a minimum of 10 ounces of water or other approved beverages while in this area.
- Smoking shall not be permitted in this area.

Section C: Medical Treatment and Transport

This Section is staffed by an ALS crew and at least one EMS transport vehicle. Personnel reporting here will receive evaluation and treatment for heat stress and other injuries or illnesses. A standard EMS patient report form should be started for each person sent to this Section. The ALS personnel assigned will advise the Rehab Group/Sector Supervisor of the necessity of medical transportation and extended medical attention requirements of personnel due to physical condition. Members who are transported to a medical facility should be accompanied by a department representative. Crews released from Section C will be released as intact crews to report to Section D. The ALS crew in this Section will pay close attention to the following:

- pulse;
- blood pressure;
- body temperature; and
- obvious injuries or illness.

After appropriate rehabilitation and medical monitoring (minimum of 20 minutes for an initial cool down and evaluation period) the pulse, blood pressure, and temperature will be reevaluated and triage members with one of the following dispositions:

- Returned to duty—adequately rehabbed and medically sound;
- Removed from duty—evidence of an illness or injury; including any person with a pulse rate greater than 100; or
- Transported to an appropriate medical facility for further evaluation and treatment of illness or injury; including any member who has a temperature greater than 101 °F (38 °C) or a blood pressure less than 100.

Section D: Reassignment

This critical Section determines a crew's readiness for reassignment. Diligent efforts and face-to-face communication with the Rehab Group/Sector Supervisor are required. Personnel staffing this Section advise the Rehab Group/Sector Supervisor of the status of all companies for reassignment and crews that are running short or without a Company Officer (CO). This information is relayed to Command by the Rehab Group/ Sector Supervisor. Crews without a CO will be assigned to another company or have a member of the crew move up to the officer's position.

The Rehab Group/Sector Supervisor will collect accountability passports from companies reporting to Section A—Entry Point. The passports will be placed on a status board and all personnel will be logged on the Rehabilitation Group/Sector Personnel Log Form. The log will indicate the assignments as directed by Command. Companies may be reassigned to operating Groups/Divisions/Sectors or released from the scene.

The Rehab Group/Sector Supervisor will update Command throughout the operation with pertinent information including the identities of companies in Rehab, the companies available for reassignment, and the status of injured personnel. All personnel leaving Rehab will retrieve passports from the Rehab Group/Sector Supervisor. COs must keep crews intact and report to the proper sections in Rehab. The Rehab Group/Sector Supervisor will direct the crew to the proper sections; however, it is the CO's responsibility to make sure crew members receive refreshments, rest, and a medical clearance.

The basic function of rehab needs to be addressed for each firefighter or emergency responder that enters rehab—drink fluids, rest, and be ready for work prior to leaving the Rehab area.

INDEX

A

B

C

D

E

N

O

P

Q

R

S

T

U

V

W